MW01593571

SLACK International Book Distributors

In the Europe, the Middle East and Africa.
  John Wiley & Sons Limited
  Baffins Lane
  Chichester, West Sussex P019 1UD
  England

In Canada:
  McAinsh and Company
  2760 Old Leslie Street
  Willowdale, Ontario M2K 2X5

In Australia and New Zealand:
  MacLennan & Petty Pty Limited
  P.O. Box 425
  Artarmon, N.S.W. 2064
  Australia

In Japan:
  Central Foreign Books Limited
  1-13 Jimbocho-Kanda
  Tokyo, Japan

In Asia and India:
  PG Publishing Pte Limited.
  36 West Coast Road, #02-02
  Singapore 0512

Printed in the United States of America

Library of Congress Catalog Card Number: 85-62643

ISBN: 0943432-61-8

Published by: SLACK Incorporated
              6900 Grove Rd.
              Thorofare, NJ 08086

Last digit is print number: 10 9 8 7 6 5 4 3 2 1

DEDICATION

*This book is dedicated
to Otto AuFranc,
an outstanding surgeon,
teacher and friend.*

Hugh P. Chandler

CONTENTS

Preface

1. **Biology of Bone Grafts**   1
   Henry J. Mankin, M.D. and Gary E. Friedlaender, M.D.

2. **Principals and Practical Applications of Bone Banking**   13
   William W. Tomford, M.D. and Henry J. Mankin, M.D.

3. **Pre-operative Planning**   19
   Hugh P. Chandler, M.D. and Brad L. Penenberg, M.D.

4. **Surgical Approaches**   41
   Hugh P. Chandler, M.D. and Brad L. Penenberg, M.D.

5. **Acetabular Reconstruction**   47
   Hugh P. Chandler, M.D. and Brad L. Penenberg, M.D.

6. **Femoral Reconstruction**   103
   Hugh P. Chandler, M.D. and Brad L. Penenberg, M.D.

7. **Post-operative Management**   165
   Hugh P. Chandler, M.D. and Brad L. Penenberg, M.D.

8. **Results and Complications**   169
   Charles P. Capito, M.D., Hillel D. Skoff, M.D., Steven A. Bohmer, M.D.,
   Hugh P. Chandler, M.D., and Brad L. Penenberg, M.D.

Index   181

PREFACE

The purpose of this book is to share our experience with bone grafts used to reconstruct bone deficiencies in the pelvis and femur prior to total hip replacement. We present methods that have proven successful for us as well as those that have failed with the hope that the reader could avoid some of the mistakes that we have made.

Few of these cases are exactly similar and the surgeon must be prepared to use new methods for new problems that are based on principles that have been proven to be succesful in the past. We apologize for the short follow-up of some of these techniques, especially in femoral reconstruction, but feel that some of these very difficult problems are virtually unsolvable without the use of bone grafts. We also believe that it is likely that these will stand the test of time, based on our longer experience with less complex grafts.

These procedures are technically demanding and should not be undertaken by the surgeon who is unwilling to spend the time to shape and secure grafts accurately. Speed is commendable if the result is excellence but the surgeon who sacrifices quality for quickness will find a high early failure rate. It is not fair to the patient to hurry the procedure and to save an hour in the operating room at the cost of adding weeks or months to the post-operative hospital stay.

We have been greatly influenced by the teachings of Otto Aufranc, whose principles of meticulous soft tissue management have proven so effective in our hands. Sharp rather than blunt dissection, careful redefining of tissue planes starting from known and working toward undefined and scarred anatomy, saving of all the potential fat planes, the use of moistened wound towels sewn into depths of the exposure to protect tissues and finally the avoidance of excessive retraction, especially with self retaining retractors, are all very important.

Although this book is about bone grafting techniques, we clearly do not advocate bone grafts if an equally effective solution is available that will not eventually result in further bone loss. Modern uncemented acetabular component are now available in low profile and in a variety of sizes including those much smaller and much larger than the components available even two or three years ago. Some of the acetabular grafts that we have presented might now not be necessry using these more modern components. On the femur however, we feel that there is actually an increasing need to reconstruct defects with bone grafts because techniques using larger, longer and stiffer components, cemented or uncemented, are likely to cause even further bone loss because of stress shielding.

We would like to express our thanks to Laurel Cook (Medical Graphics, Boston, Massachusetts), for her outstanding art work which we have found so helpful in explaining these complex techniques. We would also like to thank Deborah Scarff (The Better Light, Burlington, Massachusetts), for her excellent photographs.

CONTRIBUTORS

Hugh P. Chandler, M.D.
Visiting Orthopedic Surgeon
Massachusetts General Hospital
Boston, Massachusetts
Assistant Clinical Professor of Orthopedic Surgery
Harvard Medical School
Boston, Massachusetts

Brad L. Penenberg, M.D.
Assistant Professor of Orthopedic Surgery
University of Southern California Medical School
Los Angeles, California

William W. Tomford, M.D.
Associate in Orthopedic Surgery
Massachusetts General Hospital
Boston, Massachusetts
Associate Professor of Orthopedic Surgery
Harvard Medical School
Boston, Massachusetts
Director of Massachusetts General Bone Bank
Boston, Massachusetts

Hillel D. Skoff, M.D.
Instructor of Orthopedic and Plastic Surgery
Harvard Medical School
Boston, Massachusetts
Beth Israel Hospital
Boston, Massachusetts

Henry J. Mankin, M.D.
Chief of Orthopedic Service
Massachusetts General Hospital
Boston, Massachusetts
Edith M. Ashley Professor of Orthopedic Surgery
Harvard Medical School
Boston, Massachusetts

Charles P. Capito, M.D.
Clinical Fellow in Pelvic and Total Joint Reconstruction
University of Pittsburgh

Steven Bohmer, M.D.
Orthopedic Surgeon
Indian River Memorial Hospital
and Sebestian Humana Hospital
Vero Beach, FL

Gary E. Friedlaender, M.D.
Chief, Orthopedic Department
Yale New Haven Hospital
Chairman, Department of Orthopedics and Rehabilitation
Yale University

ONE

Henry J. Mankin, M.D.
Gary E. Friedlaender, M.D.

Bone and Cartilage Allografts: Physiological and Immunological Principles

Introduction

By the standards of the first half of the twentieth century, the past forty years has been a period of spectacular advancement in the technology of orthopedic surgery. There are now a number of methods available to reconstruct skeletal defects and restore the paitent to normal structure and function, but with the development of modern systems for the treatment of trauma, spinal disorders, arthritis, tumors, and genetic abnormalities has come the ability to create even greater defects in the skeleton for the purpose of cure. In many ways these systems seem miraculous and have enabled the surgeon to deal with many major problems of the skeleton without resorting to amputation or other procedures that result in disability or crippling. As just one example, consider the field of malignant tumors of the skeleton.[1] Without question, until 25 years ago, the only treatment offered patients with the diagnosis of osteosarcoma or Ewing's tumor or high grade chondrosarcoma of an extremity was an amputation and even if successful, their outlook for long survival was baleful at best.[1,2] Today because of improved staging systems for neoplasms,[3,4] better imaging systems,[1,5] improved techniques of surgery,[6-9] vast improvements in adjuvant radiation and especially chemotherapeutic systems,[1,2,10] the patients with these disorders are likely not only to survive, but to have a limb sparing procedure rather than an ablation.[1,8,11] Once the diseased or incompetent bony (and adjacent soft tissue) components are removed and the degree of tissue loss assessed, the patient must now have some form of reconstruction and there now are a number of alternatives. Consider the treatment possibilities for just such lesions around the proximal femur. Obviously considerable variation will be present depending on the length of resection and the magnitude of the soft tissue defect, but a review of the current literature shows that reconstruction can be achieved by insertion of nonvascular or vascularized autograft,[7,12-14] metallic implants,[6,11,15-19] autoclaved autogeneic bone,[20] turnabout procedures,[21] or as will be the subject of this review, allograft bone with or without metallic implants.[22-26]

Because of the extensive experience of our units with the last mentioned technique, we provide a chapter in this book that describes some of the background to and our experiences with the use of allografts. It is essential for the reader to understand that the allograft enthusiasts are not "in competition" with those individuals who prefer autograft or metallic implants. Further, it is not the purpose of this chapter to suggest that allogeneic bone implants are better than or worse than any other type of device or system; the most we or anyone else can say is that they are different. On the basis of an exhaustive study of the basic science of the field, review of current series in other institutions, careful analysis of over 400 such patients treated in our own series over the last 16 years we conclude that alloimplants: have unique properties; may fill certain needs that other systems cannot; and because of their differences may be associated with some unique problems that require special knowledge and concern on the part of the surgeons if they are to be successful. The purpose of this chapter is to provide general information about allograft parts, to describe some aspects of their use, and to indicate the special problems which the surgeon and the patient must face and how to deal with them.

The History of Allografts

Frozen cadaveric allografts have a long and somewhat checkered history in the annals of orthopedic science and especially in the art of bone tumor management. Although the earliest recorded attempt at an allograft implantation was believed to be in 1881,[4] the history of the procedure in legend, at least, goes far into antiquity. From time to time the suggestion has been made that Greek mythology contains a report of the transfer of parts from one human to another, but the only report that comes close is the somewhat grisly story of Pelops, whose mother Demeter ate a large portion of the young man's shoulder. In an effort to restore the function of the part, the gods, led by Zeus, constructed a shoulder joint out of ivory (perhaps the first xenograft) and performed the necessary restoration with divine skill. Similarly the wording of the Old Testament leaves unclear the nature of the procedure performed by Adam to create Eve and the status of the rib as an allograft transplant remains somewhat murky (perhaps the first isograft!). The most clearly defined legend, however, is that associated with Sts. Cosmas and Damian, twin physicians who lived in the third century AD.[27] They performed some rather extraordinary cures over their lives but somehow angered the Emperor Diocletian who had them put to death in the year 255 AD. This should have been the end of the good saints, but they returned in the fifth century to perform a major miracle. A faithful church retainer exhausted by the pain of a cancerous limb fell asleep in a temple in the Roman Forum (now known appropriately as the Basilica Cosma et Damiano) and dreamed that the twin saints came to him. The saints performed an operative procedure, removing the cancerous limb and implanting the analogous part of a Moor who had died a short time before (the first allograft!). The procedure was alleged successful and because the skin of the Moor was darker than that of the recipient, the event became known as "The Miracle of the Black Leg." The miracle was so remarkable that the twins were beatified on the basis of it; and the surgery so spectacular it served as the subject of seemingly countless renditions of the procedure among the artists of the Reformation and Renaissance.

Physicians of the modern era read of the first alloimplant as described by Macewen,[28] in which a humerus was transplanted for trauma. The initial result was reported as good, but the long term result was unknown. The event that brought the subject back into the scientific arena, however, was the report of Lexer in 1908[29] in which he described the use of both hemi-and whole joints in the reconstruction of the knee, mostly for trauma. In a followup study performed 17 years later he reported that further study of the same

group of patients showed over half of them still retained their grafted parts.[30]

Over the ensuing years, cadaveric allograft implantation waxed and waned in popularity as a clinical activity.[3,31-38] Reports appeared in the literature describing several small series of patients in whom bone was obtained from amputation specimens or recently deceased individuals. The concept of banking became a reality during and after World War II when the National Naval Tissue Bank was established in Bethesda and a number of small banks sprang up in hospitals throughout the United States.[37-42] Small fragments, either of cortical or medullary bone, from these banks were used heterotopically to augment spinal fusions, to implant into cyst cavities, or to serve as a scaffolding for repair of non-or delayed union of fractures of the long bones.[36-38,43] For unknown reasons, the banking and use of such grafts fell into disfavor; the use of massive segments became even less popular, conceivably on the basis of some bad surgical experiences.

None of these studies, however, discouraged the interest of orthopaedic scientists, and the literature of the middle years of this century is filled with descriptions of experimental studies that attempted to establish the nature of the response of animals to allogeneic bony and cartilaginous implants.[31,32,35,44-63] The efforts of many of these scientists were extraordinary, but the contributions of a few stand out. Herndon, Curtiss, Chase and coworkers at Case Western Reserve were responsible for establishing the histologic sequence of events and the remarkable fact that freezing the bone prior to implantation appeared to reduce the immunogenicity and altered the course of the immune response.[32,45,53,54,58,59]

Burwell and his coworkers,[46,47,64,65] perhaps more than any others, established the histologic and immunologic events that ultimately defined the natural history of alloimplantation. Crawford Campbell et al.[48-50] tested and compared the alloimplant system against the autograft in a variety of settings and defined the fate of bone and cartilage grafts in experimental animals.

These experimental studies set the stage, and the establishment of reliable banks such as the National Navy Tissue Bank at Bethesda[40,41,66,67] and others[34,38,68,69] provided a source of materials making it possible for clinicians around the world to reintroduce the concept of the frozen massive alloimplant as an orthotopic replacement for a traumatically lost, tumor-ridden, or diseased part of the appendicular skeleton. Large series were described by Volkov in the USSR,[70] Nilsonne in Sweden,[69] Koskinen in Finland,[72] Ottolenghi in Argentina[71,72] and Parrish of Houston[75] to whom is credited with the first long-term followup study since that of Lexer.[76] The system remained relatively infrequently used however, partly because of the complexity of the procedure, the unpredictability of the result[77] and, perhaps most importantly, the necessity of maintaining a rigorously controlled bone bank for the procurement and storage of frozen tissues.[68,69,78-80] Some patients in whom allografts were implanted did well; and others were plagued with complications such as infection, fracture, and graft dissolution, presumably for the most part as a result of some immunologic "rejection".[23,77,81-83] Although the more recently reported series continue to improve and in fact are now "acceptable" in terms of success rate,[1,23-26,84] the results are still not as good as one would like and the problems of allograft fracture[81] and infection[82] remain as major issues.

In theory, allografting has considerable appeal in the management of skeletal defects. If harvesting and banking procedures are followed the parts should be readily available and if the cryopreservation technique used has been effective, these parts should have at least partially viable and functional cartilage surfaces.[85,86] If the graft is "accepted" and if healing and revascularization takes place as it should, the graft will be converted to living tissue — certainly a desirable goal.[51,64,65,87-89] Furthermore, the graft has attachment sites for resected motors and joint stabilizers, which make it a very valuable component. As will be discussed below, the alloimplant is not as well accepted by the host as is as an autograft—(the "gold standard"),[14,90-92]—but in general the supply of such tissue is limited, it requires considerable additional surgery to obtain autograft and it is of course impossible to reconstruct a joint.[7,9,12-14,93,94]

Comparing allogeneic components with metallic and plastic implants, it is apparent that these prosthetic systems have evolved enormously over the last two decades and are now considerably improved over the earliest devices.[15] In the hands of many reconstructive surgeons, such custom implants are the main line of management for skeletal defects[6,11,15,17-19] and justifiably so, since it is now possible and indeed probable that such devices will last a number of years. However, all of the problems of these systems have not been solved. Difficulties such as stress shielding, late loosening and material failures, which can produce failure rates as high as 20% in ten years in elderly patients, must surely occur with even greater frequency in younger patients with huge, custom metallic systems.

Biology of Graft Incorporation

Autografts

The incorporation of a bone graft, whether it is autogeneic or allogeneic in origin, is a "partnership" between the transplanted tissue and the host bed into which it is placed. The graft contributions include a passive *osteoconduction* whereby the tissue acts as a trellis or scaffold for bony ingrowth of the host tissues.[43] Equally or perhaps more importantly, the graft can play a more active role and stimulate bone formation by the poorly understood but nonetheless real process of *osteoinduction*.[43,62] In fact, Ray and coworkers[62] have shown that a small fraction of the

cells survive the transplant (more cells with cancellous than with cortical and more with rapid transplant than with delayed).

The major source of bone formation, however, results from an osteoinductive recruitment of host blood vessels which invade the graft as "cutting cones" and simultaneously destroy the donor bone and lay down new host osseous tissues, a process termed *creeping substitution*.[35,49,90-92,95,96] Although the mediator(s) responsible for the invasion of the vessels is still not elucidated, the remainder of the process is quite well defined and has been the subject of numerous studies and descriptions over the years.[43,62,90,91,95,96]

The initial events in this process have a fairly characteristic pattern of occurrence but differ somewhat with the type of graft, the vascularity of the host bed, and numerous other circumstances.[43,91,96] The initial phase is one of hemorrhage and necrosis, corresponding to the surgical injury associated with implanting the graft. The hemorrhage at the site becomes a fibrin clot with entrapped cells. Within a short period of time an inflammatory response ensues, in which is noted increased vascularity in the adjacent tissues, dilatation of the blood vessels, transudation, exudation and a resultant edema. The fibrin clot is invaded by locally derived fibroblasts that tend to wall off the "foreign body," and a loose moderately vascular granulation tissue with a large number of inflammatory cells and immature fibroblastic tissues surrounds the graft and the host bone.[49,96]

At this point the events that occur are dependent on the action of a chemotactic substance or low molecular weight mediator (or perhaps piezoelectrical effect or electomagnetic fields).[43] Whatever the mediator is, it invokes the host blood vessels to proliferate and invade the graft and develop into *cutting cones*.[49,95,96] Cells originating from the endothelial cells, pericytes, blood elements, local fibroblasts, monocytes, myoblasts or some other as yet unknown cellular elements modulate or differentiate into two separate populations: the bone formers (osteoblasts) and the bone destroyers (osteoclasts). The elements escape from the blood vessel and carry on the characteristic *creeping substitution* that in a relatively short period not only replaces at least a large part of the graft with new bone but also stimulate the host to respond by increased bone formation resulting in healing of the host-donor junction sites and, in many cases, healing of a delayed or nonunion site. The duration and predictability of this phase varies widely according to the type of graft, the degree of density of the cortex, the vascularity of the host bed, the age of the patient, the presence of infection, history of prior surgery, etc.[92] In more controlled experimental animal systems depending on the species and the site, the changes occur quite rapidly, however, and vascular ingrowths may be seen in cortical grafts within a few days to one week following implantation.[35,90,95]

One of the questions that arises is whether all of the bone in a graft is completely replaced by the newly formed host tissues. One can say with certainty regarding cortical bone that if it is replaced, it certainly does not occur rapidly.[92,95] Probably the graft will be continually remodeled after incorporation, but there remains some doubt if it is ever completely replaced.

Cancellous autogeneic bone grafts are highly cellular and porous. Depending on their source and handling they behave somewhat differently from cortical. If the source of the graft is from a "red marrow" area and if transplant occurs rapidly, some of the cells survive[49,62] and revascularization occurs quite rapidly, possibly as early as several days after implantation. The osteoinductive effect is obviously greater in degree and extent with such a graft, but the osteoconductive element is probably less as is, of course, the mechanical stability.[43]

Allografts

The response of the host and donor parts to transplantation of allogeneic tissues has been the subject of a large number of animal studies for at least the past 75 years and almost regardless of experimental design, the results show that the pattern is remarkably stereotypic.[35,51,53,58,60,87,97,98] The basic sequence of repair and incorporation of allografts is qualitatively analogous to that of autogenous bone grafts as described above. There are, however, significant variations in quantitation (particularly affecting cell complements) and at times, major temporal differences. The magnitude of these variations depends partially on the degree of genetic disparity between donor and recipient[97,99-101] and partially on the nature of the preservation techniques of the graft.[45,54,66,100]

The function of the graft as an *osteoconductive system* seems to be virtually unimpaired. With allogeneic tissues, the "partnership" between the transplanted tissue and the host bed into which it is placed remains functional and the graft acts as a trellis or scaffold for bony ingrowth of the host tissues.[43,51,87,89] The variation in behavior of this system appears to be in terms of the function of the graft as a stimulator of host bone formation by the process of *osteoinduction*.[15,35,43,46,58,60,63,64,87,89,97]

Even without a significant chronic inflammatory response which one ordinarily associates with altered immunity, the allogeneic part appears to have a very limited (or perhaps almost nonexistent) stimulatory effect on the host system to promote *creeping substitution*.[35,60,63] Thus the autograft exerts a profound effect on the host to excite an osteoinductive recruitment of host blood vessels to invade the graft as *cutting cones* and simultaneously destroy the donor bone and lay down new host osseous tissues. A similar effect does not seem to be present in nearly the same magnitude of activity when allogeneic tissues are used.

The initial events in the process of host-donor response to transplantation of allogeneic tissues may differ with the type of graft, the method of preparation (fresh, frozen, frozen and dried), the vascularity of the host bed, and numerous other mitigating circumstances,[60,89,97,98,102] but by and large have a fairly characteristic pattern of occurrence. The initial phase is identical to that of the autograft consisting of hemorrhage and necrosis, corresponding to the surgical placement of the graft. The fibrin clot develops just as it does in the autograft, and within a short period, the same inflammatory response seen with an autograft ensues and increased vascularity in the adjacent tissues, dilatation of the blood vessels, transudation and exudation are noted but perhaps are greater in extent and degree.[51,64]

At this point the response appears to differ. The fibrin clot clearly of great importance to the system seems to be poorly organized; the loosely constructed granulation tissue that serves as a source of cellular elements for repair becomes filled with chronic inflammatory cells rather than fibroblasts and blood vessel elements and the numbers of lymphocytes, plasma cells and mononuclear elements that lie in juxtaposition to the graft markedly increase.[39,47,51,64]

In contrast with autogeneic tissues the factor that stimulates host blood vessels to proliferate, invade the graft and develop into *cutting cones* appears to be diminished, absent or severely suppressed. Recruitment and differentiation of cellular elements to become vascular invaders and the osteoblastic and osteoclastic elements essential to creeping substitution are reduced in extent and degree. Replacement of tissue by host bone is slow and the stimulatory effect exerted on the host or the donor part is limited in degree and repair of the host-donor junction site is also limited. Healing of a delayed or nonunion site in the host bone may respond to the mechanical aspects of the insertion of the graft, but most authorities consider that the allogeneic donor part contributes little in the form of osteoinduction.[35,43,66,100]

In this process two special patterns of healing (or lack of it) are rarely encountered. Under circumstances as yet not well defined, the host soft tissues "wall off" the allograft part for an extended period, possibly years. Study of these tissues show little or no vascular proliferation or attempt at invasion of the graft. Under other conditions, presumably immune directed, the graft is surrounded by inflammatory cells, invaded rapidly by numerous blood vessels and destroyed. Following such a "dissolution" the donor site may show no remnants of the implanted materials. Both of these responses are unusual (especially in human tissue) and presumably record opposite ends of the spectrum of reaction of the host tissue to the antigenic challenge.[77]

Knowledge remains imperfect as to whether host tissues ever completely replace an autogeneic transplant but with allogeneic no such mystery exists. Animal experiments and numerous salvage studies of human donor parts years following alloimplantation show that some parts of the bone remain dead and clearly represent the old graft.[103] Probably at least a portion of the graft eventually will be remodeled sufficiently to be considered autogenous tissue, but there is no doubt that the graft is never completely replaced and that large segments of donor tissue remain uninvaded and present in the host for years. Whether this tissue acts as a foreign body or a continuous source of antigen is not known.

Like autografts, cancellous allogeneic bone grafts are highly cellular and porous and probably, especially if frozen and dried, behave very differently from cortical bone grafts. It is likely that revascularization occurs much more rapidly, possibly as early as several weeks or months following implantation. Once again the degree to which such a graft is replaced by host tissue is not well known, but there is some evidence to suggest the graft is not completely replaced even years after implantation. It is likely that the osteoinductive effect is moderately greater in degree than that of the cortical allografts but does not approach that of the "gold standard" autografts.[43]

The use of autogeneic cartilage for transplantation is an unusual usage in clinical orthopedic surgery but is not as unusual in animal experimental protocols.[50,52] As might be expected for a tissue without a blood supply, all investigators have shown excellent survival for articular cartilage under these circumstances—not so for epiphyseal. The question is raised about the fate of allogeneic transplanted cartilage, and it has also been extensively studied.[48,57-59,98] Of considerable importance to such a system is the viability of the chondrocytes. Some evidence supports the concept that the fresh graft has good cell survival and hence remains not only alive but functional for years after implantation.[87,104] If it is necessary to freeze the graft, which may be an important consideration in relation to the need to reduce the immunogenicity of the underlying bone and to maintain an adequate supply of parts in a tissue bank, the use of cryoprotectants has been advocated as a method of maintaining chondrocyte viability.[85,86,105-107] Studies by Tomford[85,86] and Schachar[98] have supported the original suggestion by Smith[106] that glycerol or, more recently, dimethylsufoxide (DMSO) can reduce the extent of cryoinjury to the chondrocytes. The best effect, however, is noted in isolated cells;[86,106] when the system is applied to the intact cartilage, the results are far less salutory and probably less than 50 percent of the cells retain their viability.[85] The cause of the failure to translate the excellent results for chondrocyte cells suspensions to the intact tissue remains enigmatic, but probably has to do with the matrix, which not only limits diffusion of the cryoprotectant, but may in fact serve as a cold reflectant.[85] Even with successful transplant, either as fresh graft or frozen cryoprotected graft, late degenerative changes would seem to be inevitable and have been demonstrated both experimentally and clinically.[24,25,48] It should be noted, however, that "fit" of the graft appears to influence materially the rate at which the degeneration occurs and well-fitted grafts may show a long delay in appearance of such changes.[77,108,109]

The Immune Response to Bone and Cartilage Allografts

The issues raised when considering the host immune responses to bone allograft remain intriguing, not so much as to the existence of the response but rather as to the biologic consequenses. Are there really true "rejections"? Can we define some processes that could be termed either graft versus host disease or host versus graft response? Clearly animal studies have demonstrated the consequences of major mismatches in tissue typing,[97,99,100,110-112] but can we identify a similar process in the human?

Bone is a composite tissue containing a variety of cells, collagen, and matrix proteins—all of which can serve as antigens and a mineral phase that does not.[43] Collagen, the major protein constituent, can under certain circumstances serve as a weak antigen while the various other matrix components may show a variable pattern, depending on the extent to which these materials are exposed to the host system. Most of the attention at least for osteochondral allografts, centers around the cell surface antigens, surface membrane glycoproteins expressed under the control of major histocompatability complex.[87,111,113-115] These antigens appear on a wide variety of cells found in bone (including osteogenic, chondroblastic, fibroblastic, fatty and neural cells) but appear most prominently as in other tissues on the cells of the vascular system (endothelial and perithelial elements) and of the hematopoietic system.[46,47,64,65,111,113]

In the decades since the seminal work of Burwell, a number of investigators, using various animal models, have evaluated cell-mediated and humoral responses following transplantation of fresh or preserved allogeneic bone[47,87,99-102,110-114,116,117] or cartilage[55,56,104,117] segments. All have shown an evoked immune response. The response is most marked with fresh osteochondral grafts but can be significantly reduced by freezing the graft[66,97,100,102,110] and reduced even further by freezing and drying of the allogeneic implant.[66] Studies of animal species have demonstrated that antibodies may be detected in a high percentage of the recipients of grafts and these are similar to the current data for humans, which have shown that about 85% of the patients who receive a massive graft show sensitization following the procedure.[100,115,118] Class I antigens are most frequently detected but Class II can also be found and to date the significance of the response of one or both of these antigens is not understood.[67,100]

The major problem related to these issues, at least for humans, is the failure to find some biological abnormalities either retrospectively or, more importantly, those which might be predicted prospectively as a result of these host tissue antibodies. Current attempts to correlate the response of the graft with the degree or class of antibody present in the host have not been productive. Despite several animal studies which suggest in a purer system they are likely to exert an effect,[97,99,110,112] to date these findings have yet to be corroborated in humans.

Results of Experimental Studies on Bone and Cartilage Allografts

Since Macewen's[28] and Lexer's[29],[30] first experiments with the use of hemi-and whole joint transplants in man, the allograft system has stimulated an enormous number of experimental studies and continues to do so. As evidence is an entire volume published in 1983[119] and a more recent report of an invitational conference.[65] The interested reader is urged to review this information in detail to determine the current state of the science. The numerous findings can be summarized as follows:

1. Allogeneic bone appears to excite a host immune response characterized by the presence of humoral and cellular cytotoxic antibodies.[47,87,97,99-102,110-114,116,117] This response appears to be "dose dependent" and considerably, although not entirely predictably, ameliorated by freezing the graft.[45,87,97,99,102] Freezing appears to have its effect by killing the cells and disrupting their membranes but may cause the production of a blocking antibody[87,102] and also has been shown to result in marked inhibition of collagenase activity.[107]

2. The normal course of events that occur with devitalized autograft has been extensively studied and shows a specific rate of revascularization and creeping substitution, both osteoclastic and osteoblastic in nature, which may vary with a number of parameters, including the nature of the graft, the bed and the vascularity of the host bone.[35,48,51,53,58,64,87,89,97,98] The effect of the immune response on the analogous form of allograft, particularly for fresh frozen segments, appears to be principally one of a delay, sometimes extraordinarily long in the normal course of revascularization and new bone formation when compared with autografts.[15,63,91,92] Osteoclastic resorbtion appears to be more inhibited than osteoblastic activity. Some grafts appear to remain uninvaded and show failure of healing at the host-donor junction site for a very long time while others, (fortunately only a few) show a rapid dissolution.[64,117]

3. On the basis of the above, it is evident that the time of onset, rate and extent of the revascularization of the graft may vary considerably and, although to some extent dependent on immune response, remain unpredictable.[99,114,117]

4. Articular cartilage contains numerous materials that are capable of exciting the host humoral and cellular immune response and a number of studies have shown antibodies to the cartilage matrix and cells.[55,56,104,114,117] Although this immune reaction could probably be greatly reduced by freezing, cryoinjury to the matrix of the articular cartilage would probably greatly reduce the effectiveness of the tissue as a gliding and bearing surface.

5. Because the matrix of cartilage is so dense, the theoretical pore size of the tissue is miniscule and hence sharply limits the egress of large, and presumably antigenic, proteinaceous materials and at the same time markedly decreases the rate of ingress of antibodies or cells.[55,104] These data suggest that as long as the cartilage matrix remains intact the tissue is "immunologically privileged."

6. It is possible to reduce the size and number of ice crystals that form on the cell membranes and within the chondrocyte by use of the cryopreservatives 8% DMSO and 10% glycerol.[85,86,106] Cryopreservation with isolated chondrocytes is uniformly successful,[86] but similar techniques using the tissue with the intact matrix vary in the degree of viability maintained.[85]

7. Studies have shown that both fresh and cryopreserved frozen cartilage survive allogeneic transplantation, but appear to slowly deteriorate—partly on the basis of putative host immune response, but also because of the problems of joint incongruity.[48,89,98]

8. The three major complications of the allograft procedure, infection, allograft fracture and nonunion are probably all in part immunologically directed and represent various forms and degrees of "rejection".[77,81,82]

These eight points should make it clear that the system as we know it is still imperfect and that our current knowledge remains less than complete.[65] On the basis of our clinical and experimental observations, however, it is possible to state that if a frozen osteoarticular allograft (with cryoprotected cartilage) is implanted into an orthotopic site and a "good fit" is achieved, the system has a reasonable chance (70% to 85%) of success and long survival.[25,83,84] If we wish to improve on that rate and make the procedure more predictable, considerably more research must be done in basic immunology of bone and cartilage and ways of diminishing host-versus-donor reactions.

Allograft Procurement and Bone Banking

If allograft procedures are contemplated it is essential that the surgeon and his team become involved in allograft procurement and banking. Although some of the not-for-profit banks throughout the United States and Canada do sell bones to prospective users, there is really no available "off the shelf" system analogous to the accustomed system for total joints. Each part used must be procured from a "clean" donor, cultured, serologically tested, and sized; the cartilage cryopreserved; and the segment wrapped, labeled, and stored at the appropriate temperature. Records must be carefully kept and some system of followup used to be certain that no untoward events occur. Anyone using the system must assume the responsibility for either doing all this or being certain that it is done in an acceptable manner.

Procurement (harvest) is almost always done in cooperation with living organ donations.[69,80] The various state laws differ but it is now common to have anatomical gift agreements as part of drivers' registrations and some recent legislation mandates the necessity of asking for donations by hospital personnel. For the most part, donors are drawn from trauma deaths. The following rules are utilized by the Massachusetts General Hospital and other bone banks:[68,69,80,105,114]

1. Donors should be between fifteen and forty-five years of age (to be certain that the epiphyses are closed and diminish the likelihood of occult metastases and metabolic bone disease).

2. Donors should be screened by history and subsequent autopsy for infectious disease, malignant neoplastic process, or substance abuse. Because of the dangers of bone microabscesses, prolonged periods of high—dose corticosteroids or respirator support will generally exempt the individual from serving as a donor.

3. The heart blood, urine, pleural and peritoneal fluid and each of the bony parts should be cultured for both anaerobic and aerobic organisms.

4. Donors must be carefully screened by history, at autopsy and especially serologically, for evidence of acquired immunodeficiency syndrome (AIDS), the various forms of hepatitis, other viral disease and syphilis.

Assuming that all of the above criteria are met and that the tests as outlined are normal, the procurement is considered likely to yield usable bones. For such, the harvest should take place in an operating room under sterile conditions with as much attention to the details of the procedure as with any other operations. The parts should be resected through extensile utility incisions, which preserve the blood vessel for subsequent embalming. Donor blood and lymphocytes should be typed (both ABO and HLA) and several lymph nodes obtained and stored frozen after exposure to glycerol for subsequent immunological studies. Each part should be separately cultured (see above), stripped of soft tissues, but leaving the tendinous insertions and joint capsular and ligamentous structures at least 2 to 3cm. long. The cartilage should be exposed to the cryoprotectant for one or more hours, the part placed into gas sterilized polyethylene bags, wrapped in towels, labeled, radiographed in two planes and frozen to $-80°C$. Records should be maintained of the entire process and a computer system for storing of data and possibly sizing of parts (using CT and a digitizer) may be a valuable adjunct to such a system.

At the time of use of the part, sizing films should be compared against the host part (sometimes a radiograph of the opposite is necessary if there has been a distortion of normal anatomy by a tumor or loss of bone stock). After careful checking of all culture and serological data to be certain there are no contraindications to introduction into the host, the part should be unwrapped, recultured, thawed in warm (60°C) Ringer's lactate to which antibiotics have been added.[66,120] Serial radiographs, white blood cell counts, sedimentation rates, bone scans and appropriate serological studies can be performed over the ensuing months to assess the state of the graft and the status of the procedure. These data and especially information about complications should also be entered into the bank record-keeping system.

Even with such a rigorous system totally controlled by our own personnel in our own bank in our own institution, there remain concerns about quality control and the possibility that an infected graft will be implanted into a patient or that hepatitis or AIDS will be transmitted to the recipient with the bone allograft as a vector. Although we have had some bacterial infections transmitted with the graft,[77,82] neither has there been a reported case of transmission of a virus by way of the frozen osseous or cartilaginous alloimplant, nor have we any reason to believe that intracellular viruses can survive the cell death that accompanies the freezing and thawing process.

Special Problems with Allograft Surgery

As indicated above, some of the problems that arise in the course of allograft surgery seem to be unique to the system or arise in sufficiently greater frequency in such procedures to warrant special consideration and attention. The two major complications of the surgical procedure in our hands have been infection and fracture: both severely imperil the results of the surgery and in fact to some extent place the patient in some degree of jeopardy. Over the past several years, we have performed several studies which have attempted to address these complication.[77,81-83]

The first study was an analysis of a series of patients in which we demonstrated not only that infection is the principal complication of fresh frozen cadaveric allograft implantation for tumor but also that the rate is high, approaching 12% in our series of 270 cases followed for two or more years. Deep wound infection related to the surgery was usually manifest by four months following that event, although a second smaller number of patients developed their infection late in the course, usually in relation to additional surgery for fracture or nonunion or as a result of an event such as dental extraction.[82]

One possible source for the high infection rate in this group of patients has been fairly clearly ruled out. Transfer of the infection with the graft is unlikely: to date we have found only one case out of 370 (0.3%). Despite the almost 7% contamination reported for the Naval Tissue Bank[69] and the findings of a similar rate for our current hospital-based bank,[78] control of the materials as advocated by the American Association of Tissue Banks[79,105] appears effective in providing sterile tissues for use at the time of surgery.

Why then the high rate of infection? In the series of surgical procedures for tumor cited in this study a high incidence of predisposing comorbid factors were present (26 of the 33), but it seems significant that other such extensive procedures are performed routinely by our oncology unit and those of others without the high risk of infection. This suggests that some factor or factors are present in the allograft or the implantation procedure that makes it more likely to be infected. Although we have no proof for the thesis, it seems to us that the allograft procedure is quite "unforgiving" and exposure of the graft to nosocomial organisms or transient bacteremias associated with a wide variety of postoperative and rehabilitative events is much more likely to lead to disaster than with other orthopedic procedures. The graft, possibly because of its status as an antigen or conceivably as a result of the host-versus-graft response, appears to have virtually no defenses against organisms implanted at the time of surgery or those that appear in the hematoma in the immediate (and even later) postoperative period. Some factors related to the donor bone (possibly aided by the host response) seem to cause the graft to serve as locus *resistantiae minoris*, and to fall prone to infections that would under most circumstances be eliminated by the host defenses and/or the antibiotics with which the patient is treated in the postoperative phase. Once an infection is established in the region of an allograft, the result is often disastrous (in our series only six out of 33 cases responded to conservative care). Unlike hematogenous or postoperative acute or subacute osteomyelitis where one is dealing with viable, well-perfused autogenous bone, the alloimplant is dead, and has no blood supply. The host bed surrounding it is also abnormal, possibly as a result of the surgery or conceivably as a result of an immune response to the graft. The graft under these circumstances serves as a giant "dead space" that cannot be effectively perfused and is not protected by the host's cellular defense mechanisms. Using this hypothesis, it is easy to project that the infection then becomes rampant, spreads to the adjacent viable (possibly immunocompromised) host parts and rapidly becomes a problem for which the only solution in many cases is resection of the graft or amputation of the limb.

As far as the second complication, fractures, a recent study by Berrey et al.,[81] has established the incidence of this problem in approximately 16% of the patients in our tumor series. The number did not vary materially with the year of performance of the surgery, suggesting that it is likely to be inherent in the allograft system, rather than a function of the surgical technique. This observation is further enhanced by the failure to find any major distinguishing features in the allograft fracture group from an otherwise similar nonfracture cohort. The age, sex distribution, type of tumor, site of graft and stage were virtually identical for the two groups.

The study also defined a mean time and range to occurrence of the fracture. Patients do not appear to be at risk during the first six months following surgery, but then have a sharply increasing likelihood of occurrence until the peak period that falls between two and three years after implantation of the graft. By three years, over three quarters of the fractures had occurred and virtually no fractures occur after four years. We were also able to demonstrate three types of fractures, which differ considerably in presentation and in management. The first and rarest (two of 43 cases) consists of dissolution of the graft (see above). It occurs early in the course, is frightening in its rapidity and requires resection of the graft and replacement with an appropriate system. The second, shaft fracture, is the most common (22 of 43 cases) and occurs most frequently early in the second year. It is more common in males and is more frequently associated with a nonunion of the host-donor junction site. This type of fracture is difficult to treat but, for the most part, responds to open reduction, rearrangement of the internal fixation and addition of autograft. The third, intra-articular fracture, is somewhat less common (19 of 43 cases), occurs later (closer to the third year following the surgery than to the second) and occurs more frequently in women. For the most part, it requires a conventional total joint replacement for restitution.

The data provided by these analyses aided only marginally to illuminate the cause of allograft fracture. The fact that fractures are rare after four years, provides at least some tentative evidence that such a period of time is required of revascularization and competent remodeling in order to achieve the necessary resistance to the stresses of weight-bearing and/or unrestrained use of the limb. Although the demonstration that type II (shaft) fractures occur more readily in patients with slow union of the host-donor junction site suggested that a delay in vascularization is one of the predisposing causes, such a formulation is speculative and requires further proof.

A Brief Look at the Future

Although the results for the published series of patients with allograft implants seem to be not only "acceptable" but equivalent or perhaps even more suitable than many other methods used in the management of patients with major loss of bone substance as a result of tumor, failed implants or trauma, it is evident to all in the field that the system could be materially improved by continued investigation.[1,22-25,77,120-124]

Although numerous studies of graft incorporation have been performed there is an obvious need for a clearer definition of the nature of the cellular processes involved in bone vascularization and host-donor interaction at the junction site and perhaps, more importantly, their optimal rates of occurrence. A second area of research concentration should be in the field of allograft cartilage preservation and joint physiology. Although chondrocytes from fresh allogeneic grafts are more likely to survive than those from frozen segments treated with cryopreservatives, the fresh cartilage and bone appear to exert a greater immune response and may in fact invoke a much more profound graft-versus-host disease. Study of the long-term results of allograft joint replacements in our patients and in series reported by others show an only slowly progressive joint "deterioration" with relatively few of the patients demonstrating a frank osteoarthritis. To date the followup of the series have been too short to correlate the joint changes (or lack of them) with other factors such as fit, rate of host-donor junction site healing, apparent rate of revascularization on x-ray, etc., but clearly these studies as well as further understanding of the biology of transplanted cartilage and improved cryopreservation techniques will be required if we are to advocate this system as method of management of joint disease.

Finally, it should be evident that the ultimate breakthrough in the field of allogeneic transplants of all types will be the development of a safe and efficacious system of altering either the immune mechanism of the host or the immune composition of the donor part so that the allograft is treated by the host in the same manner as it would an autogeneic part. Such an approach could be part of a general alteration of the host but this has such sufficient disadvantages that it is more likely the ultimate system will be specific for each donor part or each host in relation to that donor segment. Such discoveries could ultimately lead to major contributions such as living joint transplants, microvascular anastamosis of host vessels to donor parts and transplants of viable epiphyseal plates to individuals with disturbed growth patterns. Such research is currently in its early phases and clearly has far to go. It is likely that within the next few decades the "dream" will become a reality and such transplants as are depicted in the Miracle of Sts. Cosmas and Damian will become commonplace events.

References

1. Mankin, H.J., Gebhardt, M.C.: Advances in the management of bone tumors. Clin Orthop 200:73-84, 1985.
2. Picci, P., et al.: Preoperative chemotherapy in osteosarcoma: local results and histologic evaluation of necrosis in a study of 97 patients. In Limb Salvage in Musculoskeletal Oncology. Enneking, WF (Ed.): New York, Churchill Livingstone, 1987. pp. 294-297.
3. Farrow, R.C.: Summary of the results of bone-grafting for war injuries. J Bone Joint Surg 30A:31-39, 1948.
4. Gebhardt, M.D., Mankin, H.J.: The diagnosis and staging of bone tumors. Surgical Rounds, 9:86-107, 1986.
5. Rosenthal, DI: Tumors of the musculoskeletal system: Magnetic resonance imaging and computed tomography. Bull NY Acad Med 63:493-503, 1987.
6. Kotz, R., Ritschl, P., Trachtenbrodt, J.: A modular femur-tibia reconstruction system. Orthopedics 9:1639-1652, 1986.
7. Sijbrandij, S.: Resection and reconstruction for bone tumors. Acta Orthop Scand 49:249-254, 1978.
8. Simon, M.A., et al.: Limb salvage treatment versus amputation for osteosarcoma of the distal end of the femur. J Bone Joint Surg 68A:1331-1337, 1987.
9. Wilson, P.D., Jr., Lance, E.M.: Surgical reconstruction of the skeleton following segmental resection for bone tumors. J Bone Joint Surg 47A:16291656, 1975.
10. Rosen, G.: Neoadjuvant chemotherapy for osteogenic sarcoma. in Limb Salvage in Musculoskeletal Oncology. Enneking, W.F. (Ed.): New York, Churchill Livingstone, 1987, pp. 260-268.
11. Sim, F.H., Chao, E.Y.S., Peterson, L.F.A.: Reconstruction following segmental resection of primary bone tumors of the hip. The Hip. 302-324, 1975.
12. Enneking, W.F., Eady, J.L., Burchardt, H.: Autogenous cortical bone grafts in the reconstruction of segmental skeletal defects. J Bone Joint Surg 62A:1039-1058, 1980.
13. Enneking, W.F., Shirley, P.D.: Resection-arthrodesis for malignant and potentially malignant lesions about the knee using an intramedullary rod and local bone grafts. J Bone Joint Surg 59A:223-226, 1977.
14. Weiland, A.J., Daniel, R.K.: Microvascular anastomosis for bone grafts in the treatment of massive defects in bone. J Bone Joint Surg 61A:98-104, 1979.
15. Burrows, H.J., Wilson, J.N., Scales, J.T.: Excision of tumors of the humerus and femur with restoration by internal prosthesis. J Bone Joint Surg 57B:148-159, 1975.
16. Lewis, M.C., Chekofsky, K.M.: Proximal femur replacement for neoplastic disease. Clin Orthop 171:72-79, 1982.
17. Scales, J.T.: Massive bone and joint replacement involving the upper femur, acetabulum and iliac bone. The Hip. 245-275, 1975.
18. Sim, F.H., Chao, E.Y-S.: Segmental prosthetic replacement of the hip and knee. In Tumor Prostheses for Bone and Joint Reconstruction, Chao, E.Y-S. and Ivins, J.C. (Ed.): New York, Thieme Stratton Co., 1983, pp. 247-266.
19. Takahashi, K., et al.: Functional results in patients with custom made hip and knee implants. In Tumor Prosthesis for Bone and Joint Reconstruction, Chao, E.Y.S. and Ivins, J.C. (Ed.): New York, Thieme Stratton Co., 1983, pp. 439-450.
20. Harrington, K.D., et al.: Limb salvage and prosthetic joint reconstruction for low grade and selected high grade sarcomas of bone after wide resection and replacement by autoclaved autogeneic grafts, Clin Orthop 211:180-214, 1986.
21. Winkelmann, W.W.: Hip rotationplasty for malignant tumors of the proximal part of the femur. J Bone Joint Surg 68A:362-369, 1986.
22. Borja, F.J., Mnaymneh, W.: Bone allografts in salvage of difficult hip arthroplasties. Clin Orthop 197:123-130, 1985.
23. Dick, H.M., Malinin, T.I., Mnaymneh, W.A.: Mas-

sive allograft implantation following resection of high-grade tumors requiring adjuvant chemotherapy treatment. Clin Orthop 197:88-95, 1985.

24. Jofe, M.H., et al.: Osteoarticular allografts and allografts plus prostheses in the management of malignant tumors of the proximal femur. J Bone Joint Surg in press.

25. Mankin, H.J., Doppelt, S.H., Tomford, W.W.: Clinical experience with allograft implantation. The first ten years. Clin Orthop 174:69-86, 1983.

26. McGann, W., Mankin, H.J., Harris, W.H.: Massive allografting for severe failed total hip replacement. J Bone Joint Surg 68A:4-12, 1986.

27. Danilevicius, Z.: Cosmas and Damian: The patron saints of medicine in art. JAMA 201-1021-1025, 1967.

28. Macewen, W.: Observations concerning transplantation of bones: Illustrated by a case of inter-human osseous transplantation, whereby over two-thirds of the shaft of a humerus was restored. Proc Roy Soc London 32:232,247, 1881.

29. Lexer, E.: Die Verwendung der freien Knochenplastik nebst Versuchen uber Gelenkversteifung und Gelenktransplantation. Arch Klin Chir 86:939-954, 1908.

30. Lexer, E.: Joint transplantation and arthroplasty. Surg Gynec Obstet 40: 782,809, 1925.

31. Carnesale, P.L., Spankus, J.D.: A clinical comparative study of autogenous and homogenous bone grafts. J Bone Joint Surg 41A:887-894, 1959.

32. Chase, S.W., Herndon, C.H.: The fate of autogenous and homogenous bone grafts. A historical review. J Bone Joint Surg 37A:809-841, 1955.

33. Christie, H.K.: Grafting of homogenous bone and cartilage. Australian and New Zealand J Surg 19:320-334, 1950.

34. Guilleminet, M., Stagnara, P., Dubost Perret, T.: Preparation and use of heterogenous bone grafts. J Bone Joint Surg 35B:561-567, 1953.

35. Heiple, K.G., Chase, S.W., Herndon, C.H.: A comparative study of the healing process following different types of bone transplantation. J Bone Joint Surg 45A:1593-1612, 1963.

36. Henry, M.O.: Homografts in orthopedic surgery. J Bone Joint Surg 30A:70-76, 1948.

37. Herbert, J.J.: Technique of preparing and storing bone for grafts. Summary of the use of grafts in 82 patients. J Bone Joint Surg 33B:312-322, 1951.

38. Wilson, P.D.: Experience with the use of refrigerated homogenous bone. J Bone Joint Surg 33B:301-315, 1951.

39. Bush, L.F.: The use of homogenous bone grafts. A preliminary report on the bone bank. J Bone Joint Surg 29:620-628, 1947.

40. Flosdorf, E.W., Hyatt, G.W.: The preservation of bone grafts by freeze drying. Surgery 31:716-719, 1952.

41. Kreuz, F.P., et al.: The preservation and clinical use of freezed-dried bone. J Bone Joint Surg 33A:863-872, 1951.

42. Spence, K.F., Sell, K.W., Brown, R.H.: Solitary bone cyst: Treatment with freeze-dried cancellous bone allograft. A study of 177 cases. J Bone Joint Surg 51A:87-96, 1969.

43. Urist, M.R.: Bone transplantation in Fundamental and Clinical Bone Physiology, Urist, M.R. (Ed.): Philadelphia, J.B. Lippincott Co., 1980, pp. 331-368.

44. Bonfiglio, M., Jeter, W.S., Smith, C.L.: The immune concept: Its relation to bone transplantation. Ann NY Acad Sci 59:417-433, 1955.

45. Brooks, D.B., et al.: Immunological factors in homogenous bone transplantation. IV. The effect of various methods of preparation and irradiation on antigenicity. J Bone Joint Surg 45A:1617-1626, 1963.

46. Burwell, R.G., Gowland, G.: Studies in the transplantation of bone. III. The immune response of lymph nodes draining components of fresh homogenous bone treated by different methods. J Bone Joint Surg 44B:131-148, 1962.

47. Burwell, R.G., Gowland, G.: Studies in the transplantation of bone. I. Assessment of antigenicity. Serological studies. J Bone Joint Surg 43B:814-819, 1962.

48. Campbell, C.J.: Homotransplantation of half or whole joint. Clin Orthop 87:146-154, 1972.

49. Campbell, C.J., et al.: Experimental study of the fate of bone grafts. J Bone Joint Surg 35A:332-346, 1953.

50. Campbell, C.J., et al.: The transplantation of articular cartilage. An experimental study in dogs. J Bone Joint Surg 45A:1579-1592, 1963.

51. Chalmers, J.: Transplantation immunity in bone homografting. J Bone Joint Surg 41B:160-179, 1959.

52. Chaigmyle, M.B.L.: An autogradiographic and histochemical study of long term cartilage grafts in the rabbit. J Anat 92:467-470, 1958.

53. Curtiss, P.H., Chase, S.W., Herndon, C.H.: Immunological factors in homogenous bone transplantation. II. Histologic studies. J Bone Joint Surg 38A:324-328, 1956.

54. Curtiss, P.H., Powell, A.E., Herndon, C.H.: Immunological factors in homogenous bone transplantation. III. The inability of homogenous rabbit bone to induce circulating antibodies in rabbits. J Bone Joint Surg 41A:1482-1488, 1959.

55. Elves, M.W.: A study of the transplantation antigens on chondrocytes from articular cartilage. J Bone Joint Surg 56B:178-185, 1974.

56. Elves, M.W.: New knowledge of the immunology of bone and cartilage. Clin Orthop 120:232-259, 1976.

57. Hamilton, J.A., Barnes, R., Gilson, T.: Experimental homografting of articular cartilage. J Bone Joint Surg 51B:566-567, 1969.

58. Herndon, C.H., Chase, S.W.: Experimental studies

in the transplantation of whole joints. J Bone Joint Surg 34A:564-578, 1952.

59. Herndon, C.H., Chase, S.W.: The fate of massive autogenous and homogenous bone grafts including articular surfaces. Surg Gynec Obstet 98:273-290, 1954.

60. Heslop, B.F., Zeiss, I.M., Neisbet, M.W.: Studies on Transference of bone: I. A comparison of autologous and homologous bone implants with reference to osteocyte survival, osteogenesis and host reaction. Br J Exp Pathol 41:269-287, 1960.

61. Marrangoni, A.G.: The fate of frozen homogenous bone transplants. Am J Surg 82:378-380, 1951.

62. Ray, R.D., Sabet, T.Y.: Bone grafts: cellular survival versus induction. An experimental study in mice. J Bone Joint Surg 45A:334-337, 1963.

63. Zeiss, I.M., Neisbet, N.W., Heslop, B.F.: Studies on transference of bone. II. Vascularization of autogenous and homologous implants of cortical bone in rats. Br J Exper Pathol 41:345-363, 1960.

64. Burwell, R.G.: The fate of bone grafts. In Apley, GA, Recent Advances in Orthopedics. (Ed.): London, Churchill, 1969, pp. 115-207.

65. Burwell, R.G., Friedlaender, G.E., Mankin, H.J.: Current perspectives and future directions: The 1983 Invitational Conference on osteochondral allografts. Clin Orthop 197:141-158, 1985.

66. Friedlaender, G.E., Strong, D.M., Sell, K.W.: Studies of the antigenicity of bone. II. Donor-specific anti-HLA antibodies in human recipients of freeze dried allografts. J Bone Joint Surg 66A:107-116, 1984.

67. Strong, D.M.: unpublished data.

68. Hart, M.M., Campbell, E.D., Jr., Kartub, M.G.: Bone banking. A cost effective method for establishing a community hospital bone bank. Clin Orthop 206:295-300, 1986.

69. Tomford, W.W., et al.: 1983 bone bank procedures. Clin Orthop 174:15-21, 1983.

70. Volkov, M.: Allotransplantation of joints. J Bone Joint Surg 52B:49-53, 1970.

71. Nilsonne, U.: Homologous joint transplantation in man. Acta Orthop Scandinavia 40:429-447, 1969.

72. Koskinen, E.: Wide resection of primary tumors of bone and replacement with massive bone grafts. Clin Orthop 134:302-319, 1978.

73. Ottolenghi, C.E.: Massive osteoarticular bone grafts. J Bone Joint Surg 48B:646-659, 1966.

74. Ottolenghi, C.E.: Massive osteo and osteoarticular bone grafts. Technique and results of 62 cases. Clin Orthop 87:156-164, 1972.

75. Parrish, F.F.: Treatment of bone tumors by total excision and replacement with massive autologous and homologous grafts. J Bone Joint Surg 48A:968-990, 1966.

76. Parrish, F.F.: Allograft replacement of part of the end of a long bone following excision of a tumor: Report of twenty-one cases. J Bone Joint Surg 55A:1-22, 1973.

77. Rosenberg, A.G., Mankin, H.J.: Complications of allograft surgery. In Complications in Orthopedic Surgery, 2nd Edition, Volume 2. Epps, CH, Jr, (Ed.): Philadelphia, J.B. Lippincott Co., 1986, pp. 1385-1417.

78. Doppelt, S.H., et al.: Operational and financial aspects of a hospital bone bank. J Bone Joint Surg 63A: 1472-1479, 1981.

79. Friedlaender, G.E.: Guidelines for banking osteochondral allografts. In Osteochondral Allografts, Friedlaender, G.E., Mankin, H.J., Sell, K.W. (Ed.): Little Brown and Co., Boston, 1983, pp. 177-180.

80. Tomford, W.W., Ploetz, J.E., Mankin, H.J.: Bone allografts of femoral heads: procurement and storage. J Bone Joint Surg, 68A:534-537, 1986.

81. Berrey, W.H., Jr., et al.: Allograft fractures: Prevalence, management and end results. J Bone Joint Surg, submitted for publication, 1987.

82. Lord, C.F., et al.: The incidence, nature and treatment of allograft infections: Accepted for publication in J Bone Joint Surg, 1987.

83. Mankin, H.J.: Complications of allograft surgery. In Osteochondral Allografts, Friedlaender, G.E., Mankin, H.J., Sell, K.W. (Ed.): Little Brown and Co., Boston, 1983, pp. 259-274.

84. Mankin, H.J., et al.: Osteoarticular and intercalary allograft transplantation in the management of malignant tumors of bone. Cancer 50:613-630, 1982.

85. Tomford, W.W.: Cryopreservation of articular cartilage. In Osteochondral Allografts, Friedlaender, G.E., Mankin, H.J., Sell, K.W. (Ed.): Little Brown and Co., Boston, 1983, pp. 215-218.

86. Tomford, W.W., Duff, G.P., Mankin, H.J.: Experimental freeze-preservation of chondrocytes. Clin Orthop 197:11-14, 1985.

87. Czitrom, A.A., et al.: Bone and cartilage allotransplantation. A review of 14 years of research and clinical studies. Clin Orthop 208:141-145, 1986.

88. Enneking, W.F., Spanier, S.S., Goodman, M.A.: Current concepts review: the surgical staging of musculoskeletal sarcoma. J Bone Joint Surg 62A:1027-1030, 1980.

89. Goldberg, V.H., et al.: Fate of transplanted whole joints. in Osteochondral Allografts, Friedlaender, G.E., Mankin, H.J., Sell, K.W. (Ed.): Little Brown and Co., Boston, 1983, pp. 103-113.

90. Burchardt, H.: Biology of cortical bone graft incorporation. In Osteochondral Allografts, Friedlaender, G.E., Mankin, H.J., Sell, K.W. (Ed.): Little Brown and Co., Boston, 1983, pp. 51-58.

91. Burchardt, H., Busbee, G.A., Enneking, W.F.: Repair of experimental autologous grafts of cortical bone. J Bone Joint Surg 57A:814-819, 1975.

92. Enneking, W.F., et al.: Physical and biological

aspects of repair in dog cortical bone transplants. J Bone Joint Surg 57A:237-252, 1975.

93. Johnson, J.T.H.: Reconstruction of the pelvic ring following tumor resection. J Bone Joint Surg 60A:747-775, 1978.

94. Miller, R.C., Phalen, G.S.: The repair of defects in the radius with fibular bone grafts. J Bone Joint Surg 29A:629-636, 1947.

95. Burchardt, H.: The biology of bone graft repair. Clin Orthop 174:28-42, 1983.

96. Burchardt, H., Enneking, W.F.: Transplantation of bone. Surg Clin N Amer 58:403-427, 1978.

97. Bos, G.D., et al.: The long term fate of fresh and fresh frozen orthotopic bone allografts in genetically defined rats. Clin Orthop 197:123-130, 1985.

98. Schachar, N.S., et al.: Fate of massive osteochondral allografts in a feline model. In Osteochondral Allografts, Friedlaender, G.E., Mankin, H.J., Sell, K.W. (Ed.): Little Brown and Co., Boston, 1983, pp. 81-102.

99. Bos, G.D., et al.: The effect of histocompatability matching on canine frozen bone allografts. J Bone Joint Surg, 65A:89-96, 1983.

100. Friedlaender, G.E.: Immune responses to osteochondral allografts. Current knowledge and future directions. Orthop Clin N Amer 18:241-247, 1983.

101. Goldberg, V.H., et al.: Improved acceptance of frozen bone allografts in genetically mismatched dogs by immunosupression. J Bone Joint Surg 66A:937-950, 1984.

102. Langer, F., et al.: The immunogenicity of fresh and frozen allogeneic bone. J Bone Joint Surg 57A:216-220, 1975.

103. Kandel, R.A., et al.: The pathologic features of massive osseous grafts. Hum Pathol 15:141-146, 1984.

104. Langer, F., Gross, A.E.: Immunogenicity of allograft cartilage. J Bone Joint Surg 56A:297-304, 1974.

105. Friedlaender, G.E., Mankin, H.J.: Guidelines for the banking of musculoskeletal tissues. Newsletter, Amer Assoc Tiss Banks 3:2-7, 1979.

106. Smith, A.U.: Survival of frozen chondrocytes isolated from adult mammals. Nature, 205, 782-784, 1965.

107. Tomford, W.W., Ploetz, J.E., Mankin, H.J.: Collagenase activity in banked bone. Unpublished manuscript.

108. Rodrigo, J.J., et al.: Osteocartilaginous allografts as compared with autografts in the treatment of knee joint osteocartilaginous defects in dogs. Clin Orthop 134:342-349, 1978.

109. Rodrigo, J.J.: The problem of fit in osteocartilaginous allografts. In Osteochondral Allografts, Friedlaender, G.E., Mankin, H.J., Sell, K.W. (Eds.): Little Brown and Co., Boston, 1983, pp.

249-255.

110. Bos, G.D., et al.: Immune responses of rats to frozen bone allografts. J Bone Joint Surg 65A:239-246, 1983.

111. Muscolo, D.L., Kawai, S., Ray, R.D.: Cellular and humerol immune responses analysis of bone-allografted rats. J Bone Joint Surg 58A:826-832, 1976.

112. Powell, A.E., et al.: Immune responses to bone allografts. in Osteochondral Allografts, Friedlaender, G.E., Mankin, H.J., Sell, K.W., (Eds.): Little Brown and Co., Boston, 1983, pp. 141-150.

113. Czitrom, A.A., Axelrod, T., Fernandez, B.: Antigen presenting cells and bone allotransplantation. Clin Orthop 197:27-31, 1985.

114. Friedlaender, G.E., Mankin, H.J., Langer, F.: Immunology of osteochondral allografts: Background and general considerations, In Osteochondral Allografts, Friedlaender, G.E., Mankin, H.J., Sell, K.W., (Eds.): Little Brown and Co., Boston, 1983, pp. 133-140.

115. Muscolo, D.L., et al.: Tissue typing in human massive allografts of frozen bone. J Bone Joint Surg 69A:583-595, 1987.

116. Muscolo, D.L., Kawai, S., Ray, R.D.: In-vitro studies of transplantation antigens present on bone cells in the rat. J Bone Joint Surg 59A:342-348, 1977.

117. Schachar, N.S., et al.: Immune responses to bone allografts. in Osteochondral Allografts, Friedlaender, G.E., Mankin, H.J., Sell, K.W. (Eds.): Little Brown and Co., Boston, 1983, pp. 151-158.

118. Rodrigo, J.J., Fuller, T.C., Mankin, H.J.: Cytotoxic HLA antibodies in patients with bone and cartilage allografts. Trans Orthop Res Soc 1:131, 1976.

119. Friedlaender, G.E., Mankin, H.J., Sell, K.W., (Eds): Osteochondral Allografts, Little Brown and Co., Boston, 1983.

120. Gross, A.E., et al.: The use of allograft bone in revision of total hip arthroplasty. Clin Orthop 197:115-122, 1985.

121. Gross, A.E., et al.: The use of allograft bone in revision hip arthroplasty. Hip 47-58, 1987.

122. Harris, W.H.: Autografting and allografting in aseptic failure of total hip replacement. Hip 286-295, 1984.

123. Head, W.D., Malinin, T.I., Berklacich, F.: Freeze-dried proximal femur allografts in revision total hip arthroplasty. A preliminary report. Clin Orthop 215:109-121, 1987.

124. Trancik, T.M., et al.: Allograft reconstruction of the acetabulum during revision total hip arthroplasty. Clinical, radiographic, and scintigraphic assessment of the results. J Bone Joint Surg 68A:527-33, 1986.

Two

William W. Tomford, M.D.
Henry J. Mankin, M.D.

Principles and Practical Applications of Bone Banking

Introduction

Over the past several years, Mankin[1,2] and others[3] have shown that large stored allografts can provide a very successful means of bone replacement following surgical resection for tumors. Although extensive bone loss is often encountered in failed joint replacements, such grafts have not been as popular in this type of surgery for several reasons: large stored allografts are not readily available; there is little reported experience on their use with metal and cement;[4] and, there is probably a natural tendency to think of metal and cement rather than bone grafts as tools for reconstruction following failed joint replacement.[5] In addition, with the use of uncemented components in revision surgery, small amounts of allograft bone have been used alone and to supplement autograft bone to fill cavities previously filled by cement.[6] With the current trend of an increasing number of failures of cemented joint arthroplasties, there will undoubtedly be an increasing application for both large and small bone allografts as illustrated by other chapters in this book. A knowledge of principles of storage of these bones should prove helpful to orthopedists who desire to use them. Any method that inhibits or destroys the action of degradative enzymes, such as collagenase and other proteases, will permit storage of bone. The two most popular include freeze-drying[7] and freezing.[8] Many commercial bone banks prefer to freeze-dry their bone grafts. Freeze drying requires a large initial outlay of funds for equipment, but may be less expensive over a long period, and certainly provides an effective method of stor-

age. Our bone bank has chosen to store bone by freezing because this method does not require elaborate equipment. This chapter is based on our experience in bone banking and will therefore concentrate on freezing as the method of storage.

Organization of a Bone Bank

A commercial bone bank may be organized as a single tissue bank supplying only bone, or as part of a multi-tissue bank supplying other tissues such as skin and dura. The U.S. Navy founded the first large bone bank in 1951 as part of a tissue bank[9]. Table 2-1 lists commercial bone banks from which bones may be obtained. These banks will sell large and small bone grafts to surgeons who can prove they have a legitimate need and who are willing to pay for the cost of procuring and processing the bone.

Bone banks may also be organized in hospitals for the use of surgeons within a particular hospital or medical center. Hospital-based bone banks frequently confine bone procurement and storage to femoral heads[10] although with dedicated manpower and appropriate facilities, they may also obtain and store long bones from cadavers.[8]

Regardless of the scope of a bone bank, it should be organized using the guidelines and standards published by and available from the American Association of Tissue Banks (AATB) (See Table 2-1). Founded in 1977, the AATB is composed of tissue bankers, including bone bankers, who meet annually to discuss principles and practices of

Table 2-1
Commercial Bone Banks in the United States
Providing Bones to Orthopedic Surgeons

American Red Cross
St. Paul Region
100 South Roberts Street
St. Paul, Minnesota 55107
(612) 291-4679

American Red Cross Tissue Bank
4050 Lindell Boulevard
St. Louis, Missouri 63108
(314) 658-2193

Eastern Virginia Tissue Bank
533 Newton Road
Virginia Beach, Virginia 23462
(804) 625-3171

Michigan Tissue Bank
1215 East Michigan Avenue
P.O. Box 30480
Lansing, Michigan 48909
(517) 483-2557

Northern California Transplant Bank Pacific Medical Center
P.O. Box 7999
San Francisco, California 94120
(415) 922-3100

Pennsylvania Regional Tissue and Transplant Bank
200 Adams Avenue
P.O. Box 622
Scranton, Pennsylvania 18501
(717) 343-5433

American Association of Tissue Banks
1117 North 19th Street
Suite 402
Arlington, Virginia 22209
(703) 528-0663

bone and tissue banking. The standards were written by AATB members with several years of experience in banking bones.

A bone bank's activities should be directed by a physician who serves as the medical director. The director is responsible for ensuring that the tissue is as safe as possible: that it is procured, stored, and provided to surgeons in a manner that avoids contamination. The medical director should also serve as a consultant for surgeons who desire to know more about which bones are available and how to use these bones in their practice.

Technicians are useful in bone banking. In larger banks, they may provide valuable assistance in the procurement of long bones. In smaller banks, they may provide manpower for the necessary record-keeping. Any technician who is involved in bone banking should have a thorough knowledge of sterile technique for application in procurement and storage as well as use of the bone.

Techniques of Procurement and Storage

Bone procurement can be performed in several ways

which vary according to the type of bone to be used and the method of storage. If long bones are to be procured, it is advisable to contact the local organ procurement agency and work with that group. Organ procurement agencies are usually local organizations responsible for finding donors of kidneys and other organs. Because tissue donation can frequently accompany organ donation, organ procurement agencies can provide information and assistance in obtaining tissues in addition to the organs for which they are responsible. Although tissue donation is less frequent than organ donation, the fact that bones are now used for such procedures as revision of joint replacement as well as replacement of bone destroyed by tumors suggests that the need for bone donation will increase. Because cadaver donors are in demand, it is easiest to work with, rather than in competition with, organizations that are already involved in the procurement of organs. Every hospital that has a kidney transplant service has, or works in association with, an organ procurement agency, and contacting that agency to express an interest in tissue procurement is extremely worthwhile.

If bone is to be procured sterilely and will not be sterilized prior to transplantation, it is important to follow sterile technique during procurement, to culture the bone frequently, and to maintain storage of the bone in a sterile container. Our bone bank procures bone only in an operating room under strict aseptic conditions. We have a team of three surgeons: two working simultaneously on the body and the third culturing and wrapping the bones for storage. Long bones are retrieved starting with the femur, followed by the tibia, and the upper extremity bones (humerus and distal radius). Pelvic bones are taken last because of the possibility of contamination from the pelvic contents. Ligaments and insertions of tendons are left long in order to make further reconstruction easier. The bone is removed as a whole rather than cutting it into parts because it is difficult for the surgeon to determine prior to surgery precisely what length of bone will be needed.

Long bones can be packaged in several ways. The U.S.

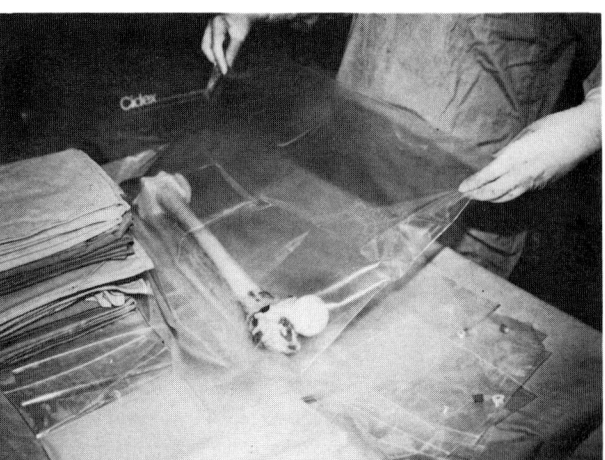

Figure 2-1. Bones to be frozen may first be wrapped in plastic bags.

Navy Tissue Bank used vacuum-packed large glass jars to store freeze-dried bones. Bones to be frozen may first be wrapped in sterile plastic bags (Figure 2-1), then in three sterile towels and finally in an outer heavy-mil plastic bag to prevent any water seeping in or out of the towels (Figure 2-2). The final plastic bag is tightly taped. Identification of the bone is written in ink on the tape and includes the name of the donor, the bone, and the date of the procurement.

Bones not sterilized but procured sterilely and packed and stored in a sterile manner must be cultured at the time of procurement. Our bone bank uses swabs to culture only the surface of the bone. We do not culture pieces of the bone. Our philosophy is that a piece of the bone represents only a small part of the bone and therefore does not provide a significant test for contamination. Systemic contamination is determined by blood cultures taken from the heart at the time of procurement or from blood cultures obtained during the donor's hospitalization.

Guidelines for assuring sterility of the bones, if the bones will not be sterilized, should be followed closely. A patient who has a history of prolonged fevers or infections is not a good donor. In addition, any patient who has a history of hepatitis or AIDS is not a good donor. Blood testing for these two diseases should be obtained at the time of procurement. Likewise, any patient with a history of osteomyelitis or other chronic infections, tumors, or diseases of unknown etiologies, is not a good donor. A patient who is healthy and who dies traumatically is the best donor, of both organs and tissues. A patient who has had a prolonged hospitalization, has been on a respirator for a prolonged period of time (generally more than three days), or dies of drug abuse, is not a good donor.

If the bones are to be sterilized, these guidelines may be amended. For example, procurement does not have to be performed sterilely. However, if the method of sterilization is not effective in killing viruses, a donor should be determined to be free of any viral diseases or diseases thought to

be caused by viruses. Culturing under these circumstances should be performed after sterilization by using a certain percentage of the tissues sterilized as a means of evaluation of all tissues.

If bone is to be stored frozen and not sterilized, procurement of tissue should be performed within twelve hours of death. Otherwise, the organisms on the skin overgrow, and it becomes difficult to sterilize the skin, even with strong antiseptic solutions such as iodine or alcohol. Likewise, the storage method (freezing) should not be delayed any longer than possible. Refrigeration of tissues, although inhibiting the growth of organisms, does not completely stop this growth, and any organisms that are on the bone may multiply and become abundant.

Storage temperature should be low enough to inhibit enzymatic action. Freezing at any temperature below zero degrees will achieve prohibition of enzymatic action. There is good evidence that the lower the temperature, the safer it is to store tissues for long periods of time.[11] The lowest temperature commercially possible is $-179°C$, or the temperature of liquid nitrogen. Storage tanks of liquid nitrogen are easily purchased, and may provide long-term, safe storage of bone; however, in order to keep enough nitrogen in large freezers, the supply must be renewed several times a month. Because of the cost involved in this endeavor, we have chosen to use electrical freezers maintained at temperatures of approximately $-80°C$. Our bone bank has employed 19 cubic foot chest-type freezers because many long bones such as femurs and tibias can be easily stored in this size of freezer.

Freezing does not kill bacteria. Therefore, culturing the bones and searching for contamination is important. Swabs from the external surface of the bones are placed into culture media (blood agar plates and thioglycolate broth) which will allow growth of aerobic organisms. Separate cultures are performed for anaerobic organisms. Cultures should be kept for 10 to 15 days after procurement of bone. In our bone bank, any bone that has cultured positively is set aside in a separate freezer to be kept for sterilization by irradiation, or it is discarded. Approximately 15% of the procured bones have positive cultures. Approximately 90% of the positive cultures grow *Staph epidermidis* that is undoubtedly the result of inadequate skin sterilization and contamination during procurement of the bone. Blood cultures obtained during the patient's demise or at the time of bone retrieval should be placed in standard blood culture media. Two to three sets of blood cultures should be obtained in order to avoid confusion over inadvertent contamination, which is quite frequent in culturing blood. If two out of three cultures are positive, suggesting systemic contamination, use of the bones is contradindicated.

Bones should be x-rayed prior to use to check for possible fractures or lesions and to assess size. Several methods are available for sizing, including the use of a radiopaque ruler laid beside the bone. If a ruler is not available, magnification by x-ray may be minimized by laying the bone on

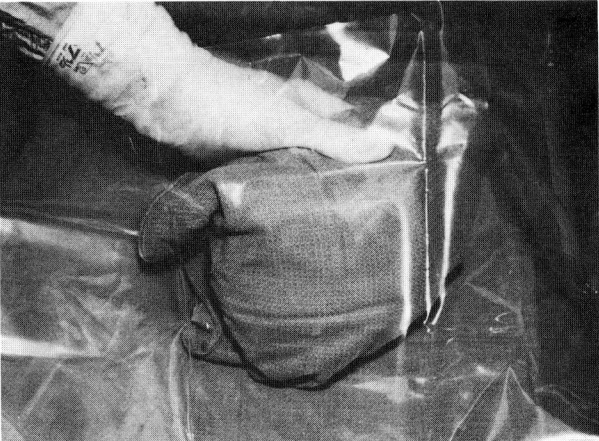

Figure 2-2. Bones are then wrapped in three sterile towels and then in an outer heavy-mil plastic bag to prevent any water seeping in or out of the towel.

the x-ray cassette and placing the source of the beam as far away as possible before shooting.[12]

We recommend that a culture of the bone also be obtained by the surgeon at the time of transplantation. Although the result of this culture is not known until a few days after the surgical procedure, this practice affords another evaluation of the sterility of the bones in the bank. It also provides information that may be useful in choosing an antibiotic should an infection occur postoperatively, although there does not appear to be an increased incidence of infection with the use of banked bone.[13]

Procurement and storage of femoral heads follow guidelines and techniques similar to the above. A donor should be reviewed for any history of hepatitis, AIDS, cancer and any diseases of unknown origin. Blood tests should be performed to rule out the possibility of hepatitis, AIDS, and syphilis. In addition, because patients who are on steroids for long periods may have chronic infections without clinical evidence, osteonecrosis due to chronic steroid ingestion is, in our bank, a contraindication to bone procurement. Our donor of femoral heads is usually a patient in good health who fractures a femoral neck or has a primary hip replacement for osteoarthritis. Cultures are performed at the time of procurement, and any culture that is positive results in the femoral head being discarded.

Femoral heads may be stored in several ways. One method has employed the use of two sterile jars, one inside the other, with the femoral head inside the innermost jar. Our bone bank has used only one jar with a screw-on lid (Figure 2-3). This jar is wrapped by the scrub nurse in three sterile towels (Figure 2-4) and then placed into a plastic bag which is taped, and labeled with a tag which identifies the donor, provides an estimate of size made by the surgeon at the time of procurement (small, medium, large), and records the date of procurement. This method has proven to be successful in storing femoral heads over the course of four years' experience.[10]

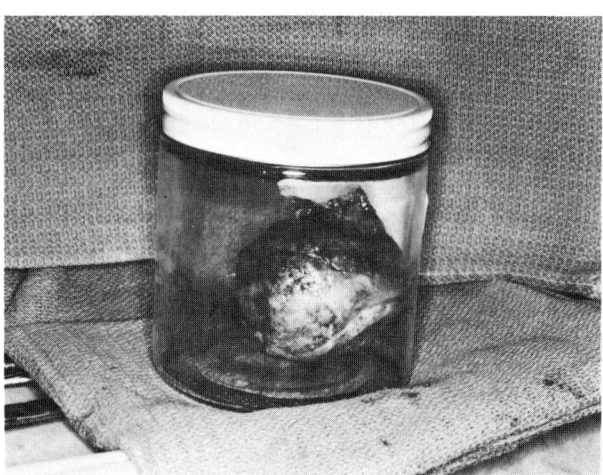

Figure 2-3. The femoral head is placed within one jar with a screw-on lid.

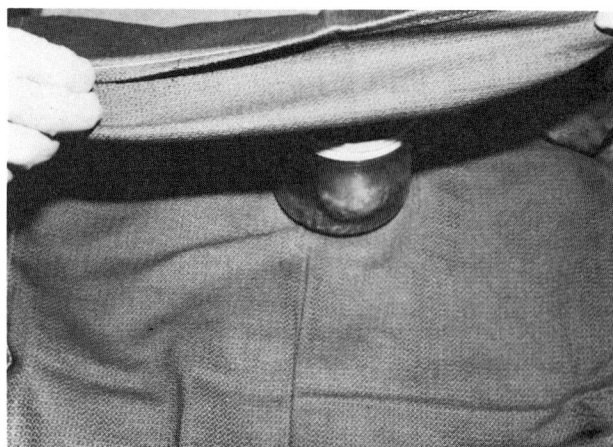

Figure 2-4. The jar is wrapped in three sterile towels and then placed into a plastic bag.

Record Keeping and Billing

Record keeping is an extremely important part of bone banking. Should infection occur postoperatively, a record of which bone was implanted into which recipient is mandatory to determine the possible source of the infection and if other bones from the same donor are contaminated. A record of the bone graft should begin at the time of the procurement and should include the name of the donor, the date of procurement, results of cultures, location in storage, and recipient. Other information that may be added includes diagnoses of the donor and the recipient and the donor's blood and tissue type. There is evidence that the results of cases using bone grafts in humans are not affected by immune responses,[14] and therefore matching tissue types may not be important. There is also evidence, however, that sensitization to an Rh antigen may be produced by a femoral head graft,[15] and it therefore appears worthwhile to match Rh types in patients who are at risk for the adverse effects of sensitization, such as females of childbearing age.

A charge is included on the patient's hospital bill to cover the costs of processing the bones which includes procurement, culturing, storage and handling. These charges help the hospital recover the prorated costs of freezers, electricity and rental space as well as the cost of operating room time for procurement. A charge slip is generated at the time of transplantation that includes the type of bone as well as the name of the donor. This practice provides a check on the supply of bones in the bank as well as a record of the donor.

Networking of Bones

If an in-house hospital bone bank decides to bank long bones, it is advantageous to join with other similar banks to exchange bones to gain access to a larger range of sizes. For the past four years, the Massachusetts General Hospital Bone Bank has been part of a collaborative effort to exchange bones with three other hospital bone banks (Mayo Clinic, University of Florida (Gainsville) and Yale University). By joining in a network with other bone banks that employ similar banking methods, access to many bones is possible.

Use of Banked Bones

Banking bone places a responsibility on the banking personnel to provide surgeons with the best possible bone for their needs. We strongly recommend consultations between the medical director of the bank and the surgeons who use the bones well in advance of the date of their surgical procedures. These meetings allow the bank personnel to understand what is needed and the surgeons to understand what can be supplied. Review of the surgical procedure to be performed as well as the planned use of the graft helps the medical director determine which size and type of bone would be best.

A professional relationship should be fostered between surgeons and the bank so bank personnel can procure bones that satisfy surgical needs. For example, if the bank has a limited number of certain bones, but these bones are frequently used, it is important for the bank personnel to be aware of this so that at the next bone bank procurement a particular type of bone can be obtained. There is a time limit on sterile cadaveric bone procurements because the use of operating rooms is extremely costly. It is therefore helpful to the bank personnel to know which bones are in demand so that procurements may be concentrated on the most needed bones. The best use of banked bone occurs when the bank understands how the surgeon uses it and can supply bone that is the correct size, Rh type, etc. This can be easily achieved with preoperative reviews between the medical director of the bank and the surgeon. Under these circumstances, a relationship will occur that will provide mutual satisfaction for everyone involved, and the bone bank can provide a very valuable service to the surgeons in the hospital or community.

References

1. Mankin, H.J., et al.: Osteoarticular and intercalary allograft transplantation in the management of malignant tumors of bone. Cancer 50:613, 1982.
2. Mankin, H.J.: Allograft replacement for the management of skeletal defects incurred in tumor surgery or trauma. In: The Design and Application of Tumor Prostheses for Bone and Joint Reconstruction. Chao, E., (Ed.): 1982, New York, Thieme-Stratton, Inc.
3. Gross, A.E., et al.: Surgical techniques and clinical experience with articular allografts at the knee. In: Osteochondral Allografts. Friedlaender, G.E., Mankin, H.J., Sell, K.W. (Ed.): 1984, Boston, Little, Brown and Co., p. 289.
4. McGann, W., Mankin, H.J., Harris, W.H.: Massive allografting for severe failed total hip replacement. J Bone Joint Surg 68A:4, 1986.
5. Harris, W.H.: Allografting in Total Hip Arthroplasty. Clin Orthop 162:150, 1982.
6. Engh, C.A., Bobyn, J.D.: Biological fixation in total hip arthroplasty. Thorofare, New Jersey, Slack, Inc., 1985, p. 89.
7. Malinin, T.I., Martinez, O.V., Brown, M.D.: Banking of massive osteoarticular and intercalary bone allografts—12 years experience. Clin Orthop Rel Res 197:44, 1985.
8. Tomford, W.W., et al.: 1983 Bone banking procedures. Clin Orthop 174:15, 1983.
9. Friedlaender, G.E.: U.S. Navy tissue bank. J Am Podiat Assn 67:38, 1977.
10. Tomford, W.W., Ploetz, J.P., Mankin, H.J.: Bone allografts of femoral heads: Procurement and storage. J Bone Joint Surg 68A:423, 1986.
11. Karow, A.M., Jr.: Cryopreservation: Pharmacological considerations. In: Organ Preservation for Transplantation. Karow, A.M., Jr., Abouna, G.J.M., Humphries, A.L. Jr. (Eds): 1974, Boston, Little, Brown and Co., p. 86.
12. Gorski, J.M., Schwartz, L.: A device to measure x-ray magnification in pre-operative planning for cementless arthroplasty. Clin Orthop Rel Res 202:302, 1986.
13. Tomford, W.W., Starkweather, R.J., Goldman, M.H.: A study of the clinical incidence of infection in the use of banked allograft bone. J Bone Joint Surg 63A:233, 1981.
14. Friedlaender, G.E., Strong, D.M., Sell, K.W.: Studies on the antigenicity of bone. II. Donor-specific anti-HLA. Antibodies in human recipients of freeze-dried allografts. J Bone Joint Surg 66A:107, 1984.
15. Johnson, C.A., Brown, B.A., Lasky, L.C.: Rh immunization caused by osseous allograft. N Engl J Med 312 (2):121, 1985.

THREE

Hugh P. Chandler, M.D.
Brad L. Penenberg, M.D.

Preoperative Planning

Reconstructive hip surgery in the face of bone deficiency is more complex and of considerably longer duration than routine total hip replacement. To be surprised at surgery as to the extent of bone deficiency is potentially quite costly. Not only can anesthesia time be unnecessarily prolonged while waiting for a different type of prosthesis or bone graft, but the most unfortunate situation for the patient would be the need to compromise or abandon the planned reconstruction because appropriate materials are unavailable at the time of surgery.

In order to avoid such complications, meticulous preoperative planning must be carried out. This may be divided into three major areas. The first relates to a thorough patient evaluation; the second to a detailed radiographic analysis of the bone defects; and the third to the proposed surgical reconstruction.

Patient Evaluation

Orthopedic Assessment

Incorporating pertinent aspects of the patient's history and physical examination, the Harris hip rating system is used to provide an objective assessment of the severity of the patient's hip problem and is helpful in making the decision whether the patient is incapacitated enough to require a long and potentially dangerous operation.

A detailed orthopedic history should be obtained. In addition to questions concerning the patients' ambulatory capacity, their ability to climb stairs, to sit and to dress their feet, specific attention should be given to the patients'

descriptions of their pain as this singular complaint has such a major bearing on the decision whether or not surgery is indicated. It is important to be sure that subjective complaints of pain in the hip region are caused by hip pathology and are not referred from the lumbar spine, the retroperitoneum, inguinal hernias or from femoral neuropathies. Subjective reports as to the severity of pain must be interpreted with regard to the psychological make up of individual patient. It is also of value to assess whether pathology in joints other than the hip or impairment of cardiac, pulmonary or neurologic systems might independently compromise the result, even if hip reconstruction was technically successful.

A thorough orthopedic physical examination should be performed. In addition to assessing range of motion and gait, specific attention should be given to previous skin incisions, leg length discrepancies and hip musculature.

Extension of old incisions or the addition of new incisions should be carefully planned to avoid necrosis.

True and apparent lengths are measured as closely as possible. A series of lifts of known thickness may be tried beneath the shoe until the iliac crests are level. Scanograms are helpful for more precise measurements. At the time of surgery, reference points should be established on the pelvis and femur so intraoperative measurements can be made. The amount of discrepancy that can be safely corrected varies considerably. A discrepancy that has existed since childhood can usually be corrected to slightly greater than one inch but beyond this, there is significant risk of neurologic injury. However, if a patient had equal leg lengths at skeletal maturity and subsequently required a resection arthroplasty with a leg length discrepancy of up to three inches, leg lengths can usually be equalized at the time of revision surgery without major risk.[1]

In assessing musculature about the hip, abductor weakness should be specifically noted. Weakness of the abductors could result in a limp or instability despite an otherwise successful reconstruction. The etiology of the weakness should be established. Mechanical weakness secondary to proximal migration of the greater trochanter can be addressed at surgery. Weakness secondary to neurologic problems such as polio might require the use of an inherently more stable, bipolar-type prosthesis. A spastic muscle imbalance such as might be seen with the residual of a cerebral vascular accidebt (CVA) or Parkinson's disease, should influence the surgeon to use an approach that leaves the posterior structures intact.[2]

Medical Assessment

All patients undergoing a lengthy and complex operative procedure with the potential for major blood loss and fluid replacement should have a thorough preoperative medical evaluation. Ideally this is done as an outpatient one month prior to anticipated surgery. In this way, the preoperative hospital stay is kept to a minimum, and any unexpected abnormalities can be further investigated or treated prior to admission.

Although a complete review of systems is a routine part of the medical assessment, pathology referable to the gastrointestinal (GI), Genitourinary (GU) and venous systems is specifically sought. Regarding the GI tract, patients may deny having ulcer symptoms but may more readily admit to frequent antacid use. The stress of major surgery may be enough to precipitate a major bleed or perforation in a patient with very subtle GI symptoms. An appropriate GI work-up should be obtained in these patients. Pre-existing ulcer disease is of particular significance because the anticoagulants warfarin and salicylates are commonly used for thromboembolic prophylaxis.[3,4]

Reports in the literature have described a significant incidence of cholecystitis following hip and other types of major surgery.[5] If a history of gall bladder symptoms is reported, appropriate studies should be obtained to rule out a diagnosis of cholelithiasis. Treating a diseased gallbladder prior to total hip replacement could prevent a potentially fatal attack of acute cholecystitis and also lessen the risk of a devastating joint infection secondary to gram-negative bacteremia.

The GU system is of particular concern because of the threat of bacteremia and possible hip sepsis as a result of infection. Many patients, especially elderly women, have asymptomatic urinary tract infection. A urine culture is therefore routinely obtained at the time of the preoperative evaluation one month before admission. A positive culture can be treated with appropriate antibiotics prior to admission for the elective surgery. Men with prostate enlargement may give a history of voiding problems that should be

evaluated preoperatively to avoid postoperative urinary retention.

A previous history of phlebitis, pulmonary embolus or clinical evidence of peripheral venous disease is also of great importance and the surgeon should strongly consider the use of warfarin prophylaxis in these patients.[3]

Because of an increasing concern with blood-borne diseases, the majority of our patients participate in an autologous blood-donor program. For a primary hip replacement, four units of red cells are preserved. For a major revision, most patients donate five to eight units. A healthy young patient can often give a unit of blood every seven to ten days. Supplementary iron (ferrous gluconate — 300 mg., t.i.d.) is given between donations. Even elderly patients can give a unit of blood every two to three weeks. The hematocrit is checked prior to each donation and if below 34, further donations are delayed. Very elderly or frail patients, those with chronic anemia or those with significant cardiac disease may not be able to donate blood. Family members are often willing to be designated donors if the patients cannot give blood.

Because of their effect on platelets, anti-inflammatory medications are discontinued ten days prior to surgery. A preoperative bleeding time should be checked in patients who have continued to ingest these medicines up to the time of surgery.

Any patient who is contemplating hip surgery deserves to be informed of its potential complications. Compared with the risks usually associated with primary total hip arthroplasty, the special risks associated with major hip revision surgery are both more common and more severe. These include a higher incidence of sepsis, loosening, dislocation, phlebitis, pulmonary embolus, and both vascular and neurological injury.[1,6,7,8] When massive allograft reconstruction is necessary, the patient must be aware that failure could result in hind quarter amputation.

Radiographic Assessment

The radiographic options include:
1. AP of the pelvis with hips in neutral rotation and neutral abduction;
2. Obliques of the pelvis;
3. True lateral of the involved hip;
4. AP and rotational views of the femur;
5. Hip aspiration and arthrogram;
6. Scanograms;
7. Tomograms;
8. Computer assisted tomography; and
9. Computer assisted modeling of the acetabulum and pelvis.

AP of the Pelvis with Hips in Neutral Rotation and Neutral Abduction. A true AP x-ray of the pelvis with both hips in neutral rotation and zero degrees of abduction should be obtained on every patient. Consistent

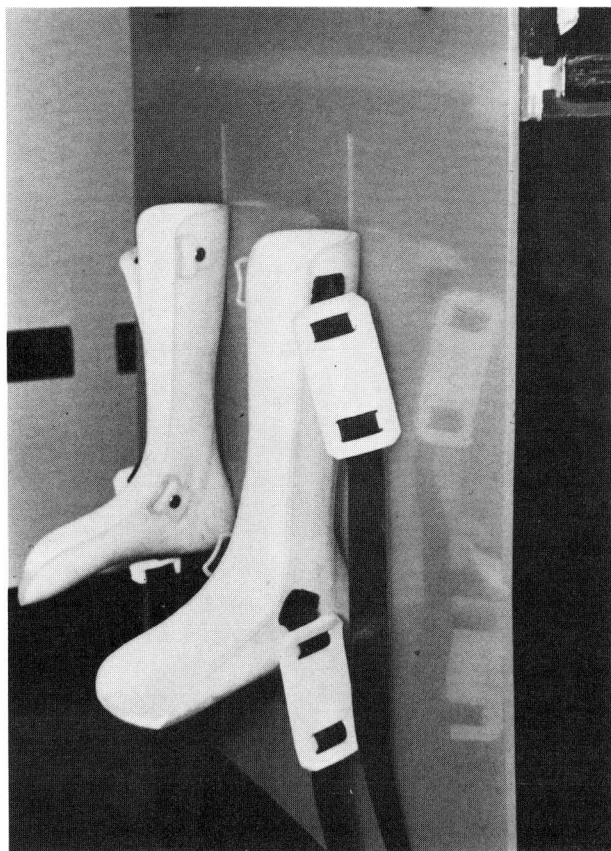

Figure 3-1A. The frame is constructed so that it can be placed at the end of a standard x-ray table. Plastic polypropylene orthoses are secured to a plastic backboard through a vertical slot. A wing nut allows adjustment for various leg lengths. Rotation and abduction remain constant.

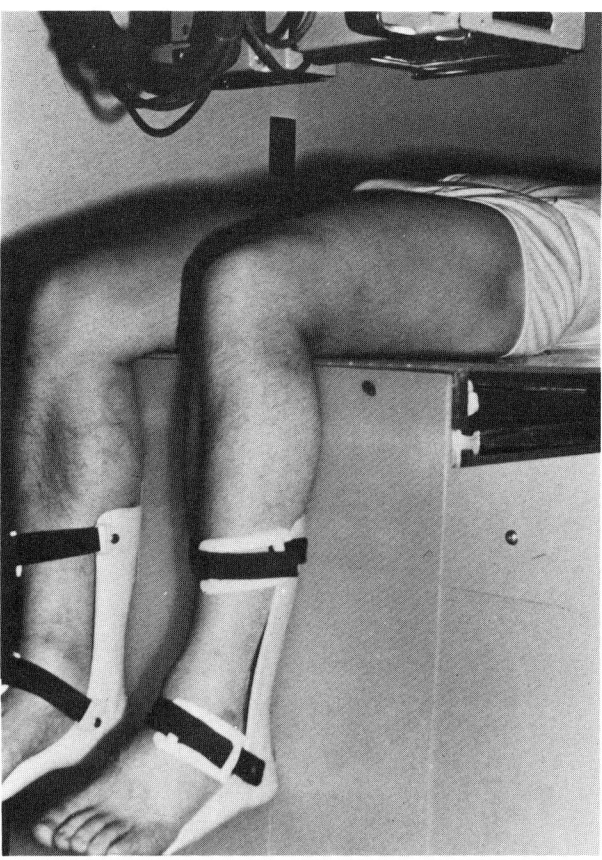

Figure 3-1B. The patient lies supine on an x-ray table with knees flexed. Feet and legs are secured in the orthoses.

patient positioning is assured by the use of an x-ray frame (Figures 3-1A and 3-1B). This frame is also used for serial postoperative x-rays since it allows more precise comparison from one film to another.

It is important to include the contralateral hip to allow comparison between the two hips. Preliminary assessment of leg length discrepancy can be made (Figure 3-2). A transverse line may be drawn across the pelvis just below the lower borders of the inferior pubic rami. This will serve as a reference line when assessing the relative difference in the levels of the lesser trochanters.

The AP pelvis x-ray allows assessment of the superior rim, the superior intra-acetabular segment of the acetabulum and often, the integrity of the medial wall. Subtle as well as large medial wall defects can usually be identified on the AP films (Figures 3-3A and 3-3B). In addition, the quality of the bone stock can be evaluated in comparison with the other hip.

If there is marked superior migration of an acetabular component on the AP view, anterior and posterior wall deficiency should be anticipated because the ilium becomes very thin above the area where the true acetabulum should be (Figure 3-4).

A true AP of the acetabulum also allows accurate

acetabular templating (Figure 3-5). However, patients with significant flexion deformities will often end up with an inlet view if the standard AP x-ray is taken with the hips in extension (Figure 3-6). This view can be misleading when templating the acetabulum and it is better to flex the hips the

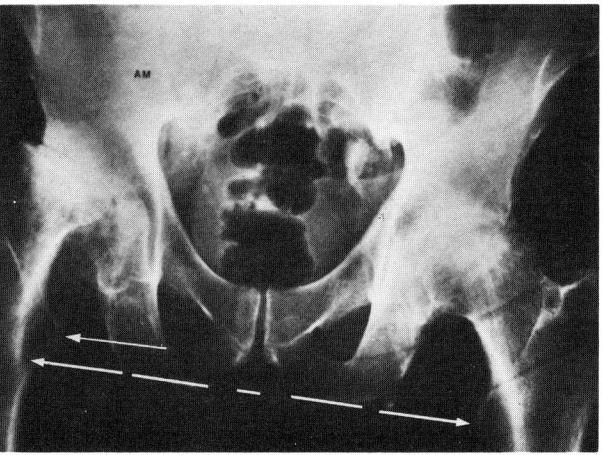

Figure 3-2. Superolateral migration of the right femoral head is present. The relative levels of the lesser trochanters allow estimation of leg length discrepancy.

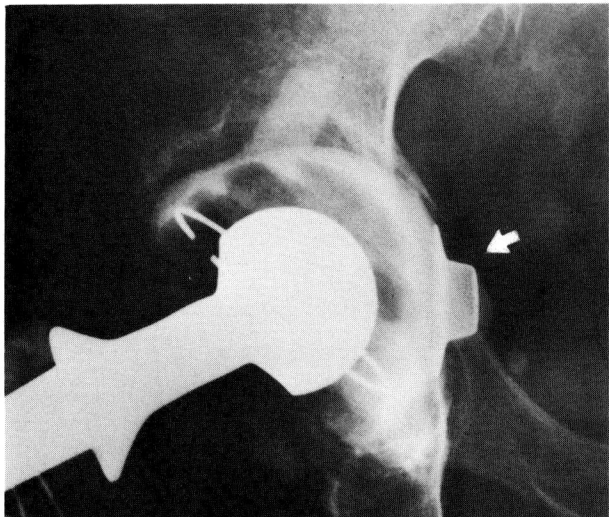

Figure 3-3A. The presence of a cement restriction andor intra-pelvic cement indicates at least a small medial wall defect.

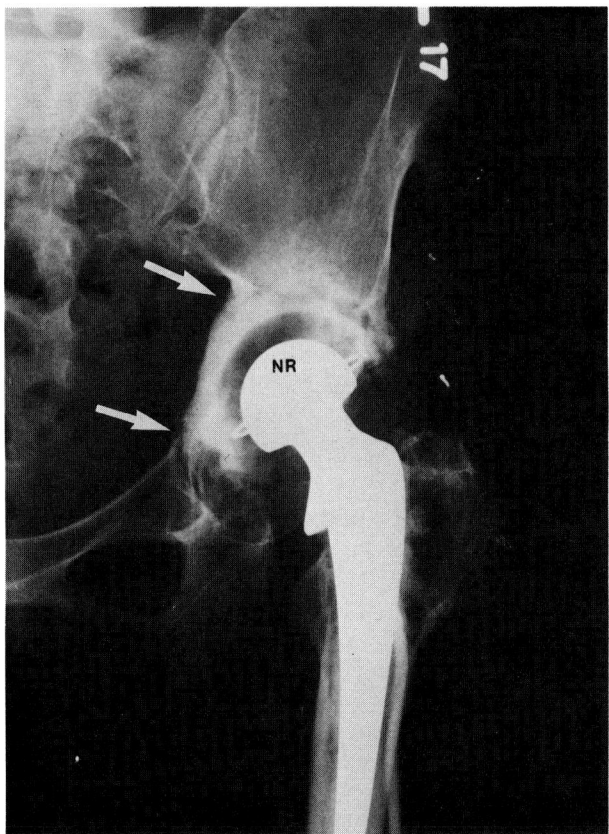

Figure 3-3B. There is no bone visible medial to the cement mantle (between the arrows). This correlated with a medial wall defect measuring 5cm. in diameter.

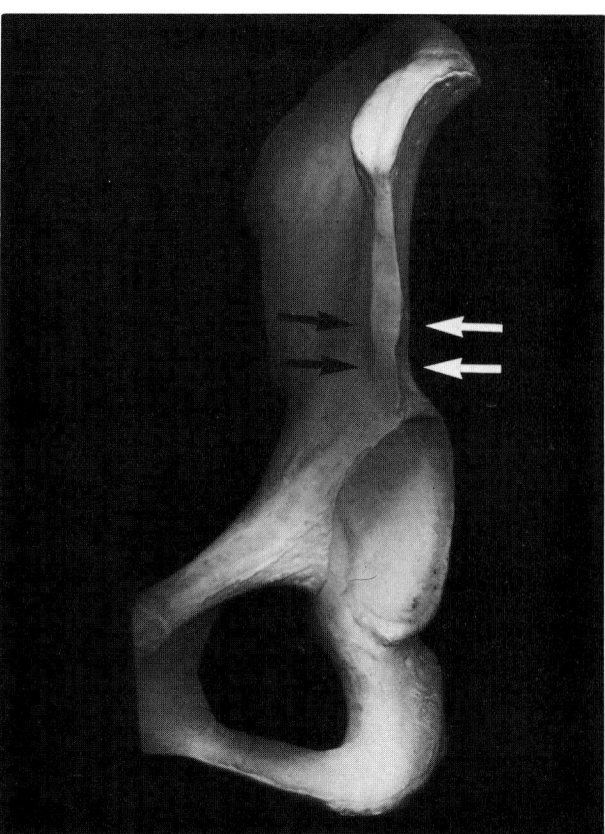

Figure 3-4. The ilium becomes extremely thin just above the true acetabulum.

necessary amount to allow a normal AP of the pelvis to be taken.

Obliques of the Pelvis. Iliac and obturator oblique views can often provide additional important information. The AP x-ray may suggest that there is adequate lateral coverage of the acetabular component as seen in Figure

3-7A. However, superior migration in this case should make one suspicious of a posterior wall deficiency. An obturator oblique view can reveal the extent of the superior rim or posterior wall deficiency (Figure 3-7B). An AP film may suggest some degree of superior rim deficiency (Figure 3-8A), an iliac oblique view may be of value to demonstrate superior coverage anteriorly but may be misleading in estimating acetabular volume (Figure 3-8B). The obturator oblique film should help to reveal the true magnitude of the superior and posterior rim deficiency (Figure 3-8C).

True Lateral of the Involved Hip. A true lateral film of the involved hip can be quite helpful in assessing bone stock on both the acetabular and femoral sides.

On the acetabular side, this view allows assessment of the thickness of the posterior intra-acetabular segment (Figure 3-9A). This segment is defined on x-ray by the apex of the sciatic notch and the mid-posterior arch of the subchondral bony condensation. Even in the presence of extensive erosion, the AP view does not demonstrate this segment (Figures 3-9B and 3-9C). An extruded cement mass can sometimes be more accurately localized when the true lateral is viewed in conjunction with the AP x-ray.

On the femoral side, the true lateral view is helpful in targeting areas of potential difficulty in cement removal. The orientation of the femoral stem can be analyzed with respect to its anterior-posterior position, proximity to cor-

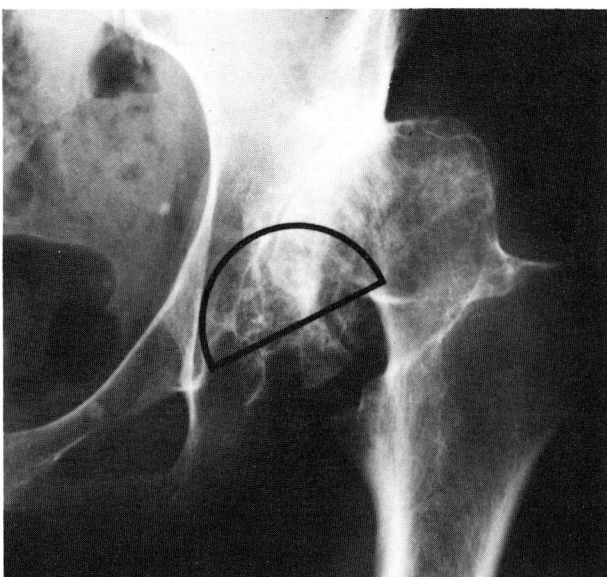

Figure 3-5. The acetabular template is usually placed at the level of the normal center of hip rotation.

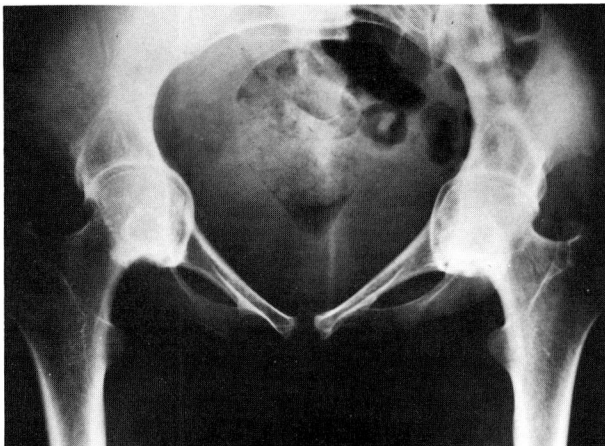

Figure 3-6. The inlet view (note slit-like obturator foramina and a large AP pelvic diameter) distorts the acetabular contour. Flexing the patient's hips at the time of x-ray will provide a more standard AP view of the pelvis.

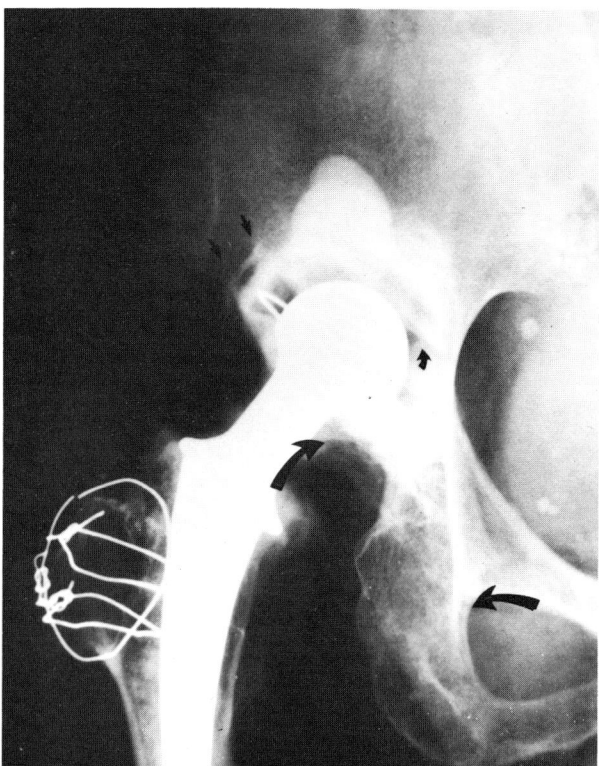

Figure 3-7A. This acetabular component is well above the true acetabulum. The large curved arrows show marked disruption of Shenton's line. Although the acetabular component appears to be well covered by a strong bony rim (two small arrows) one should be suspicious that the posterior wall will be deficient with this much superior migration.

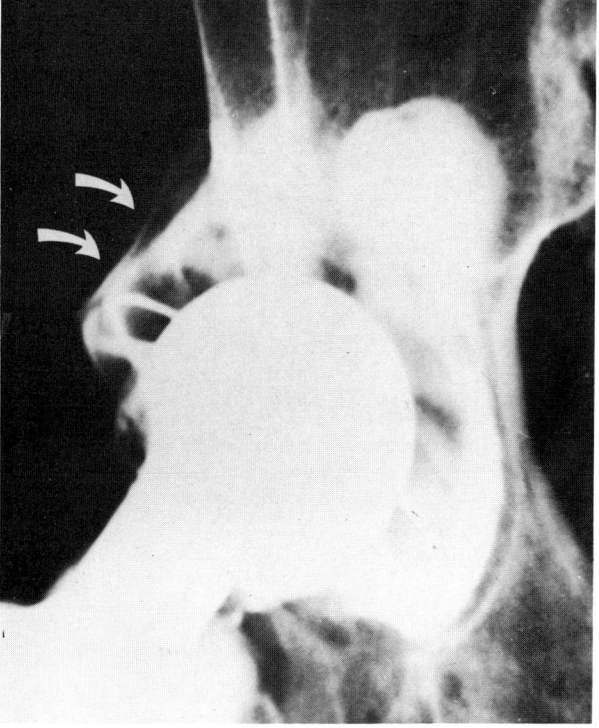

Figure 3-7B. Obturator oblique (note foreshortened ilium of the same patient as in Figure 3-7A) shows the very thin shell of the superior and posterior rim.

tical bone, or penetration through the cortex. On the AP view, the femoral component can appear to be in neutral alignment and well centered in the canal but a true lateral can often reveal cortical thinning or perforation (Figures 3-10A, 3-10B, 3-11A, and 3-11B).

AP and Rotational Views of the Femur. Internal and external rotation x-rays can often fill in the conceptual gaps with regard to the integrity of the femur and the quality of the bone. The AP x-ray of the proximal femur of the patient seen in Figure 3-12A shows evidence of bone deficiency in the region of the calcar. Internal rotational views preoperatively would have revealed the true extent of the proximal lateral cortical defect that surprised the surgeon at the time of exploration (Figures 3-12A and 3-12B).

The frog lateral view (external rotation) can also allow

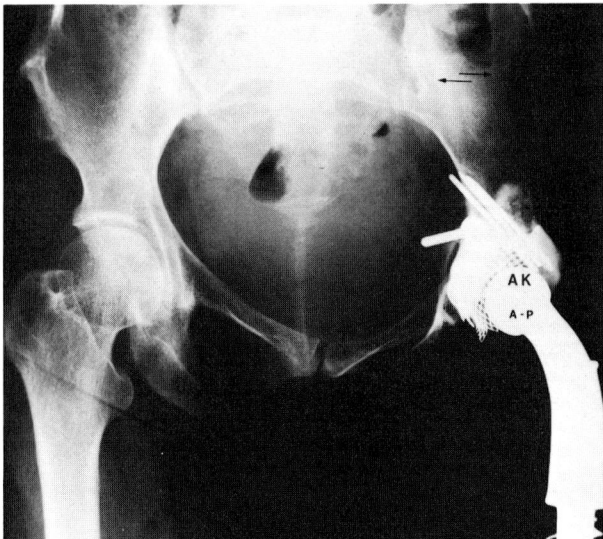

Figure 3-8A. The standard AP x-ray shows a minor rim deficiency.

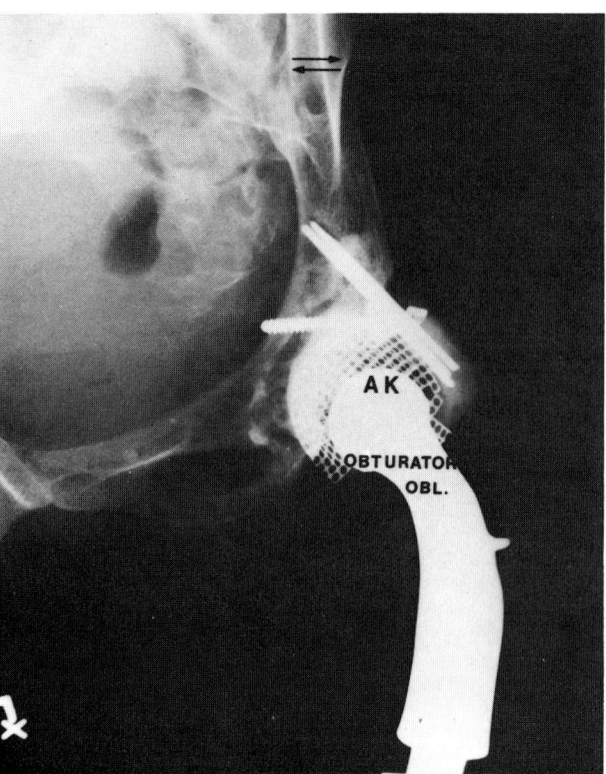

Figure 3-8C. The obturator oblique x-ray (obturator foramen clearly visible, iliac wing seen end on), should reveal the true magnitude of the superior and posterior rim deficiencies.

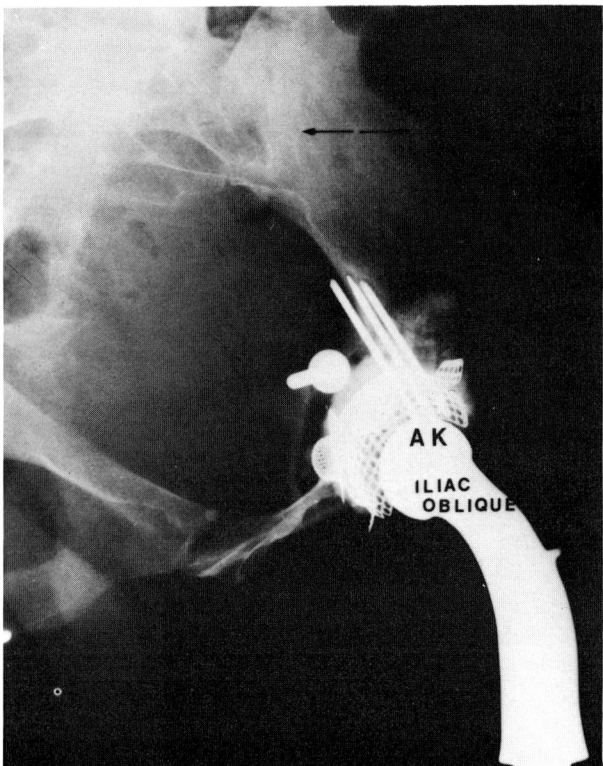

Figure 3-8B. The iliac oblique x-ray (broad iliac wing and foreshortened obturator foramen) demonstrates superior coverage anteriorly but may be misleading in estimating acetabular volume.

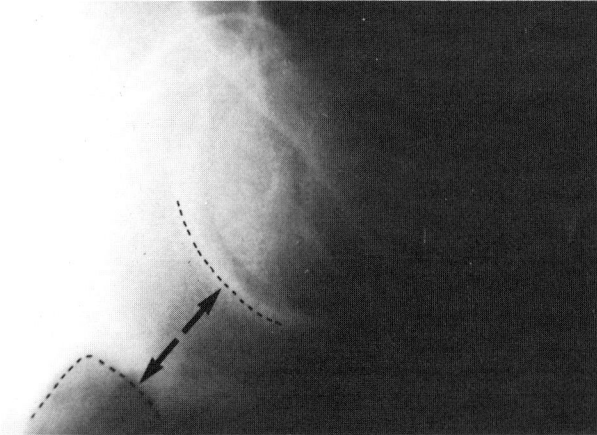

Figure 3-9A. On the true lateral x-ray, the distance between the arrows represents the thickness of the posterior intra-acetabular segment. The dotted lines (lower left) outline the sciatic notch. The upper dotted line outlines the normal subcondral acetabular bone.

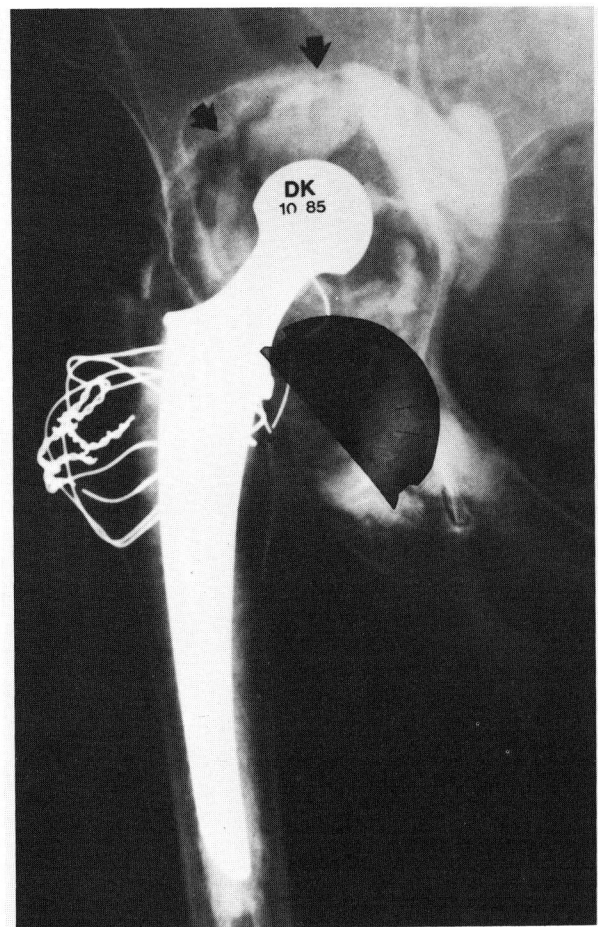

Figure 3-9B. Marked superior migration of the femoral head, cement fragmentation and bone resorption are evident on this routine AP view.

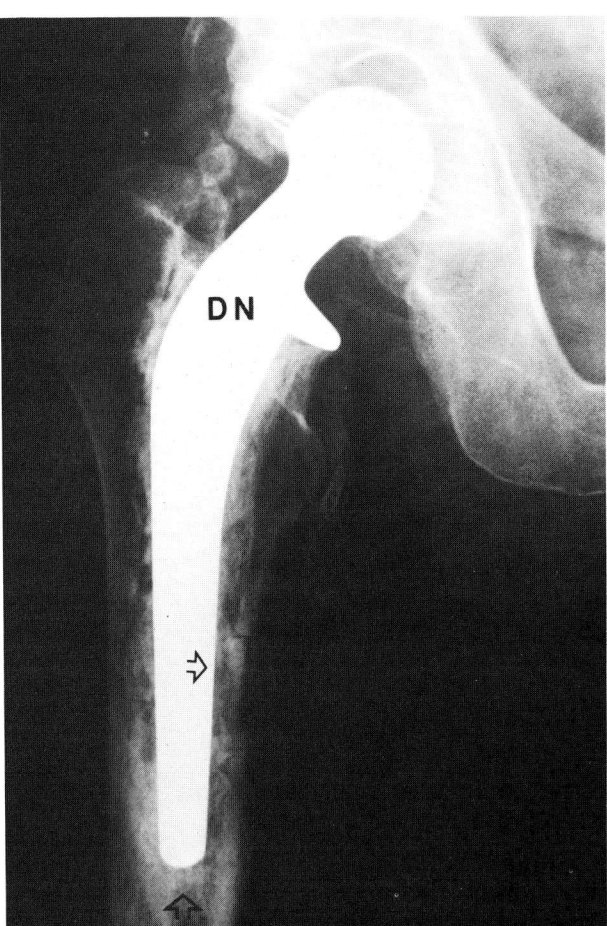

Figure 3-10A. On the AP view, the femoral component may appear to be in neutral alignment with a suspicion of cortical loss medially.

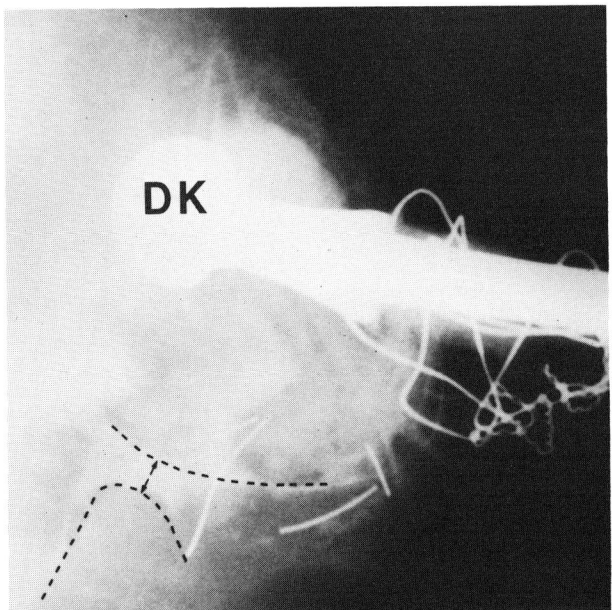

Figure 3-9C. This true lateral view shows the extent of posterior intra-acetabular erosion. Note the narrow segment between the arrows.

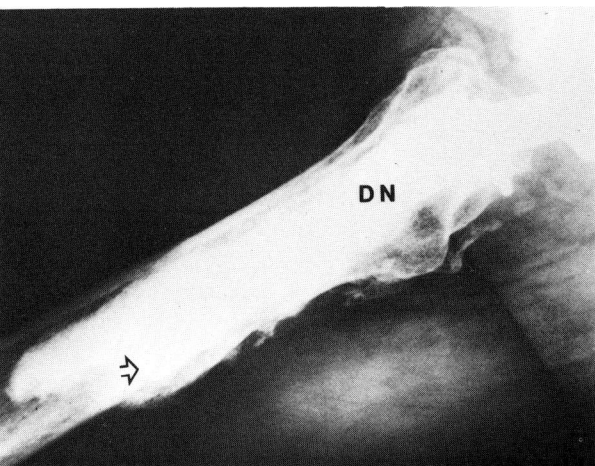

Figure 3-10B. A true lateral may show that the prosthesis is not well aligned and that the shaft has been perforated.

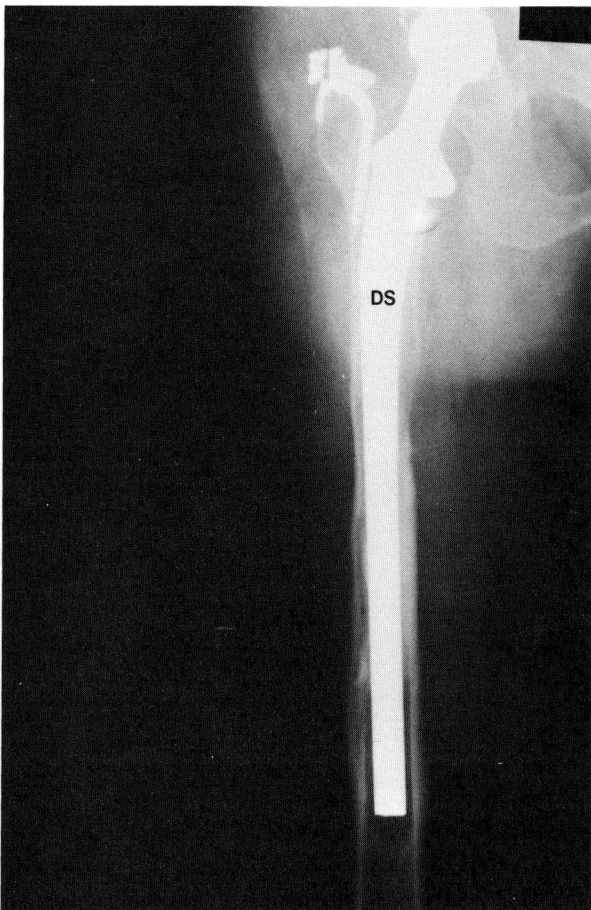

Figure 3-11A. The AP x-ray suggests some thinning of the cortex (non-barium impregnated cement is present).

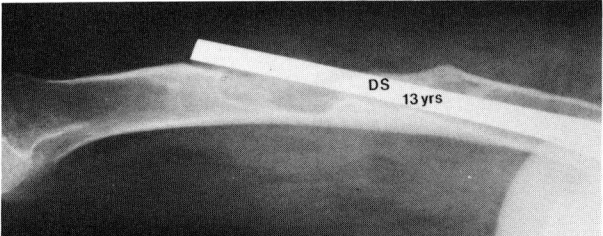

Figure 3-11B. The true lateral x-ray shows major areas of cortical thinning as well as a significant anterior bow with protrusion of a long stem prosthesis.

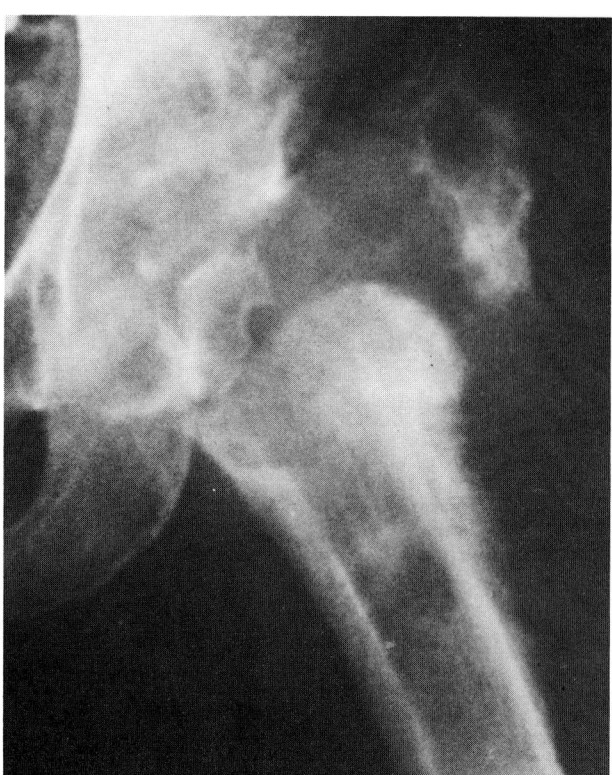

Figure 3-12A. The standard and frog lateral x-rays (external rotation) did not reveal a major defect except some deficiency of the calcar.

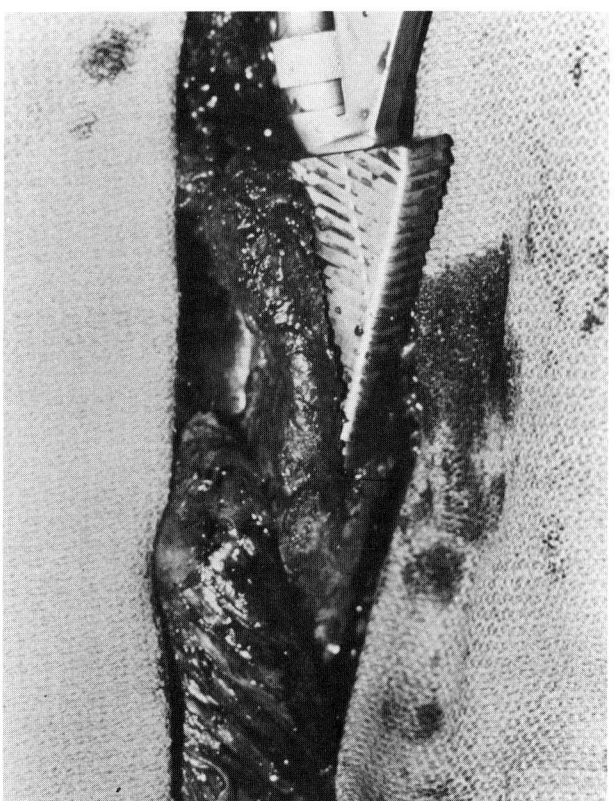

Figure 3-12B. A preoperative x-ray with the femur internally rotated would have revealed the significant proximal femoral deficiency that surprised the surgeon at the time of exploration.

assessment of the alignment of the femoral canal which can be distorted following an osteotomy (Figures 3-13A and 3-13B).

Hip Aspiration and Arthrogram. Hip aspiration is essential in any patient who has had prior intra-articular procedures, particularly if a metallic device has been inserted. Aspiration should always be carried out under strict aseptic technique. Although the procedure can be performed in an x-ray facility, it should still be considered an operative procedure with the same considerations given to sterile technique as in the operating room (Figure 3-14).

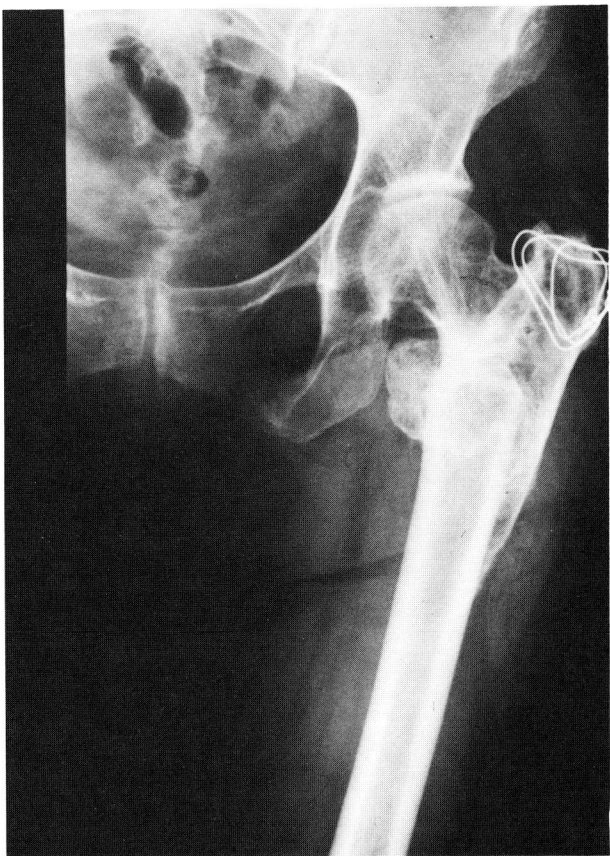

Figure 3-13A. Following a subtrochanteric osteotomy, distortion of the femoral canal may not be obvious on the AP view.

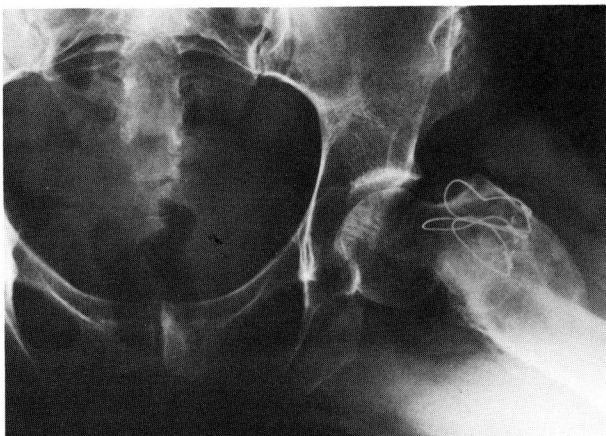

Figure 3-13B. External rotation of the femur (frog lateral) reveals that there is significant distortion of the femoral canal and insertion of the femoral component may be difficult.

Prior to revision total hip replacement, an arthrogram may be helpful in assessing acetabular loosening. In a review by Harris and O'Neil, the detection of loose acetabular components was accurate in 63% of the cases by plain x-ray and was increased to 87% accuracy with an arthrogram. However, the arthrogram is much less reliable with femoral components and in their study, there was no advantage of an arthrogram over plain radiographs in

detecting femoral loosening.[9] Our experience supports these findings.

Arthrographic techniques vary widely, but we prefer taking a plain x-ray with a needle in the joint and a catheter in place (Figure 3-15A). This is followed immediately by injection of contrast and repeat x-rays in the identical position (Figure 3-15B). These two x-rays can then be compared line for line. After the initial two AP radiographs, oblique views are taken. The patient is then asked to walk and x-rays are repeated. The pumping action of weightbearing and joint motion can aid in the distribution of contrast. It is important to remember that the coned down AP films on the arthrogram will be magnified and therefore are inappropriate for use with standard preoperative acetate templates.

A small percentage of arthrograms are falsely negative, and in any revision hip the surgeon should be prepared to change either component, despite a negative arthrogram. The bone cement interface should be cleared of all soft tissues and the component should be stressed in both tension and compression and observed for any signs of motion. Gross motion, no matter how slight, should be interpreted as loosening. Extrusion of blood at the interface between bone and cement, even without obvious motion in relationship to bone, is also evidence of loosening. Component revision should be carried out if either of these two signs of loosening is seen.

Scanograms. Preoperative clinical measurement is usually adequate but radiological measurement is more precise. Although this can be performed by means of a CAT scan, we prefer to use plain films using a calibrated grid.[10]

In the presence of significant flexion deformities, it may be necessary to flex the patient's trunk in order to nullify hip flexion deformities and allow the extremity to be flush with the x-ray film.

Tomograms. Tomograms can be helpful in the presence of hip dysplasia, resection arthroplasty, total hips with nonmetal backed acetabular components or post-traumatic

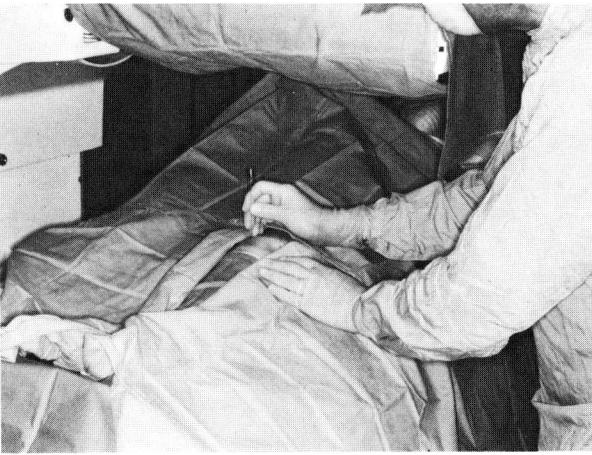

Figure 3-14. Aspiration and arthrogram of the hip may be done in the x-ray department but sterile techniques must be as meticulous as those used in the operating room.

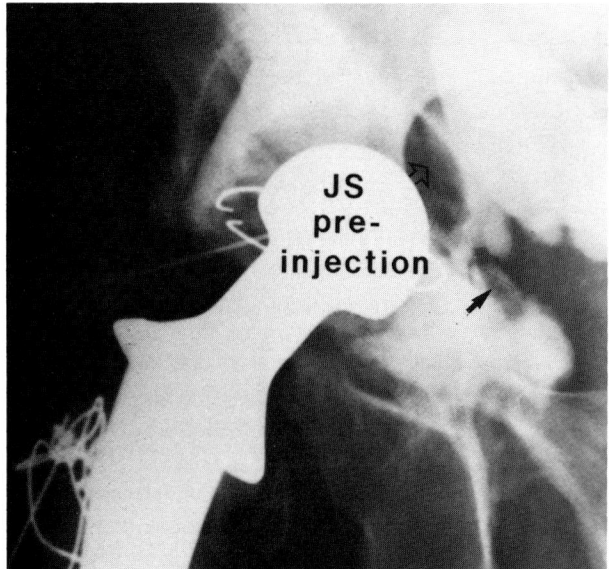

Figure 3-15A. An x-ray is taken with the needle in the joint before the contrast is injected.

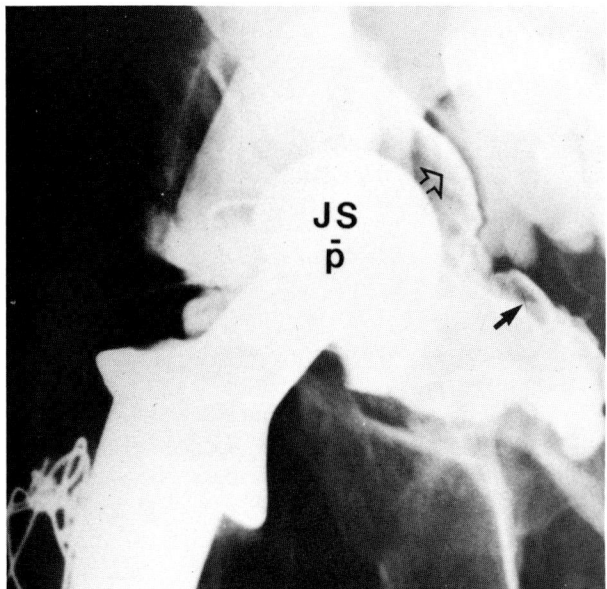

Figure 3-15B. Without noving the leg, contrast is injected and an x-ray is taken that can be accurately compared to the pre-injection study. The arrows point to dye outlining the cement.

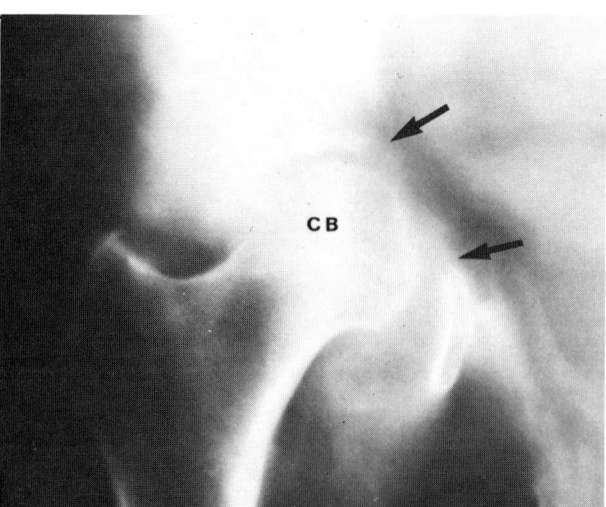

Figure 3-16. In the absence of metal, tomograms can clearly show the extent of central acetabular defects.

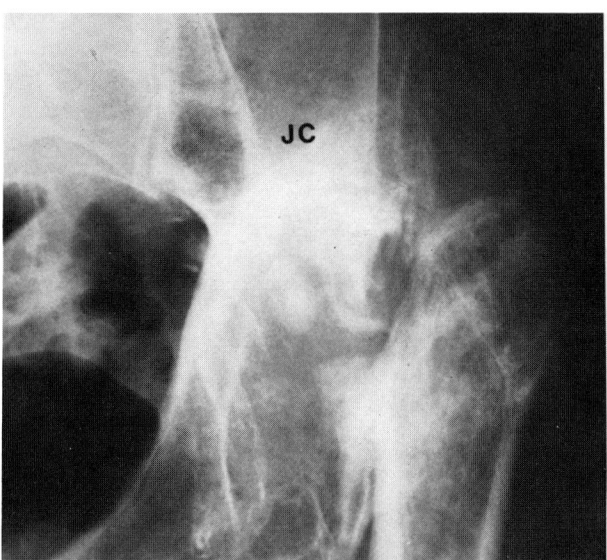

Figure 3-17A. The AP x-ray provides information concerning the superior rim and suggests that there is no posterior acetabular bone available.

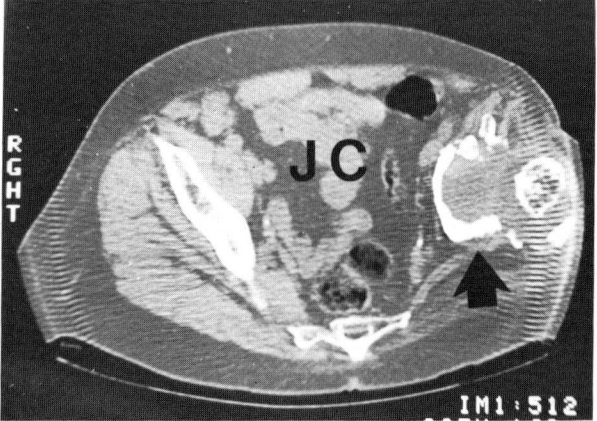

Figure 3-17B. The CAT scan demonstrates that there is adequate posterior acetabular bone.

arthritis (Figure 3-16). However, since tomograms are affected by metal scatter, they are not accurate in the presence of a metal-backed acetabular component or if a femoral stem is in place.

Computer Assisted Tomography. The CAT scan can be very valuable in assessing the bone stock available for reconstruction (Figures 3-17A and 3-17B), but, as with tomograms, metal scatter can cause significant distortion. However, with a nonmetal backed acetabular component, despite the proximity of the head of a femoral component, the CAT scan can still be helpful (Figure 3-18).[11]

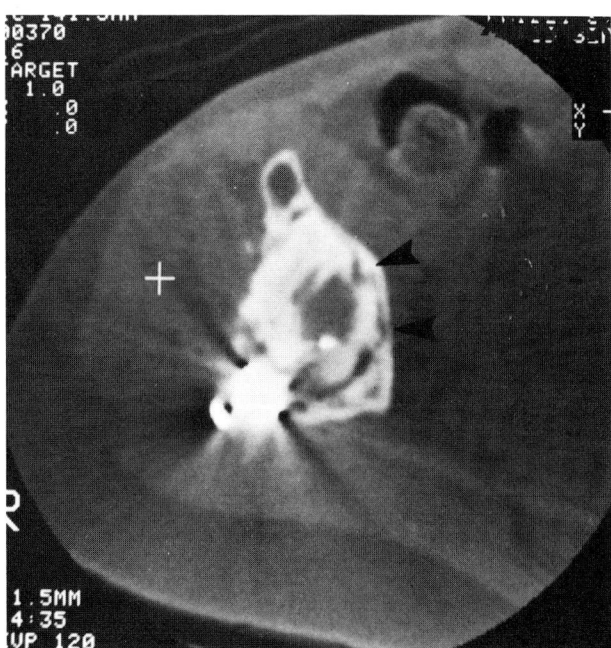

Figure 3-18. With a nonmetal backed acetabular component, despite the presence of a femoral component, bone stock and radiolucent lines can still be identified.

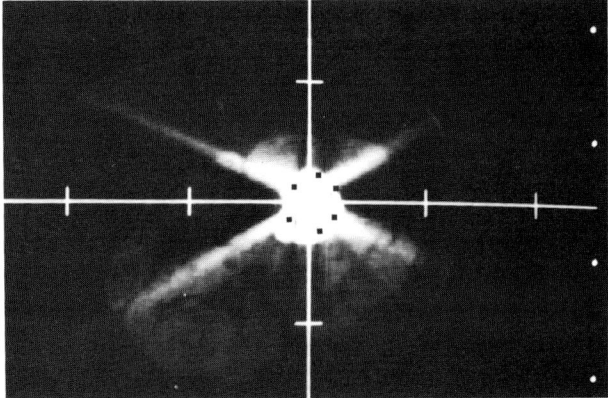

Figure 3-19. The CAT scan allows some assessment of canal diameter and cortical thickness. Despite metal scatter, the interface is visible within the areas outlined by the dots.

CAT scan techniques are disappointing on the femoral side because of metal scatter but newer scanners allow some assessment of canal diameter and of cortical thickness in the femur as well (Figure 3-19).

Computer Assisted Modeling of the Acetabulum and Pelvis. Computer assisted prosthetic designs have been available for several years. Improved algorithms have allowed startling advances in computer-generated three dimensional imaging (Figure 3-20). More recently we have been using accurate plastic models of the acetabulum and pelvis that are fabricated on the basis of CAT scan data (Figure 3-21).[11] These models are not only helpful for preoperative planning but also can be gas-sterilized so that they are available at surgery. Although we have not yet

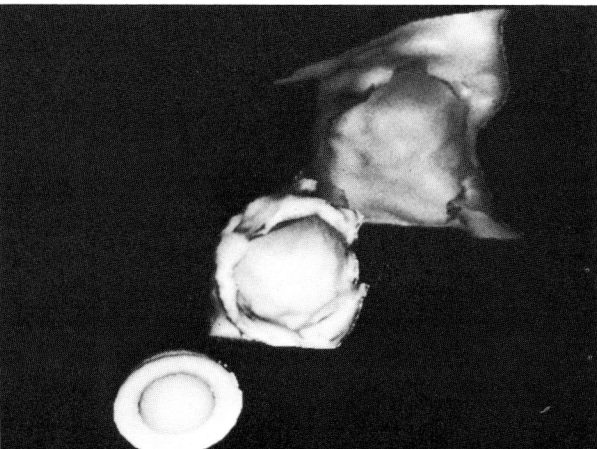

Figure 3-20. Computer assisted imaging can be very helpful and can be viewed from a variety of angles. At the bottom is the polyethylene cup, in the center is the cement and at the top is the defect in the acetabular bone.

prepared allografts preoperatively under sterile conditions using such models, we anticipate doing this in the near future. If allografts could be accurately shaped to match the defects of the patient preoperatively, prolonged anesthesia time could be avoided.

Surgical Reconstruction

Special Equipment

Because these operations are lengthy and frequently involve revision surgery, the risks of infection are higher. We therefore prefer to perform all major bone grafts in operating rooms that have either vertical laminar flow with a body exhaust system or that have ultraviolet lights.[12-15]

In addition to the standard extensive orthopedic kit, it is helpful to have extra tables to provide additional working space. This enables a second team to prepare the bone grafts while the primary team is working on the surgical exposure. A table vise is helpful to secure bone grafts while they are being shaped (Figure 3-22). A conventional oscillating saw is remarkably effective in shaping grafts and is used not only to cut the grafts into segments but also to shave off bone in the process of contouring the surface of the grafts as well (Figure 3-23). The Midas Rex (Midas Rex Institute, Fort Worth, TX) with all its various accessories is extremely helpful (Figure 3-24). A bone hook with a hole drilled transversely through the tip can be used to pass cerclage wires around the femur (Figure 3-25). Smooth 3/32nd diameter Kirshner wires are used to hold acetabular grafts in place temporarily (Figure 3-26) and final fixation for the majority of these grafts is achieved with 6.5mm.. cancellous screws and washers. Although stainless steel screws can be used, it is our preference to use chrome cobalt screws (Howmedica, Inc., Rutherford, NJ) (Figure 3-27) because the prostheses

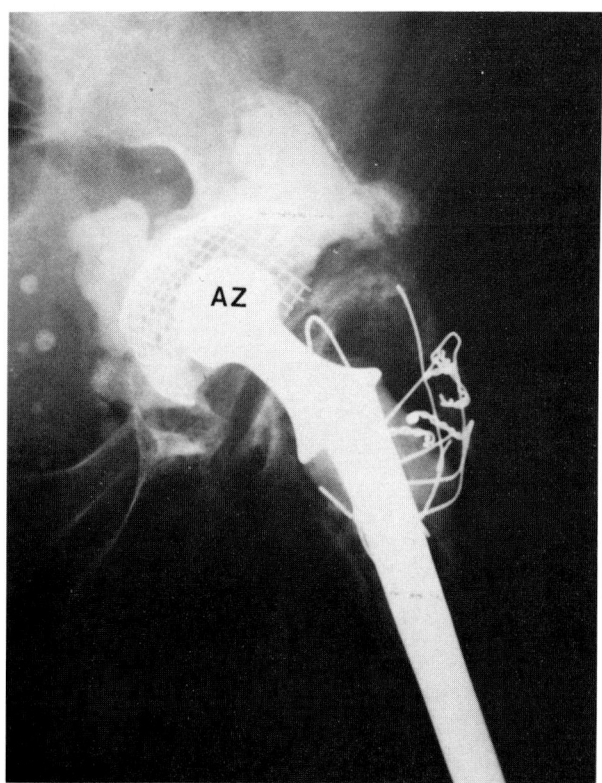

Figure 3-21A. The AP x-ray is helpful but not as accurate as the computer model in assessment of the acetabulum.

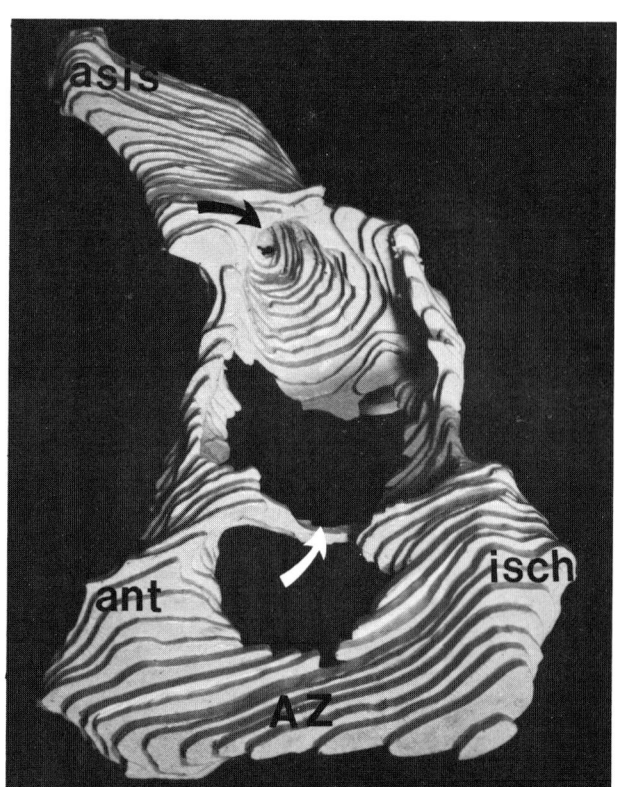

Figure 3-21C. The same model shown in Figure 3-21B, viewed from below and rotated to show the superior intra-acetabular defect.

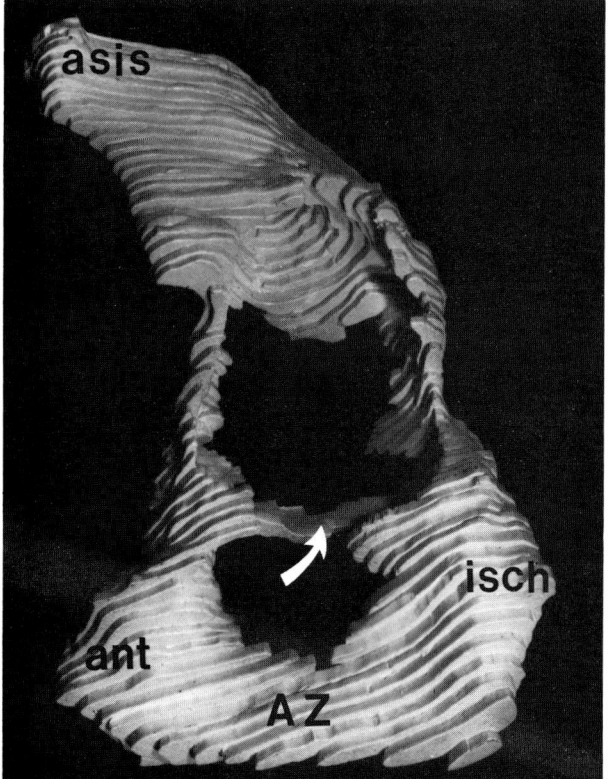

Figure 3-21B. The computer generated model of the acetabulum of the patient seen in Figure 3-21A. Note the large central defect and the thin inferior bridge between the anterior and posterior columns.

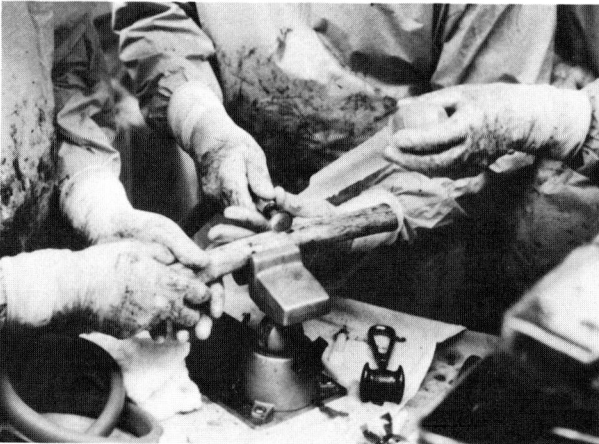

Figure 3-22. A table vise is helpful to secure bone grafts while they are being prepared (Midas Rex Institute, Fort Worth, TX).

that we prefer are made either of chrome cobalt or titanium. Stainless steel screws in conjunction with such prostheses could theoretically cause electrolysis. Although some surgeons have advocated the use of bolts, we have found that screws provide adequate fixation in even the most severe cases.[16] The advantage of screws over bolts is that they are easier to use and therefore the surgeon is less likely to avoid adding additional screws if necessary. Extensive intrapelvic dissection (in order to secure the bolts with nuts) is also unnecessary and there is less risk of injuring intrapelvic or neurologic structures. Intra-operative x-rays should be

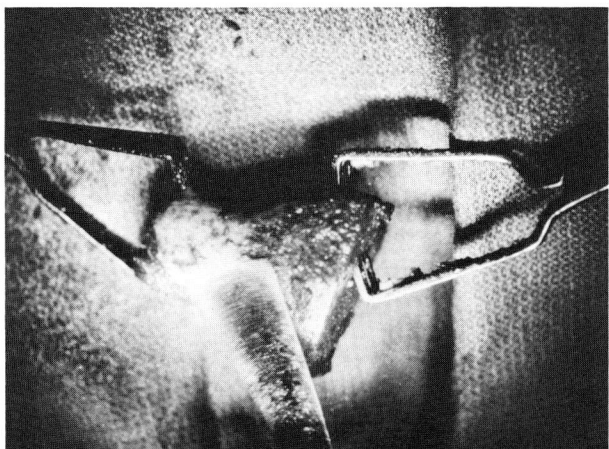

Figure 3-23. An oscillating saw is effective in cutting the grafts but can be used to shave off bone or cartilage as well.

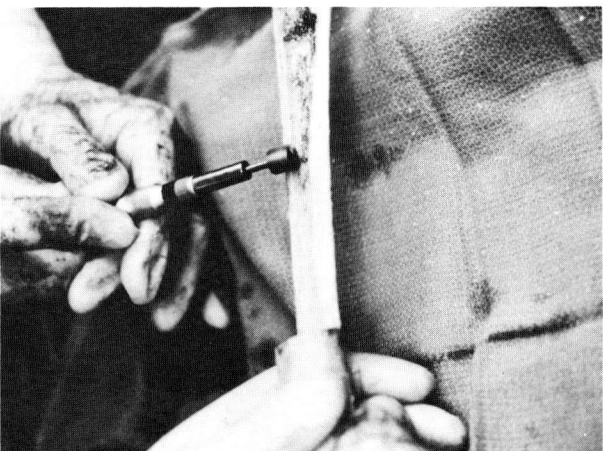

Figure 3-24. The Midas Rex is helpful in contouring bone grafts (Midas Rex Institute, Fort Worth, TX).

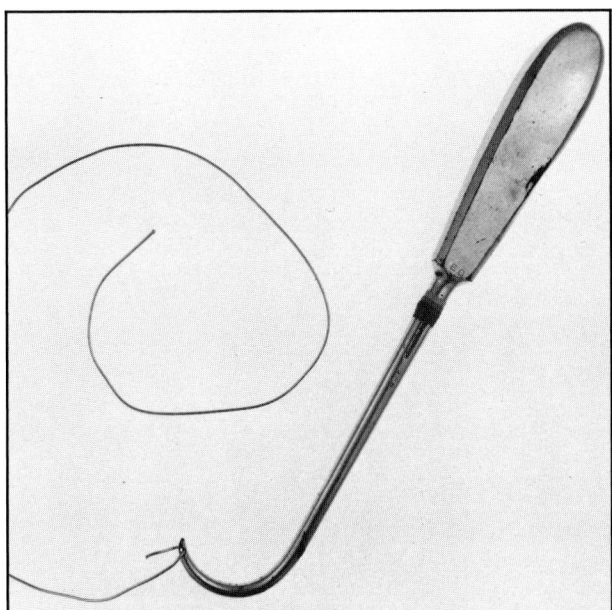

Figure 3-25. A bone hook with a transverse hole drilled through the tip is helpful when passing cerclage wires around the femur.

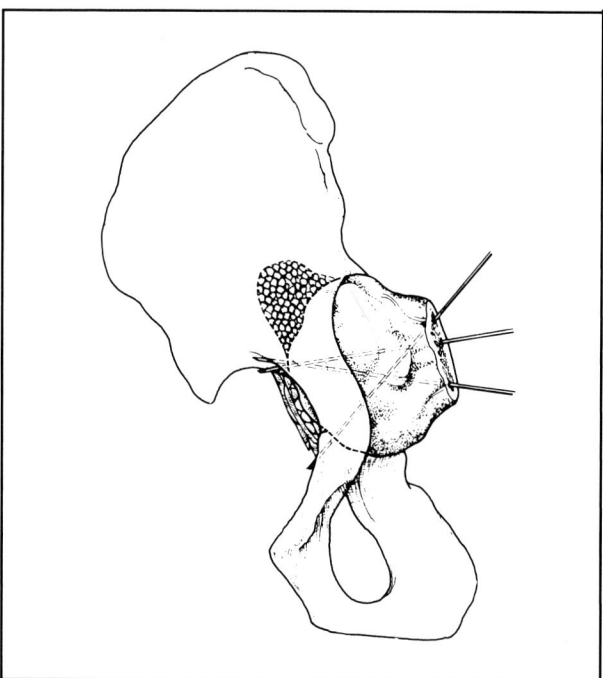

Figure 3-26. ³⁄₃₂nd smooth K-wires are used to temporarily hold acetabular grafts in place.

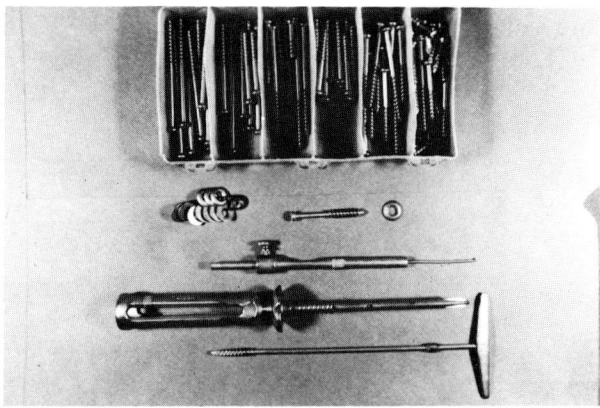

Figure 3-27. The majority of grafts are permanently fixed with Vitallium cancellous screws and washers (Howmedica Inc., Rutherford, NJ).

taken before closure to be sure that the screws are of appropriate length and do not threaten vascular or neurologic structures.

Although our longest clinical experience with major bone grafting has been in association with cemented devices and the clinical and radiographic results of these devices are generally satisfactory, we are now using uncemented devices in the majority of cases.

Acetabular Component. Cemented acetabular components have proved to have a high rate of fixation failure and in revision surgery require a complete seal of the acetabulum to avoid cement intrusion intrapelvically or between host and graft.[6-8,21,22] For these reasons, we prefer uncemented acetabular components. The time required to

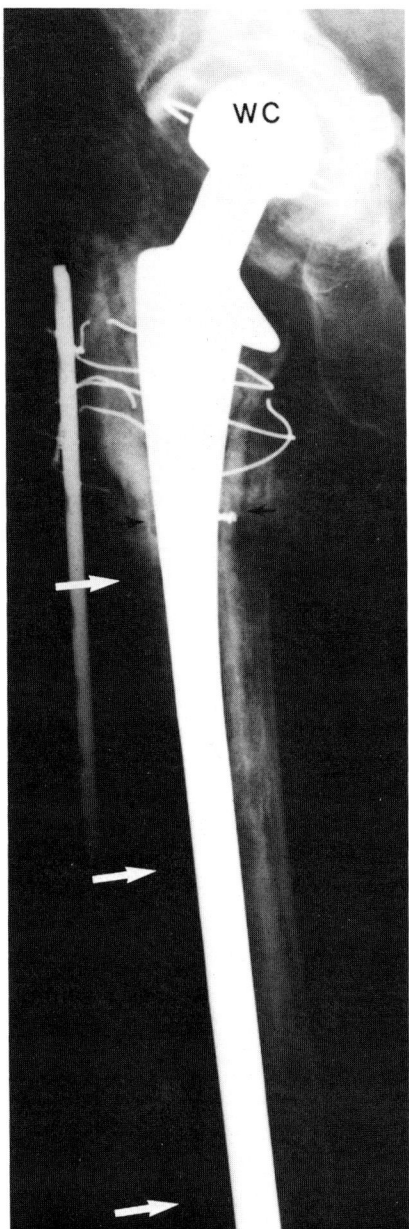

Figure 3-28. This 58 year old man had a long stem component inserted six years prior to this x-ray when a standard length stem was revised. At six years note the dramatic stress shielding of the femur. The lateral cortex has almost disappeared.

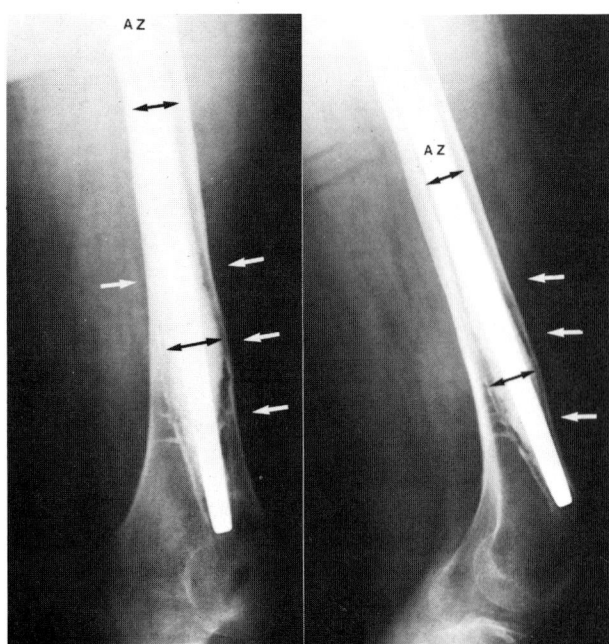

Figure 3-29. This 74 year old woman had a long stem cemented component inserted for revision of a failed total hip replacement 12 years ago. Note the stress shielding (white arrows) and the fact that the distal cement mass is wider than the isthmus making extraction difficult.

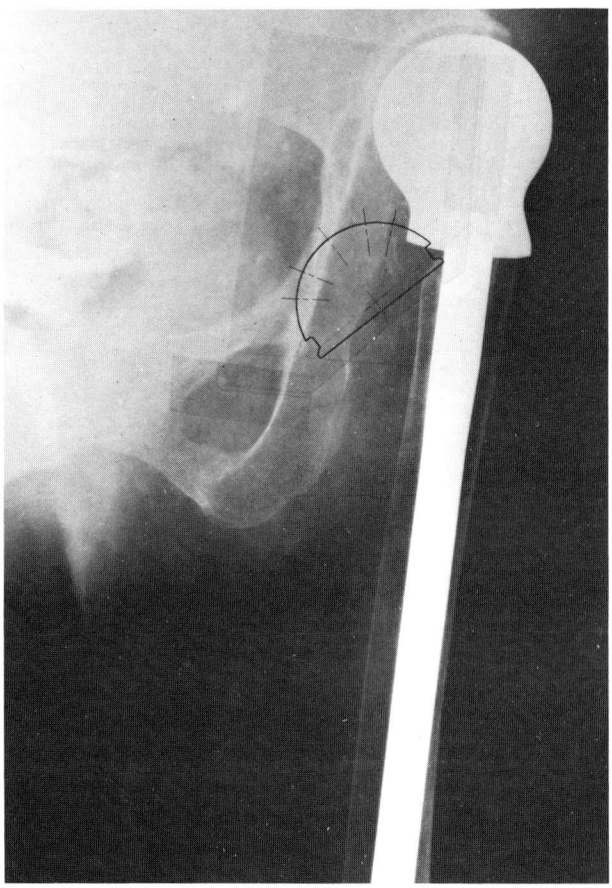

Figure 3-30. This 64 year old woman had this uncemented custom long stem prosthesis inserted 18 years ago. Note the very thin cortices.

insert a noncemented acetabular component is not excessive and the failure rate thus far is minimal.[17,18] Since the early clinical results in our hands are excellent, we prefer to use these devices in essentially all primary or revision cases. Although bipolar prostheses are frequently used in other centers,[19,20] we have not found that the exercise tolerance of our patients with such devices is comparable with that of patients with a fixed acetabular component. We therefore do not use bipolar prostheses. The one exception is in those patients with significant weakness around the hip. In this instance the bipolar prosthesis offers the advantage of greater inherent stability.

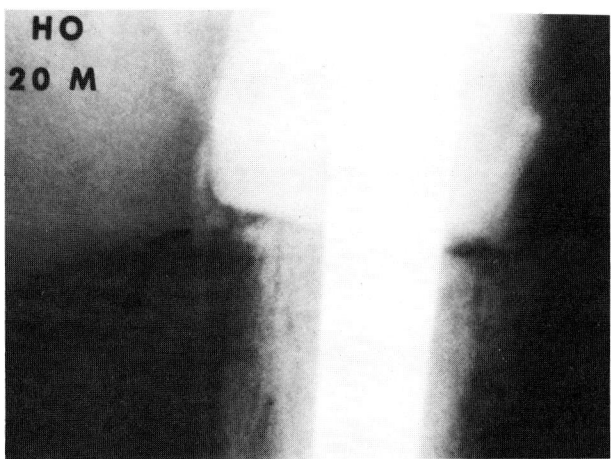

Figure 3-31. A cemented long stem prosthesis that extends beyond the junction of an allograft with the distal bone of the femur may prevent impaction and result in delayed union as is seen in this patient at 20 months.

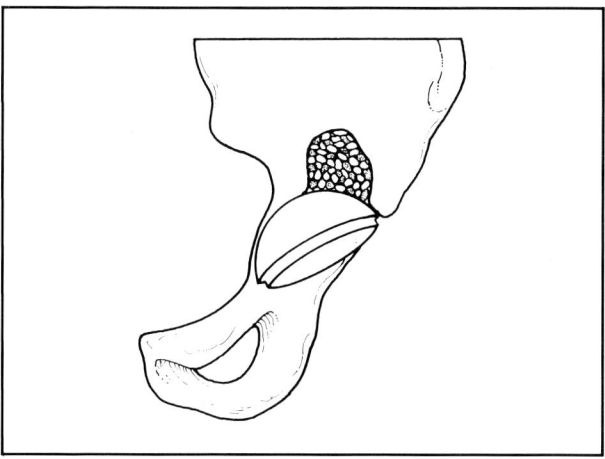

Figure 3-32. Even significant intra-acetabular defects can be managed by morsellized bone if it is contained and is not required for structural support.

Femoral Component. Although we used cemented long stem prostheses early in our experience with revision surgery, we no longer feel that these devices are necessary or advisable because of femoral stress shielding (Figure 3-28) and because of the difficulty of extracting a stem that has cement extending distal to the isthmus (Figure 3-29). Even uncemented long stem devices can cause stress shielding (Figure 3-30). Cemented stems that bridge the junction of an allograft proximal femoral replacement and the host bone have an additional disadvantage in that they can prevent impaction and lead to nonunion (Figure 3-31). We now our prefer to use standard length uncemented femoral components in virtually all femoral revisions, even when the sintered surface is entirely in contact with nonviable allograft bone. At present it is impossible to determine when or if a massive allograft will be revascularized enough to allow potentially bony ingrowth but even if this never occurs, press-fit devices such as the Moore or Thompson prosthesis or the original nonsintered Osteonics femoral component (Osteonics Corp., Allendale, NJ) have proved successful in the past. If cement is used in conjunction with a major bone graft, fixation of the component could theoretically be at risk if the graft does revascularize and the usual process of membrane formation begins.

Bone Grafts

Autogenous Bone

We prefer to use autogenous bone when available because it readily incorporates in most instances.[20] The sources of autogenous bone, however, are basically limited to the patient's femoral head (if this is available) or to the iliac crest. Theoretically, the fibula or ribs could be used, although we have no experience with these sources.

Autogenous cancellous bone (morsellized with a rongeur), can be used alone or mixed with morsellized allograft cancellous bone to fill intra-acetabular defects (Figure 3-32) or central defects with minor protrusio (Figure 3-33) as long as structural support is not needed and the bone is contained. Such coarse morsellized bone can be impacted to provide some structural support. When available, finely morsellized bone obtained from acetabular reamers and mixed with autologous blood to make a paste is routinely used in conjunction with sintered prostheses and is frequently helpful between graft and host bone. Autogenous strips are ideal to fill central wall defects as long as the uncemented acetabular component is supported by mechanically sound peripheral bone (Figure 3-34).

Full thickness iliac crest grafts can be used for central wall defects (Figure 3-35) without risk of herniation of the pelvic structures through the donor site if mandibular mesh (Howmedica, Rutherford, NJ) is used (Figure 3-36).

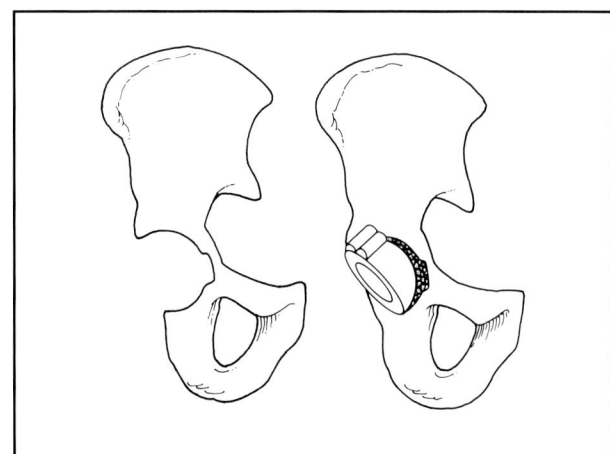

Figure 3-33. With minor protrusio acetabulum, morsellized bone from the iliac crest or from the patient's femoral head can be used to fill the central defect.

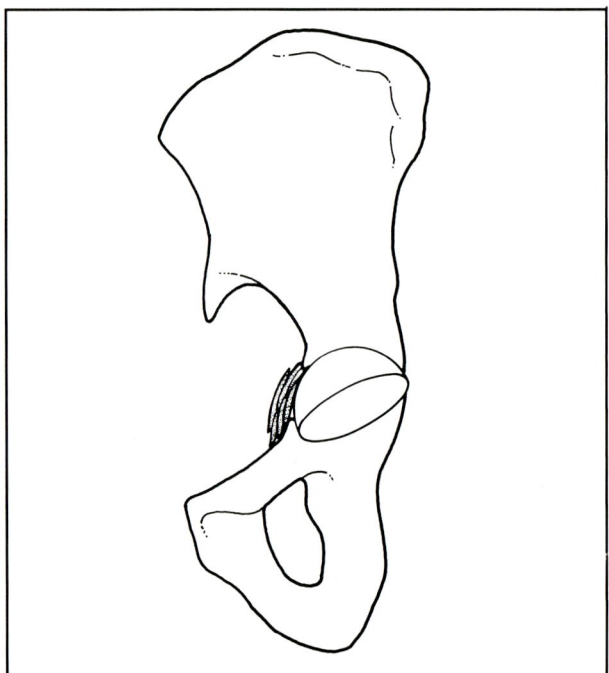

Figure 3-34. Central wall defects of the acetabulum can be grafted by means of autogenous cortical and cancellous strips from the iliac crest if a noncemented acetabular component is used.

The patient's femoral head is the optimal graft for rim (Figure 3-37) or for major central or superior intra-acetabular defects where structural support is important (Figure 3-38).

Allograft Bone. When autogenous bone is not available or not of sufficient volume or bulk, allograft bone can be used. We prefer to use autogenous morsellized bone, or strips in conjunction with all allografts (Figure 3-39).

The most readily available type of allograft is a femoral head, harvested at the time of total hip replacement or hemiarthroplasty. Such heads can be used for structural support with superior acetabular rim defects or for major intra-acetabular defects (Figure 3-40) or they can also be used to seal central defects if cement is used (Figure 3-41). Femoral head allografts can also be used for intramedullary calcar replacement (Figure 3-42) or for trochanteric augmentation (Figure 3-43).

The distal femur provides the largest graft for major acetabular defects (Figure 3-44) and the individual condyles can be used for smaller structural grafts (Figure 3-45). An inverted proximal tibia (with its proximal end facing inferiorly) can also provide significant bone stock for major acetabular reconstruction (Figure 3-46).

We have had an entire hemipelvis available on several occasions when massive acetabular defects were noted pre-

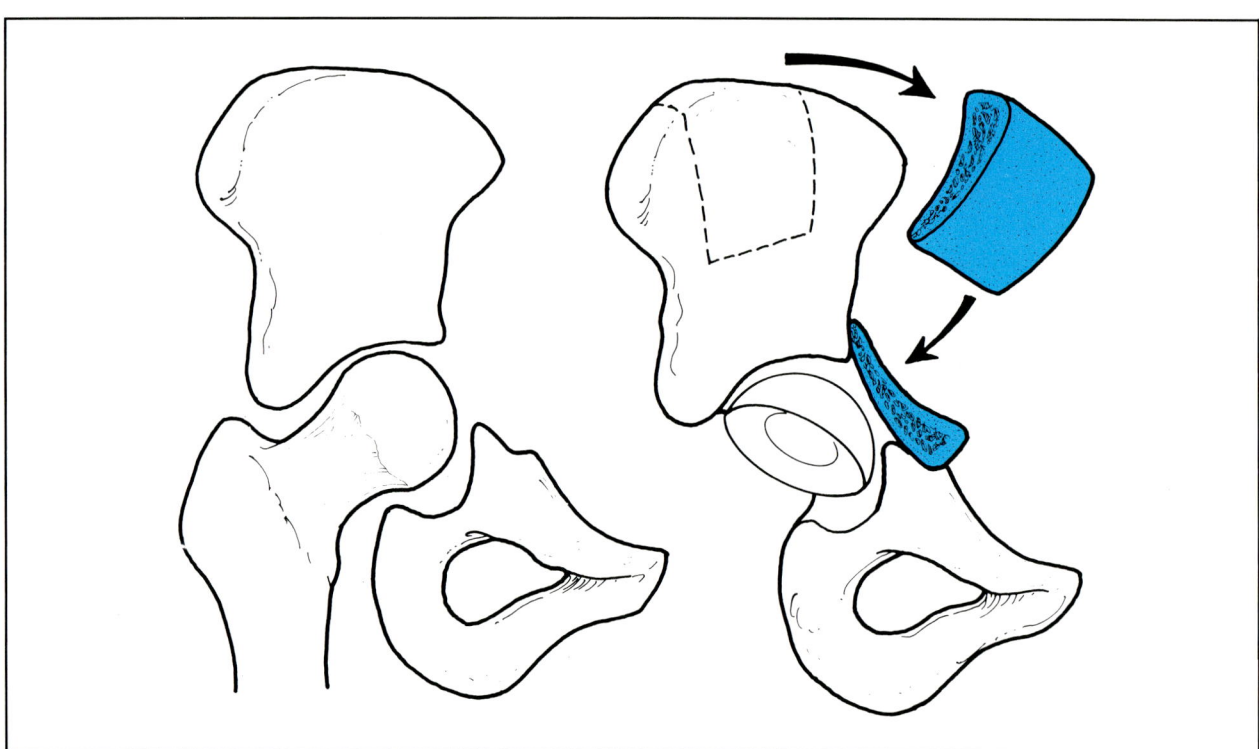

Figure 3-35. Large full thickness iliac crest grafts can be used to fix central acetabular defects.

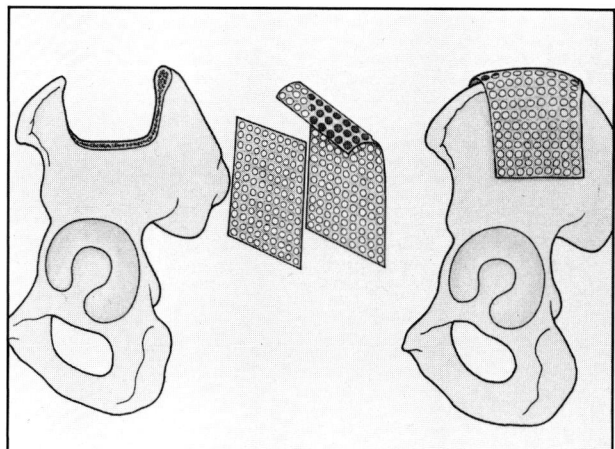

Figure 3-36. Mandibular mash (Howmedica, Rutherford, NJ) may be used to repair very large full thickness defects of the ilium.

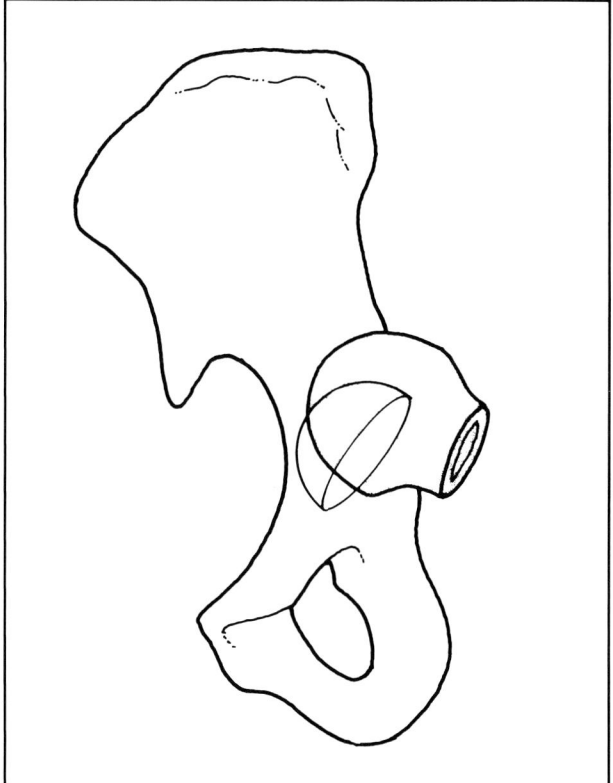

Figure 3-37. The patient's femoral head is the idea graft for large superior rim defects where structural support is necessary.

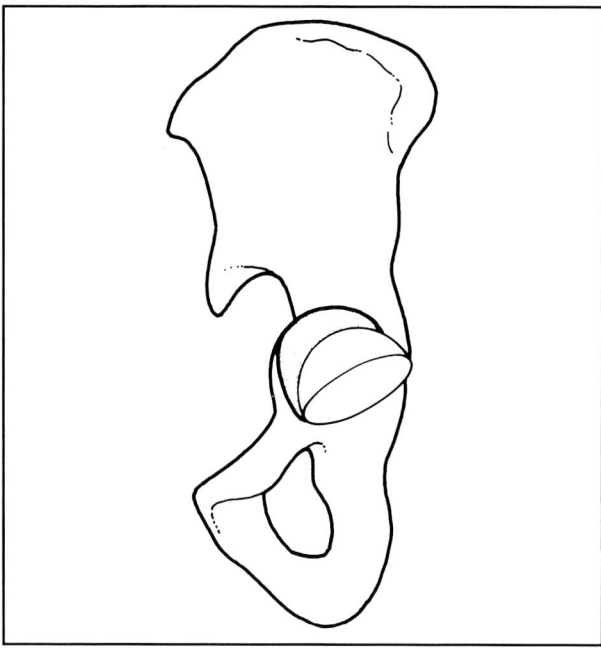

Figure 3-38. Large central or superior intra-acetabular defects may be filled by the patient's femoral head when structural support is necessary.

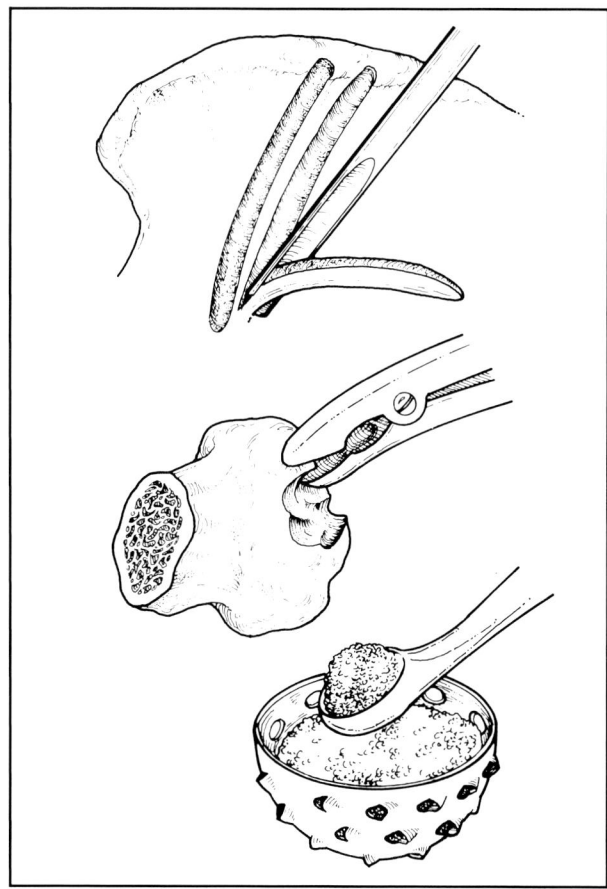

Figure 3-39. Autograft cortical and cancellous strips from the ilium or coarse morsellized bone should be used in conjunction with all allografts. Finely morsellized bone from a reamer, mixed with autologous blood to form bone paste, is helpful to fill small defects.

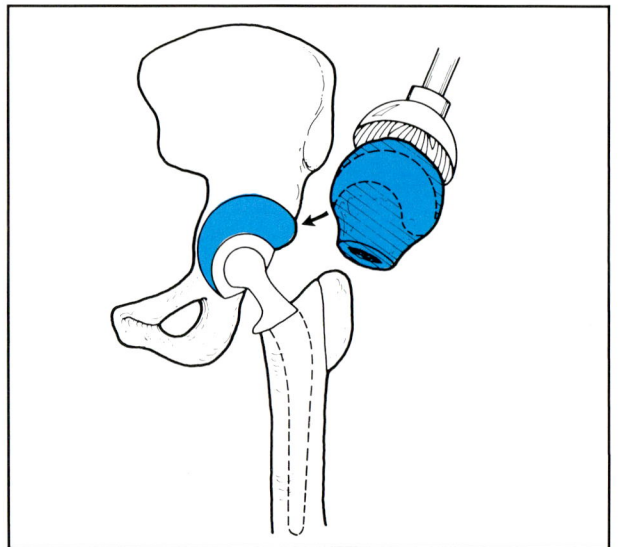

Figure 3-40. Femoral head allograft bone can be used to reconstruct major intra-acetabular defects when structural support is necessary.

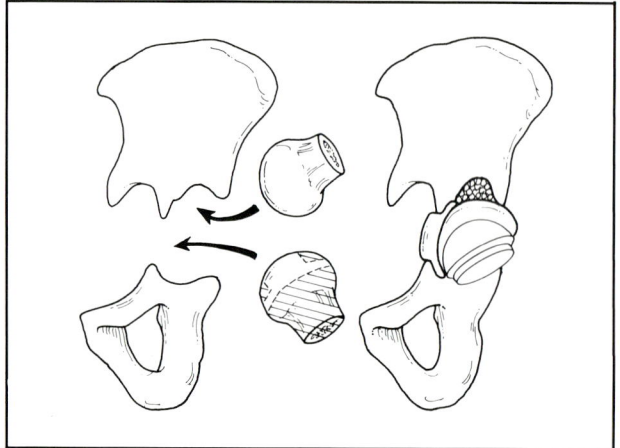

Figure 3-41. A femoral head can be shaped like a hat to seal a central acetabular defect if cement is used.

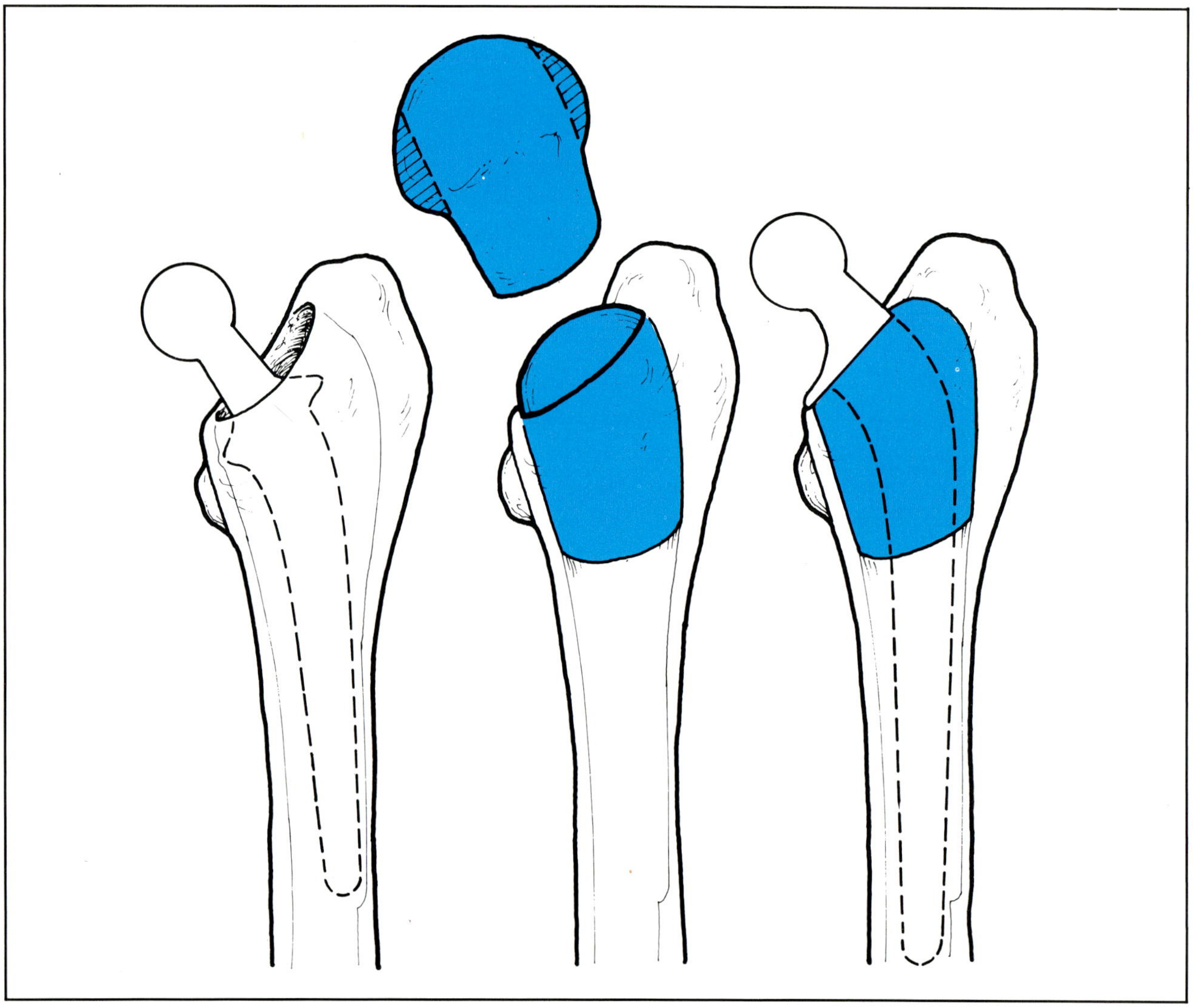

Figure 3-42. Allograft femoral heads can be used for calcar intramedullary augmentation.

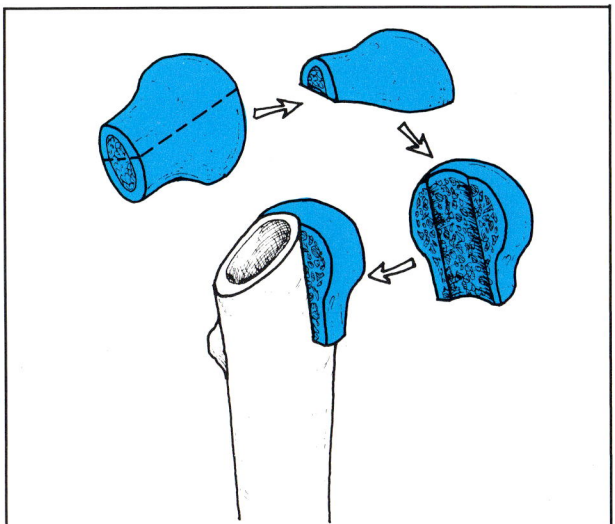

Figure 3-43. An allograft head can be used for trochanteric augmentation.

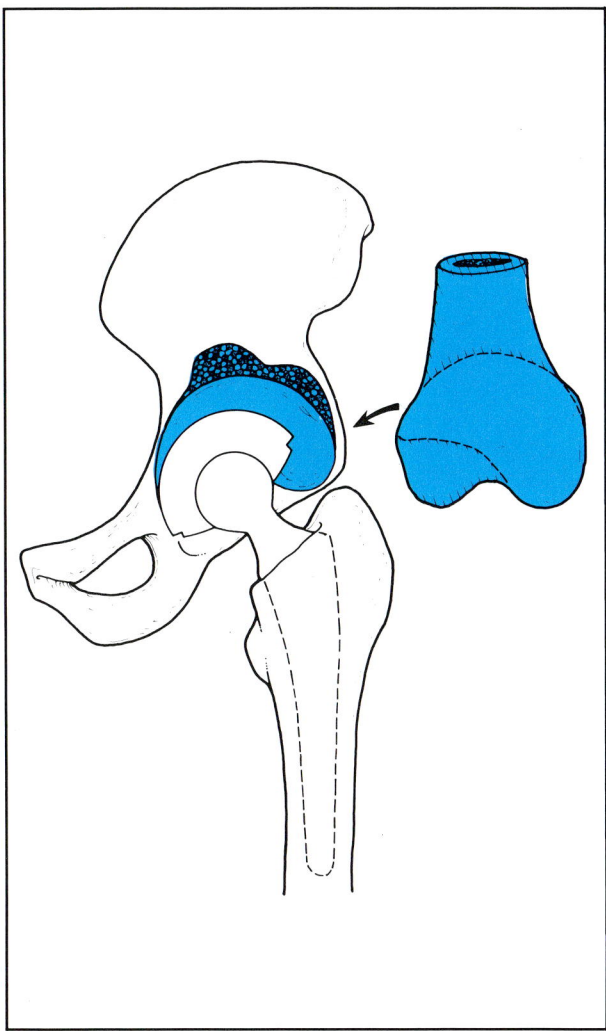

Figure 3-45. The individual femoral condyles can be used fo smaller structural grafts.

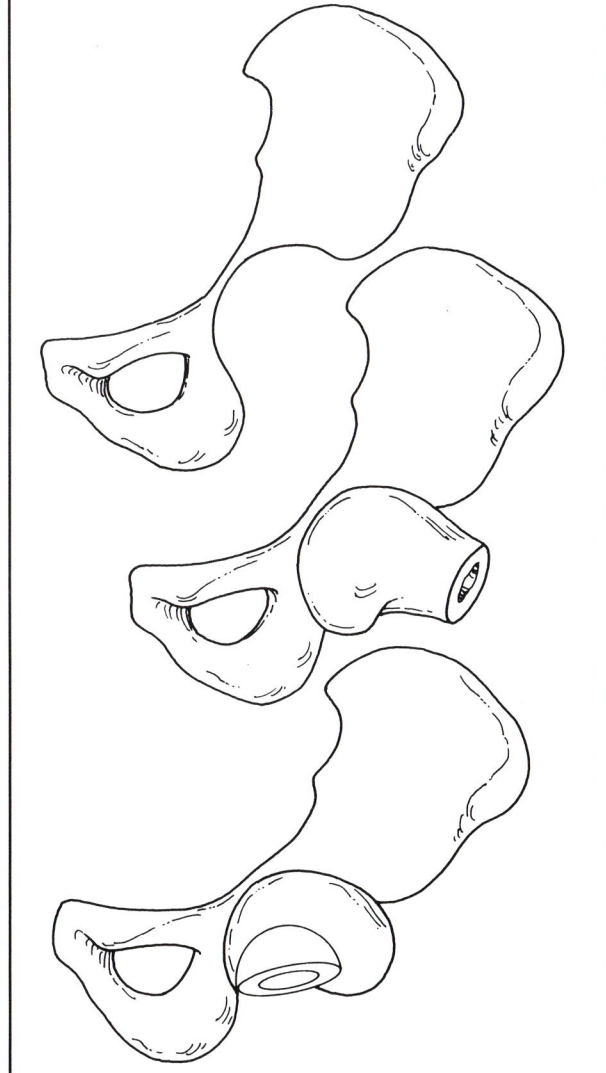

Figure 3-44. The largest acetabular defects may require allograft distal femoral condyles for reconstruction.

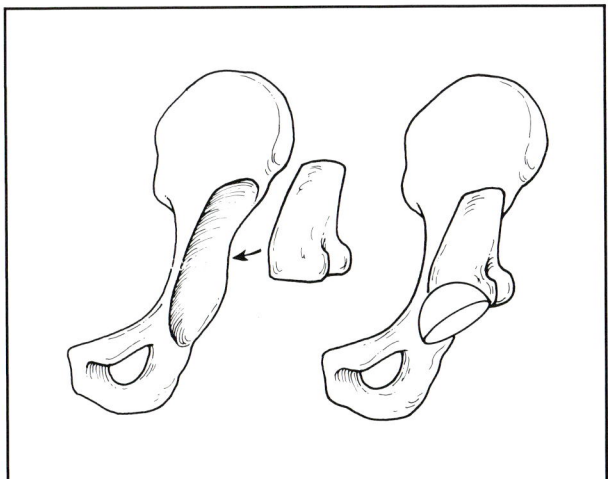

Figure 3-46. A proximal tibial allograft used with the articular sur face oriented inferiorly can provide bone stock for the reconstruc tion of the entire rim and intra-acetabular aspects of the acetabu lum.

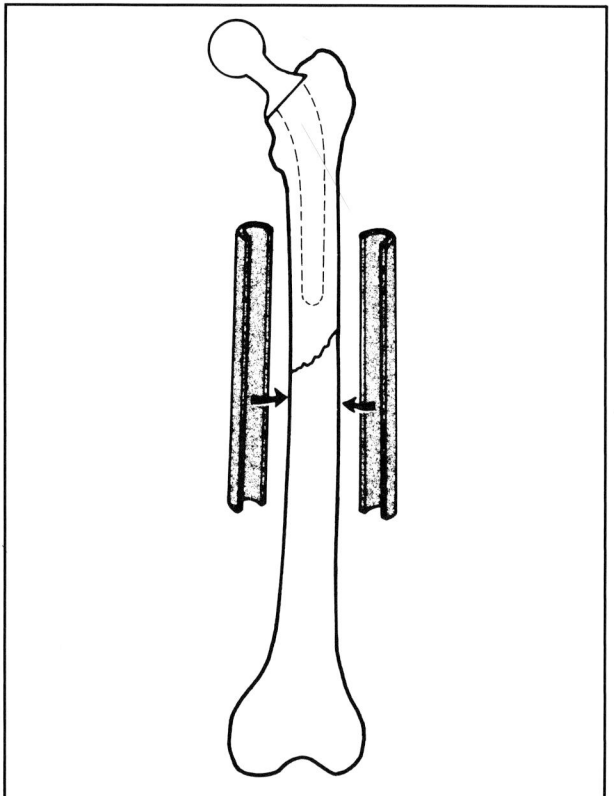

Figure 3-47. Cortical onlay grafts can be used for fracture fixation.

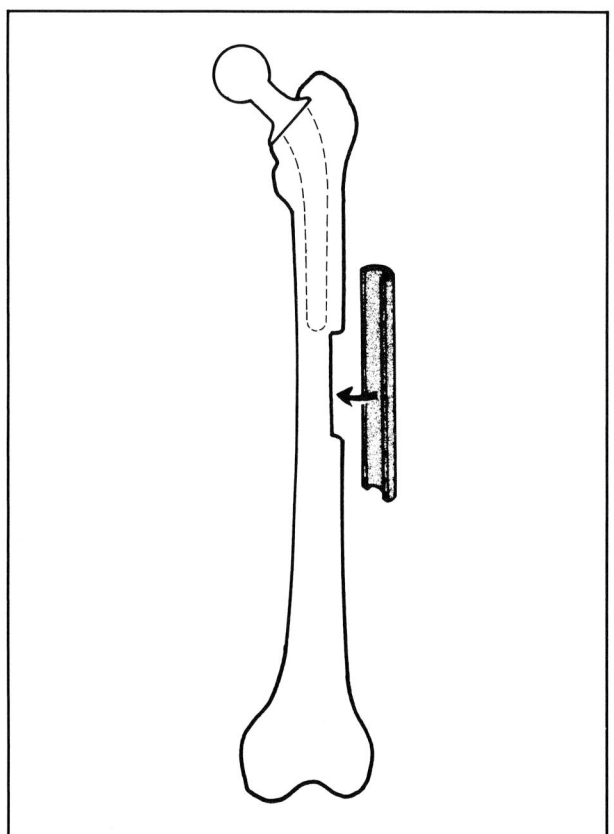

Figure 3-48. Cortical onlay grafts can be used to reconstruct cortical defects of the femur.

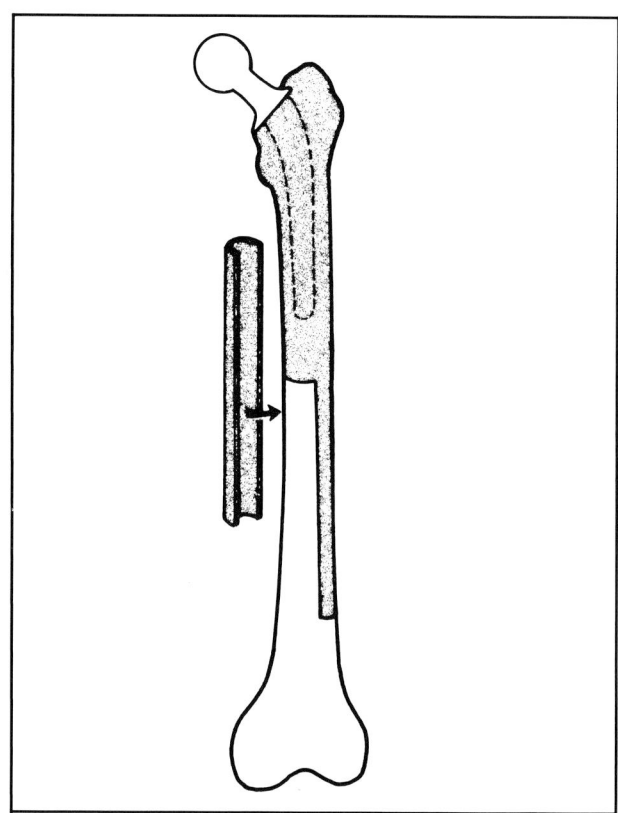

Figure 3-49. In massive proximal femoral bone loss, allograft replacement may be necessary.

operatively but have not had to use them thus far. Theoretically, such grafts would be of particular value if both columns and the central wall of the acetabulum were missing.

Massive cortical struts from the femur or tibia are helpful for fracture fixation (Figure 3-47) or to repair femoral perforations (Figure 3-48). Such struts should cover at least one half the circumference of the recipient bone.

Massive bone loss in the femur can require massive allograft proximal femoral replacement of various lengths, either in subsegments or circumferentially (Figure 3-49).

Whenever an allograft is potentially required, it is important to have a backup graft available as contamination of the original graft could leave the surgeon without adequate materials to finish the procedure. Ideally, neither allografts nor autografts should be resterilized by autoclaving as their potential capacity for incorporation is significantly impaired by these methods.

References

1. Edwards, B.N., Tullos, H.S., Noble, P.C.: Contributory factors and etiology of sciatic nerve palsy in total hip arthroplasty. Clin Orthop 218:136, 1987.
2. Fackler, C.D., Poss, R.: Dislocation in total hip arthroplasties. Clin Orthop 151:169-178, 1980.
3. Harris, W.H., et al.: High and low dose aspirin prophylaxis against venous thromboembolic disease in

total hip replacement. J Bone Joint Surg 64A:63-66, 1982.

4. Parement, G., et al.: New advances in the prevention, diagnosis and cost effectiveness of venous thromboembolic disease in patients with total hip replacement. In The Hip: Proceedings of the Fourteenth Open Scientific Meeting of the Hip Society, The C.V. Mosby Co., St. Louis, MO 1986.

5. Camer, S.: Surgical complications in revision arthroplasty. In Turner, R.H., Scheller, A.O. (ed): Revision Total Hip Arthroplasty. Grune and Stratton, Inc., NY, 1982.

6. Amstutz, H.C., et al.: Revision of aseptic loose total hip arthroplasties. Clin Orthop 170:21, 1982.

7. Pellicci, P.M., et al.: Revision total hip arthroplasty. Clin Orthop 170:34, 1982.

8. Pellicci, P.M., et al.: Long term results of revision total hip Replacement: A follow-up report. J Bone Joint Surg 67A:513, 1985.

9. O'Neil, D.A., Harris, W.H.: Failed total hip replacement: Assessment by plain radiographs, arthrograms and aspiration of the hip joint. J Bone Joint Surg 66A:540-546, 1984.

10. Helms, C.A., McCarthy, S.: CT Scanograms for measuring leg length discrepancy. Radiology 151:802, 1984.

11. Murphy, S.R., et al.: Computer aided simulation, analysis and design in orthopedic surgery. Orthop Clin N America, 17(4):637-649, 1986.

12. Charnley, J.: Post-operative infection after hip replacement with special reference to air contamination in the operating room. Clin Orthop 87:167, 1972.

13. Lidwezl, et al.: Effects of ultraclean air in operating rooms on deep sepsis in the joint after total hip or knee replacement: A randomised study. Br Med J 285:10, 1982.

14. Eftekhar, N.: Infection in joint replacement surgery: Prevention and Management. The C.V. Mosby Co., St. Louis, MO, 1984.

15. Goldner, J.L. and Allen, B.L.: Ultraviolet light in orthopedic operating rooms at Duke University: Thirty-five years experience 1937-1973. Clin Orthop 96:195, 1973.

16. Harris, W.H., Crothers, O., Oh, I.: Total hip replacement and femoral head bone grafting for severe acetabular deficiency in adults. J Bone Joint Surg 59A:752-759, 1977.

17. Hedley, A.K., et al.: Two year follow-up of the PCA noncemented total hip replacement. In The Hip: Proceedings of the Fourteenth Open Scientific Meeting of the Hip Society, The C.V. Mosby Co., St. Louis, MO, 1986.

18. Harris, W.H.: Current status of noncemented hip implants. In The Hip: Proceedings of the Fourteenth Open Scientific Meeting of the Hip Society, The C.V. Mosby Co., St. Louis, MO, 1986.

19. Scott, R.D, et al.: Two to four year follow-up of bipolar revision hip arthroplasty using morsellized acetabular bone graft. AAOS Scientific Session, San Francisco, CA, Jan 1987.

20. Murray, W.: Bipolar prosthesis and bone grafting for acetabular reconstruction. Presented at Problems in Total Joint Replacement Symposium, Palm Springs, CA, Dec. 1986.

21. Stauffer, R.N.: Ten year follow-up study of total hip replacement: With particular reference to roentgenographic loosening of the components. J Bone Joint Surg 64A:983, 1982.

22. Beckenbaugh, R.D., Ilstrup, D.M.: Total hip arthroplasty: A review of 333 cases with long term follow-up. J Bone Joint Surg 60A:306, 1978.

FOUR

Hugh P. Chandler, M.D.
Brad L. Penenberg, M.D.

Surgical Approaches

Exposure must be more extensive in these complex operations than in primary or standard revision surgery.

Dealing with Old Incisions

After the skin is prepped, a sterile marking pen should be used to outline all existing scars before a sterile plastic drape is placed over the skin, because it is very difficult to identify scars once the operative site is covered. This becomes important if an old incision must be extended or if a second incision is necessary to harvest bone, remove plates, etc. Although the hip is more forgiving than the knee, small skin bridges still may become necrotic and lead to serious complications. If it is necessary to make an extension either anterior or posterior to a segment of an old incision, it is safer to make this new incision at right angles to the old one in order to leave skin flaps with the broadest base for potential blood supply. It is also important to leave a broad base when extending an old incision proximally or distally (Figure 4-1A). Extending the new incision at a narrow angle to the old one may look appealing from the aesthetic point of view but could jeopardize the thin bridge of skin in between (Figure 4-1B).

The Posterior Approach

This approach involves division of the short external rotators from their trochanteric attachment and excision of the posterior capsule.[1] The hip is dislocated posteriorly in flexion, adduction and internal rotation. This approach pro-

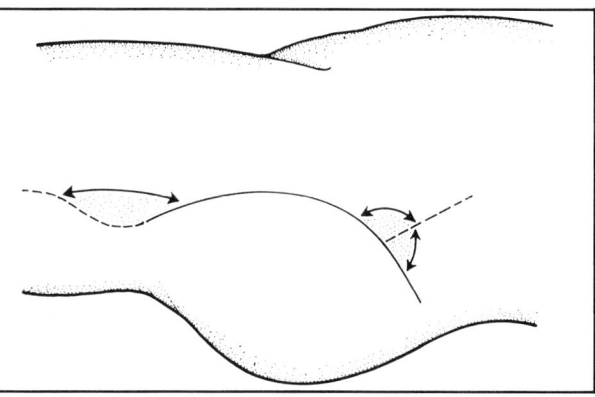

Figure 4-1A. When it is necessary to make another extension either anterior or posterior to a segment of an old incision, it is safer to make this incision at right angles to the old one in order to leave flaps with the broadest base. It is also important to leave a broad base when extending an old incision proximally or distally.

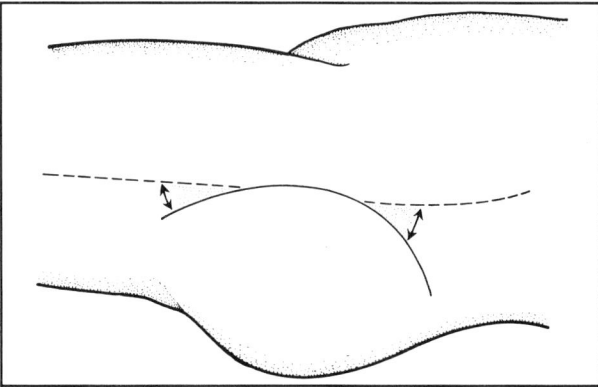

Figure 4-1B. New incisions at acute angles to old ones can potentially cause skin slough.

vides good exposure of the posterior wall of the acetabulum but limited exposure of the superior rim. Although we have had extensive experience with this approach, it is no longer our method of choice because of limited access to the superior rim and because of potential instability in flexion and internal rotation.

The Anterior Approach

Smith-Petersen Approach

This approach develops the interval between the muscles supplied by the femoral and gluteal nerves.[2] It provides good exposure to the anterior acetabulum and moderate exposure to the superior acetabulum but femoral exposure is more limited. The incidence of heterotopic bone is high and we feel that it has no advantage in these major reconstructions.

The Watson-Jones Approach

This approach develops the interval between the gluteus medius and the tensor fascia femoris.[3] It provides adequate exposure of the anterior aspect of the acetabulum but limited exposure of the superior and posterior aspect of the acetabulum and is not our preference for major grafting procedures.

The Direct Lateral Approach

This approach was first described by Hardinge.[4] It involves development of an anterior cuff comprised of the gluteus medius, gluteus minimus, the anterior capsule and the vastus medialis and intermedius (Figure 4-2A). These structures are retracted anteriorly and the hip is dislocated anteriorly in flexion and external rotation.

This approach provides adequate anterior and superior exposure of the acetabulum. It has the additional advantage that stability of the hip is enhanced because the posterior musculature is left undisturbed and the anterior musculature can be repaired anatomically. It is also possible to repair the superior capsule in all primary and in many revision cases. The direct lateral approach is our choice for all routine primary total hips and allows adequate exposure for grafting of small defects involving the anterior and superior aspects of the acetabulum.

With the direct lateral approach, firm anatomic reattachment of both the anterior cuff of capsule, gluteus minimus and gluteal medius, is critical if abductor weakness is to be prevented. In this closure, we prefer to decorticate the anterior trochanteric bed with an oscillating saw and to reattach the cuff of the anterior capsule and gluteus minimus together anatomically with five to eight mattress sutures through drill holes (Figure 4-2B). These sutures are

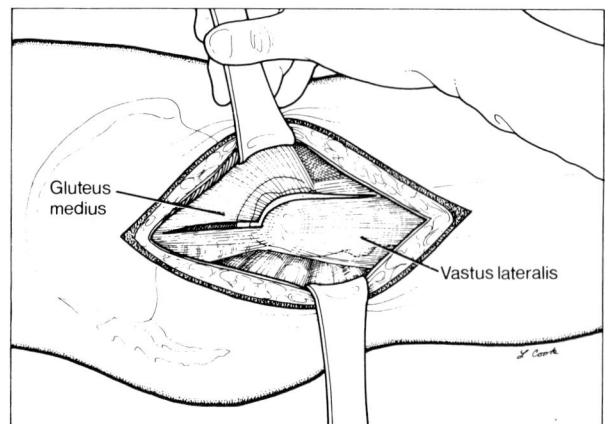

Figure 4-2A. The direct lateral approach provides excellent exposure for primary cases and adequate exposure to graft small anterior and superior acetabular defects.

tied from proximal to distal with the hip abducted and internally rotated. The gluteus medius cuff and the vastus medialis fascia are then closed as a separate layer using a running #1 absorbable suture (Figure 4-2C).

The Vastus Slide

The vastus slide is the authors' modification of the direct lateral approach which involves development of the same proximal anterior cuff comprised of the gluteus medius, gluteus minimus and anterior capsule, but at the distal aspect of the greater trochanter, the incision in the quadriceps fascia is directed posteriorly (leaving a ¼ inch cuff of the vastus origin attached to the greater trochanter for later closure). At the posterior border of the greater trochanter, the fascial incision is again directed distally (Figure 4-3A), and the entire quadriceps musculature is dissected from the femur. As with any approach to the femoral shaft, we prefer to completely sweep all quadriceps fibers anteriorly, initially separating them from the vastus fascia, then from the intermuscular septum, and finally from the femur. Perforating vessels are divided and ligated between clamps. The quadriceps is mobilized anteriorly in continuity with the proximal cuff of the gluteus medius, gluteus minimus, and anterior capsule (Figure 4-3B). The hip is dislocated anteriorly in flexion and external rotation.

This approach provides the same acetabular exposure as the direct lateral approach but also allows exposure of the femoral shaft. It is our choice when it is necessary to gain access to the superior and anterior aspect of the acetabulum as well as to the lateral, anterior, and medial aspect of the femur. As with the direct lateral approach, the vastus slide has the added advantage of increased stability of the hip. Closure of the proximal anterior cuff is the same as with the direct lateral approach. The longitudinal split in the vastus fascia is closed with a heavy resorbable running suture, and the transverse portion is reattached to the cuff at the greater trochanter with interrupted pulley stitches.

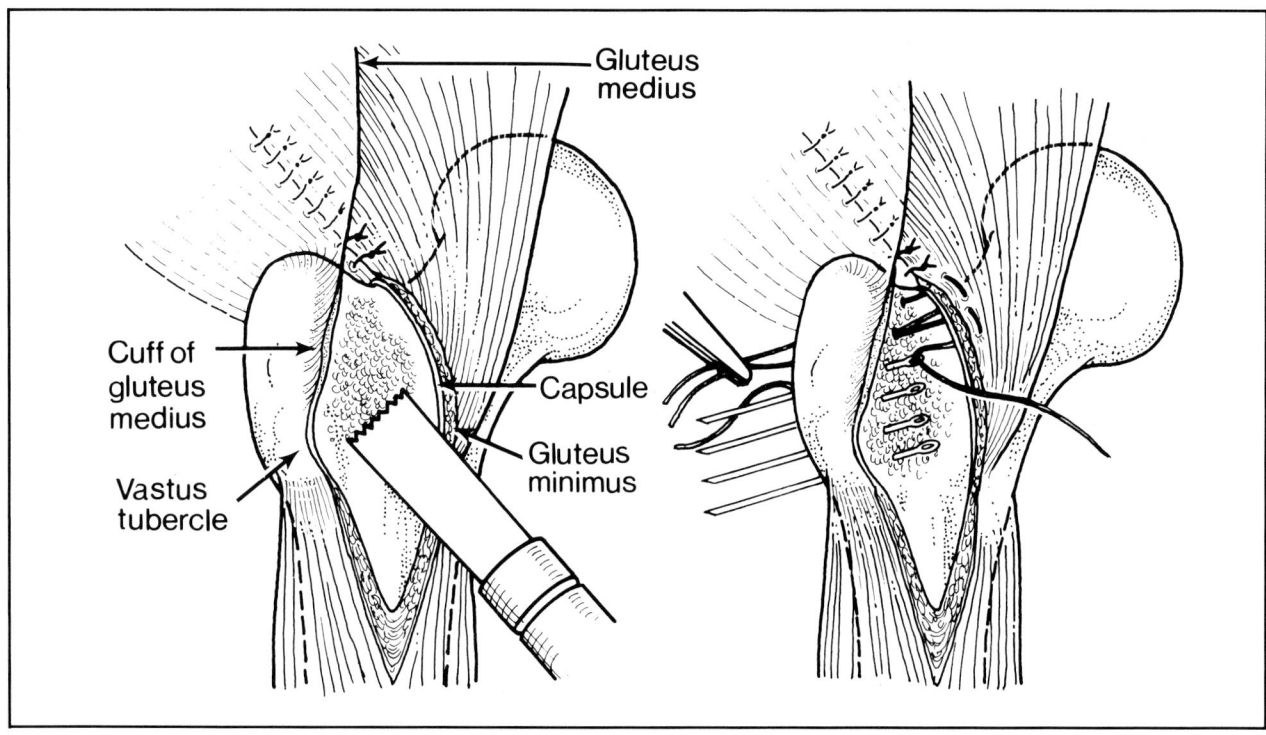

Figure 4-2B. The trochanteric bed is decorticated to bleeding bone and interrupted mattress sutures through drill holes anchor the anterior cuff of the capsule and gluteus minimus anatomically to the greater trochanter. Five to eight mattress sutures are placed through the combined anterior cuff of the gluteus minimus and the capsule, and are then passed through drill holes in the greater trochanter by means of Keith needles.

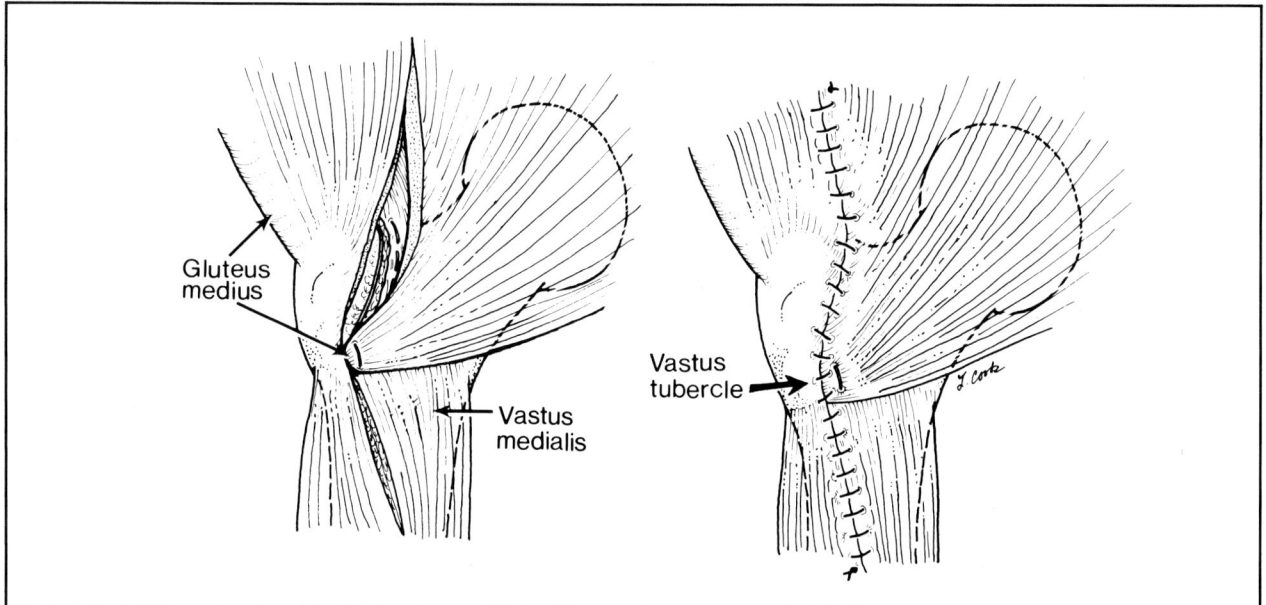

Figure 4-2C. At the vastus tubercle, the gluteus minimus, gluteus medius and vastus medialis blend together and are included in the lowest suture. The gluteus medius and vastus medialis fascia are then closed with a heavy running absorbable suture.

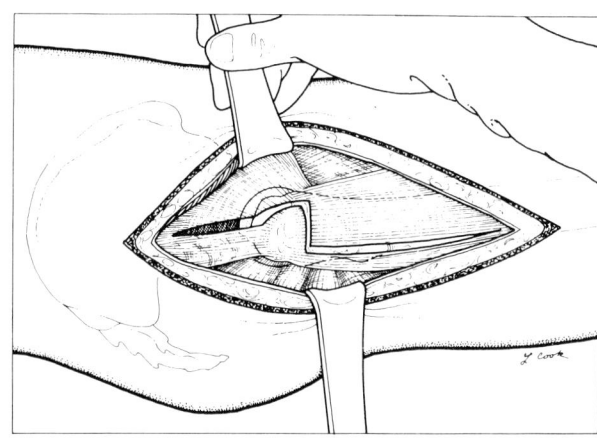

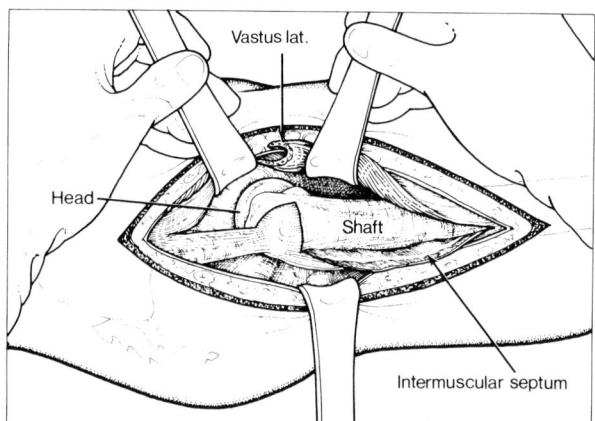

Figure 4-3A. (From Chandler, H.P. and Penenberg, B.L.: In Burke (ed.): Trauma Management, In Press. Courtesy of YearBook Medical Publishers, Inc.) The vastus slide is a modification of the direct lateral approach. Proximally the dissection is the same but at the distal aspect of the greater trochanter, the incision in the quadriceps fascia is directed posteriorly (leaving a ¼ inch cuff for reattachment) and the incision then extends distally at the posterior.

The Transtrochanteric Approach

In this approach, the tendon of the piriformis, the obturator internus and the obturator externus are identified (Figure 4-4A), divided from their trochanteric insertion and are tagged for later reattachment (Figure 4-4B).[5] The origin of the quadriceps is divided from the greater trochanter (leaving a ¼ inch cuff on the greater trochanter for future reattachment). An osteotomy of the greater trochanter is made from distal to proximal using a broad flat osteotome (Figure 4-4B). A complete capsulectomy is performed and the hip can be dislocated anteriorly or posteriorly. The tagged external rotators protect the sciatic nerve from potential injury by retraction (Figure 4-4C). This approach provides the most extensive exposure of all aspects of the acetabulum and of the lateral ilium. It is our choice for major intra-acetabular or rim grafts when it is not necessary to expose the femur.

Although there are many techniques for reattachment of the greater trochanter,[6,7] we prefer a four-wire, double-tension band technique (Figure 4-5) using #18 Vitallium

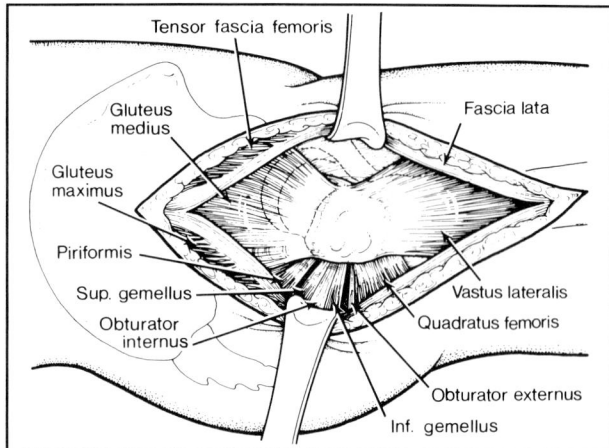

Figure 4-4A. With formal trochanteric osteotomy, the tendons of the piriformis, the obturator internus, and the obturator externus are identified. The superior and inferior gemellus muscles share the obturator internus tendon.

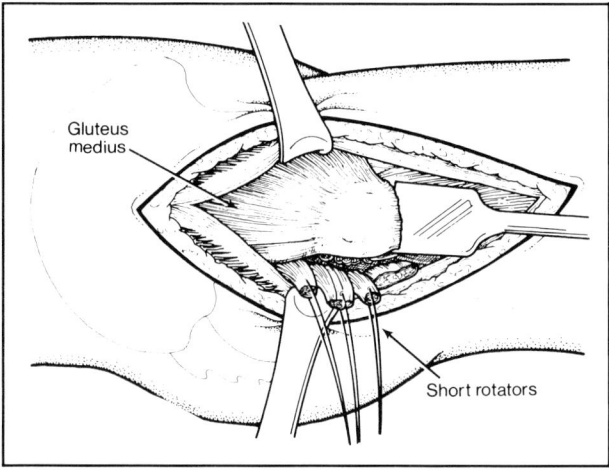

Figure 4-4B. The vastus lateralis is divided from the greater trochanter, leaving a ¼ inch cuff for reattachment. The tendons of the piriformis, obturator internus, and obturator externus are tagged for later reattachment.

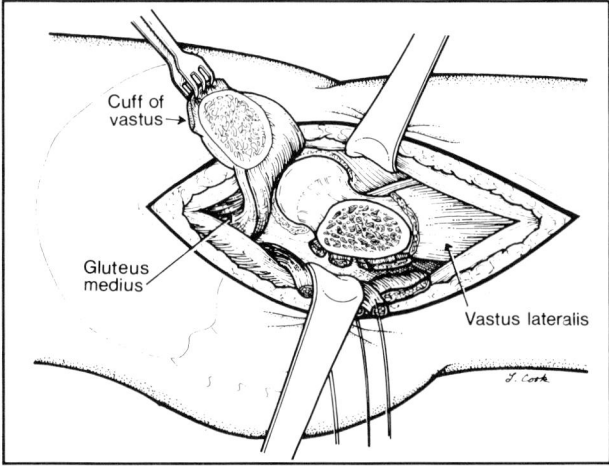

Figure 4-4C. The transtrochanteric approach provides the widest exposure to all aspects of the acetabulum. The tagged short rotator tendons protect the sciatic nerve from injury by retraction.

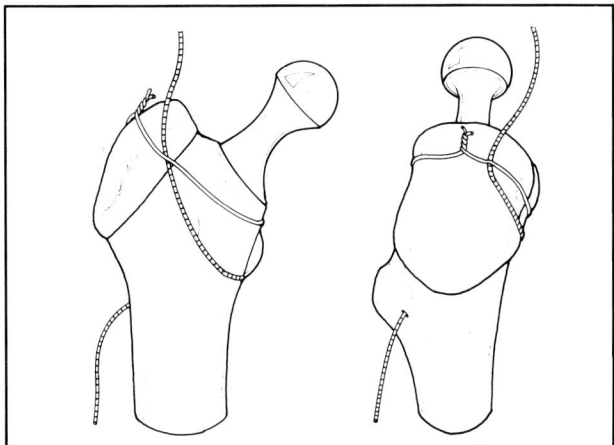

Figure 4-5A. Two of the four wires are transverse. The distal wire should pass through a drill hole in the lesser trochanter. The more proximal wire can pass through bone or around the calcar. Before tightening the proximal wire, one limb of the distal wire is placed beneath it. The proximal wire is then maximally tightened. We prefer to use a Harris wire tightener (Codman and Shurtleff, Inc., Randolph, MA) and to twist the wire rather than to tie it. The twisted ends should be buried to avoid irritation of the surrounding tissues.

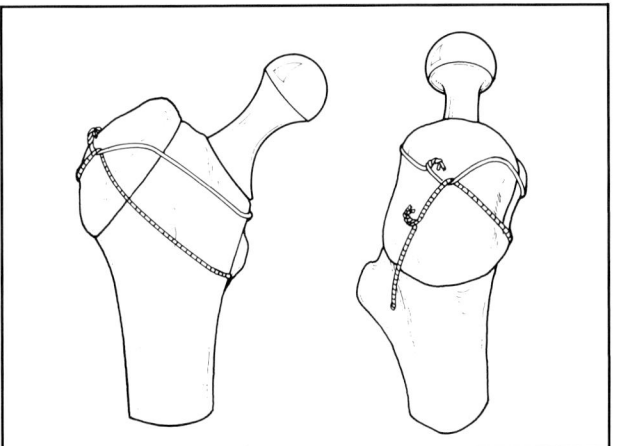

Figure 4-5B. The second wire is then tightened maximally and twisted. The first wire is placed under additional tension by the second. Both wires are now maximally tight and the trochanter is secure.

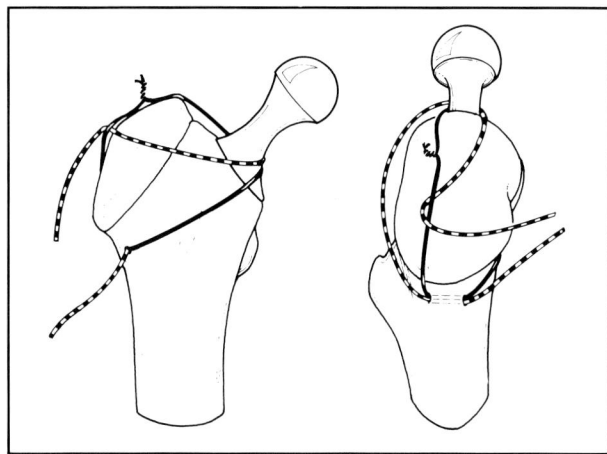

Figure 4-5C. The two vertical wires are placed through a transverse drill hole just distal to the trochanteric bed. Each is passed beneath the calcar or the neck of the prosthesis. Before tightening the first wire, one limb of the second wire is passed beneath it. The first wire is then tightened and twisted.

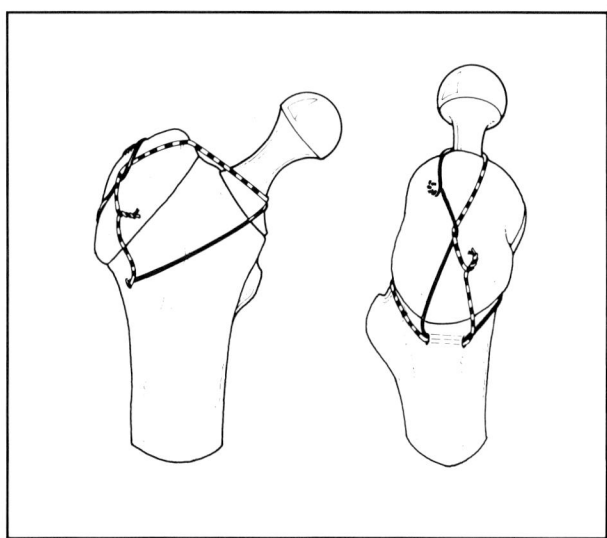

Figure 4-5D. When the second vertical wire is maximally tightened, it places the first under even greater tension.

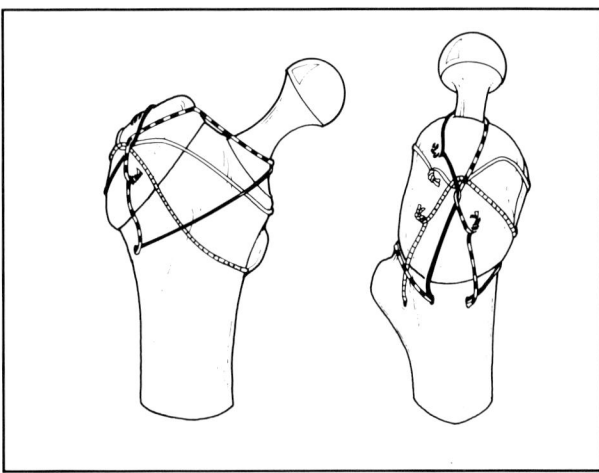

Figure 4-5E. The trochanter is extremely secure when all wires have been tightened.

wire (Howmedica, Rutherford, NJ). All four wires are placed in position but the two transverse wires are tightened first and maximally compress the greater trochanter to its bed. The two vertical wires are then added and provide extra security. There are two advantages of this technique. The first is that maximum compression of the greater trochanter to its bed is achieved as soon as the second transverse wire is tightened. If individual nonlinked wires are used, trochanteric fixation can be compromised as each successive wire adds further compression of the trochanter to its bed, effectively making the previous wire loose. In this situation, final fixation is often determined by the last single wire that is tightened. If this wire breaks, fixation is provided by the previously tightened wire. The sequence may be that the fourth, then the third, then the second and finally the first wire breaks and the trochanter migrates proximally. The second advantage of the four-wire, double-tension band technique is that wires pass around rather than through the trochanteric fragment. Cerclage of this type maximizes contact of the wires with cortical bone and decreases the likelihood of wires cutting through the trochanter.

The Trochanteric Slide

We first used this approach in 1976 for revision total hip replacement and in recent years have used it with increasing frequency. Recently described by Glassman et al.[9] it is a combination of the standard transtrochanteric approach with a modification of the myofascial slide proposed in 1954 by McFarland and Osborne.[5,8] The tendons of the short rotators are identified, divided from the greater trochanter, and tagged for later reattachment (Figure 4-4A and 4-4B). The vastus lateralis is mobilized from the posterior femur, and a trochanteric osteotomy is made starting from the posterior and inferior aspect of the greater trochanter using a broad flat osteotome (Figure 4-6A). The greater trochanter is left attached to the quadriceps and to the gluteus medius and minimus and is retracted anteriorly (Figure 4-6B). A complete capsulectomy is performed. The hip is dislocated anteriorly in flexion and external rotation, and the femur is retracted posteriorly. The greater trochanter becomes a double pedicle graft with a blood supply proximally and distally. The vastus lateralis also tethers the greater trochanter distally and helps prevent proximal migration. The greater trochanteric fragment can be thinner than with conventional trochanteric osteotomy and if the greater trochanter is absent (secondary to previous surgery), the abductors and the vastus lateralis can be left in continuity.

In the presence of a bony fragment of the greater trochanter, the four-wire, double-tension band technique is used (Figure 4-5) for reattachment. If there is no trochanteric bone available, a chair staple and/or suture can be used to prevent anterior or posterior displacement of the abductors and the quadriceps.

The trochanteric slide provides excellent exposure of the superior and posterior aspects of the acetabulum and of the femur; whereas the vastus slide is more helpful if the superior and anterior aspects of the acetabulum and of the femur require exposure. The trochanteric slide is also helpful if the trochanteric fragment is small or absent or when the greater trochanter must be attached to an allograft.

References

1. Osborne, R.P.: The approach to the hip joint: A critical review and a suggested new route. Br J Surg 18:49, 1930-31.
2. Smith-Petersen, M.N.: Approach to and exposure of the hip joint for mold arthroplasty. J Bone Joint Surg 31A:40, 1949.

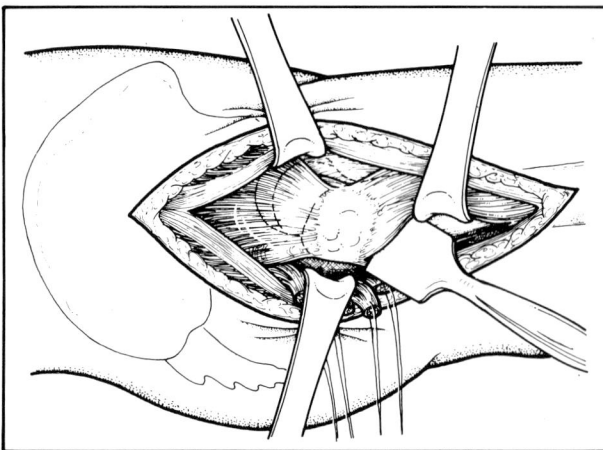

Figure 4-6A. The quadriceps is mobilized from the posterior aspect of the femur and an osteotomy of the greater trochanter is made starting from its posterior and inferior aspect.

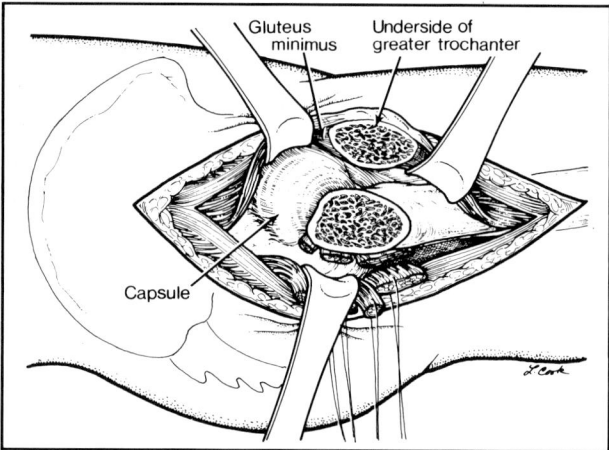

Figure 4-6B. The greater trochanter is left attached to the quadriceps and to the gluteus medius and minimus and is retracted anteriorly.

3. Watson-Jones, R.: Fractures of the neck of the femur. Br J Surg 23:787, 1935-36.
4. Hardinge, K.: The direct lateral approach to the hip. J Bone Joint Surg 64B:17, 1982.
5. Charnley, J., Ferrera, A.: Transplantation of the greater trochanter in arthroplasty of the hip. J Bone Joint Surg 46B:191, 1964.
6. Harris, W.H., Crothers, O.D.: Reattachment of the greater trochanter in total hip replacement arthroplasty. J Bone Joint Surg 60A:211, 1978.
7. Boardman, K.P., Bocco, F., Charnley, J.: An evaluation of a method of trochanteric fixation using three wires in the Charnley low friction arthroplasty. Clin Orthop 132:31, 1978.
8. McFarland, B., Osborne, G.: Approach to the hip: A suggested improvement on Kocher's method. J Bone Joint Surg 36B:364, 1954.
9. Glassman, A.H., Engh, C.A., Bobyn, J.D.: A technique of extensile exposure for total hip arthroplasty. J of Arthroplasty 2:11, 1987.

FIVE

Hugh P. Chandler, M.D.
Brad L. Penenberg, M.D.

Acetabular Reconstruction

In the past, major acetabular defects have been filled with large amounts of cement, cement and wire mesh, or "protrusio" shells. Such reconstructions have resulted in early failure and subsequent revisions are considerably more difficult than the first operation. We are now seeing an increasing number of failed total hip replacements that require revision and many of these have some degree of bone loss. It is becoming clear that it is often better to reconstruct acetabular bone defects with bone grafts rather than with more cement.

Materials

Our experience now consists of a total of 76 acetabular grafts in seventy-three patients. 49 hips required acetabular grafts alone. 27 additional hips required both acetabular and femoral grafts. There were 43 females and 30 males. The average age was 56 years (range 23 to 80 years). The average followup is 3.2 years (range 6 months to 15 years). Initial diagnoses included congenital hip dislocation or dysplasia (23), osteoarthritis (21), trauma (19) and a variety of other non-neoplastic processes in 13.

Fifty-two of these operations were for revisions of previously failed surgery. Thirty-two revisions were for failed total hip replacements, seven for failed cup arthroplasties, five for resection arthroplasties, five for failed surface replacements and three for failed Moore prostheses.

Methods

Autogenous bone was used in 26 hips (25 femoral heads and one iliac crest). Allograft bone was used in 50 cases (38 femoral heads and 12 formal harvests). Allografts were frozen at $-80°$. In the past three years, all allografts have been supplemented with autogenous bone which was taken either from the patient's femoral head, from the iliac crest, or from both. Whenever possible, a bone paste was made from acetabular reamings mixed with autologous blood and any surface irregularities at the interface between the graft and the host were filled with this material.

Smooth $\frac{3}{32}$nd K-wires provided provisional fixation for solid grafts. Bolt fixation was used in some of our early cases but permanent fixation is now achieved by means of cancellous screws or press (geometric) fit.

Postoperative Management

Postoperative management was modified only by the extent of the soft tissue dissection and not by the size or complexity of the graft. All patients were placed in balanced suspension with five pounds of Buck's traction. The average time in suspension was five days. The hospital stay averaged 14 days. Crutch protection with 50 to 60 pounds of weight bearing was encouraged for eight weeks, followed by weightbearing as tolerated. The average time on crutches was nine weeks and those patients who were able to discard their cane, did so at an average of four and one half months.

Classification of Acetabular Defects

There are an increasing number of reports in the literature concerning reconstruction of acetabular defects. A variety of bone grafting techniques have been used in association with many different acetabular components. In the past however, there has been no consistent, integrated classification of the many types of defects that are encountered.

It is therefore difficult to discuss specific types of problems and to compare one technique of reconstruction with another. With this in mind, we devised a classification system, which we have been using for the past three years, based on acetabular anatomy.

The acetabulum can be divided into three major anatomic zones—the rim, the medial wall, and the intra-acetabular area, which lies between the rim and the medial wall.

The rim and the intra-acetabular zones can each be subdivided into three segments: these are the anterior, the superior, and the posterior segments. Clinical defects can

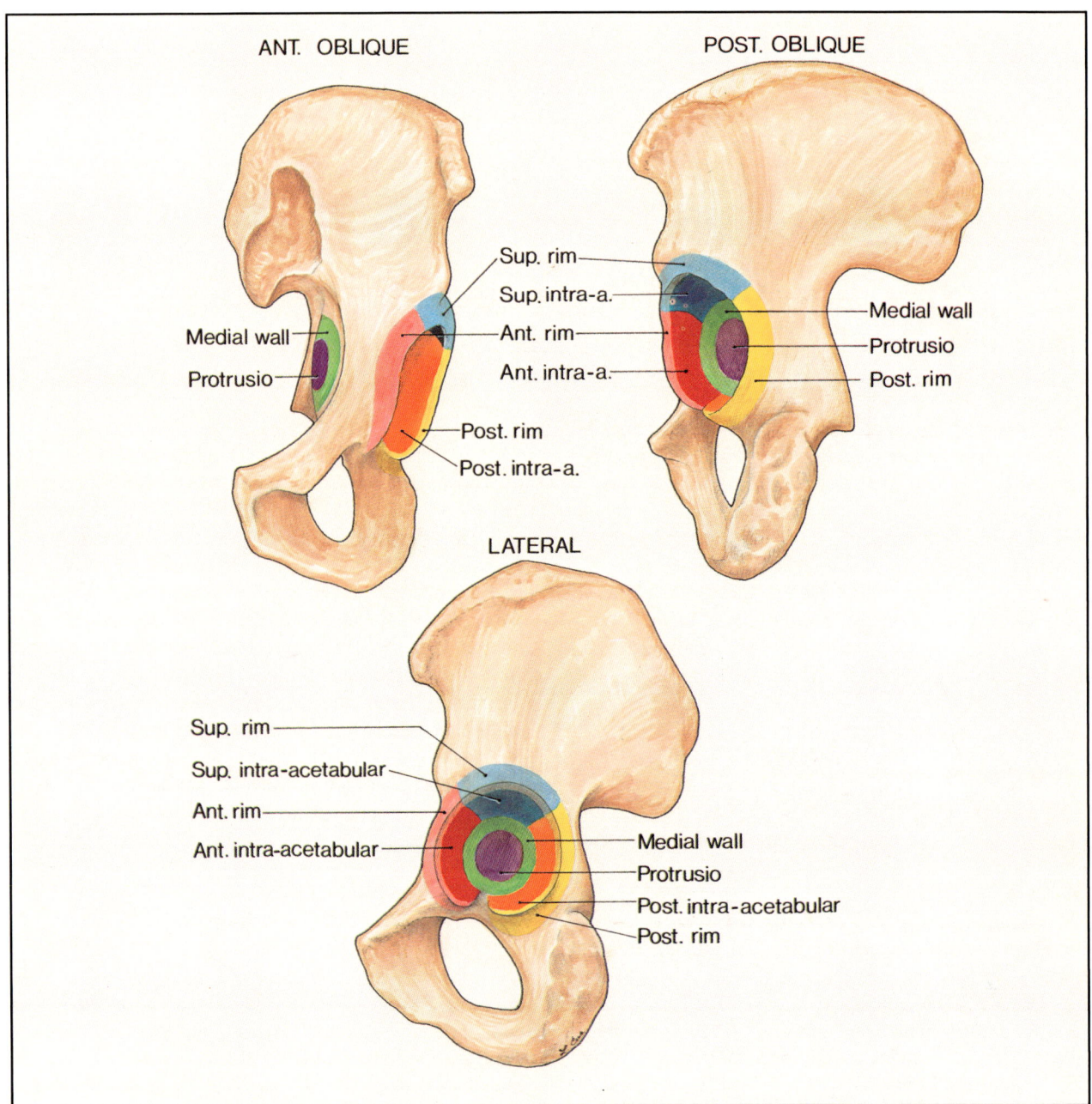

Figure 5-1. The acetabulum consists of a rim, a medial wall and the intra-acetabular area which lies between the rim and the medial wall. Defects of the rim or the intra-acetabular area can involve the anterior, superior or posterior segments. The medial wall is subject to protrusio or perforation problems.

involve one or more of these segments. The medial wall is subject to protrusio and/or to perforation.

In January of 1987, the AAOS Committee on the Hip introduced the AAOS Classsification System of Acetabular Deficiencies.[1] With all due respect to the committee members, we believe that our system of classification is simpler and more versatile than that which they propose. In the Committee's system, rim defects are called "Peripheral Segmental" (Type IA) while full thickness medial wall deficiencies are termed "Central Segmental" (Type IB). Intra-acetabular problems as well as protrusio are classed as "Cavitary" (Type II). We believe that our system more clearly defines these areas by referring to their anatomical names.

The classification system that we prefer is illustrated in Figure 5-1. The anterior acetabular rim is depicted in pink, the superior in blue, and the posterior in yellow. The anterior intra-acetabular segment is depicted in red, the superior intra-acetabular area in turquoise and the posterior intra-acetabular area in orange. The medial wall, where protrusio can occur, is depicted in purple. The area where medial perforation can occur is shown in green. Based on the anatomic sub-divisions outlined above, we have been able to categorize all 76 acetabular defects in our series. New variations may be added as they are encountered.

The four basic types of acetabular deficiencies and various combinations of deficiencies encompass our entire clinical series and are shown on Table 5-1.

In the discussion that follows, we will present examples of each type of problem and describe methods of reconstruction.

Table 5-1

1. Rim defects
2. Intra-acetabular defects
3. Protrusio of the medial wall of the acetabulum
4. Perforation of the medial wall of the acetabulum
5. Combined acetabular defects
   A. Protrusio and perforation of the medial wall of the acetabulum
   B. Superior rim and superior intra-acetabular defects
   C. Superior rim, superior intra-acetabular defects and perforation of the medial wall
   D. Superior acetabular defects and perforation of the medial wall
   E. Global deficiency (complex deficiency of the anterior, superior and posterior rim, and the anterior superior and posterior intra-acetabular area)
   F. Column defects (anterior or posterior rim and intra-acetabular defects in conjunction with major medial perforation or discontinuity between the iliac and the pubic and ischial segments)

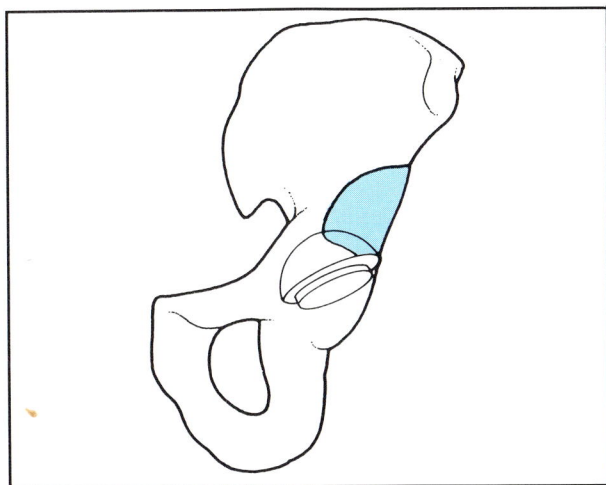

Figure 5-2. Superior rim defects.

Basic Acetabular Defects — Rim Defects (Figure 5-2)

Superior Rim Defects (Fig. 5-2)

Rim defects were the most frequently encountered defects in our series of acetabular grafts. There were 26 hips with isolated rim defects (34 percent) and another 20 hips that had combined rim and other acetabular defects, making a total of 46 (61%) with rim problems.

The etiology of the isolated rim defects was congenital hip dysplasia in 17, subluxation related to osteoarthritis (8), and subluxation related to rheumatoid arthritis (1). The remainder of the isolated rim defects, as well as all of the combined defects involving the rim, were secondary to failed previous surgery.

Review of Literature. In 1977, Harris, Crothers and Oh first described their technique of bolting autogenous femoral heads into the false acetabulum of dysplastic hips to provide superior rim coverage.[2] In 1982, Harris reported his experience with allograft femoral heads used to reconstruct the superior rim.[3] The use of femoral head autografts and allografts for this purpose is now widely accepted. Some authors have advocated fixation with bolts alone,[2,3] screws combined with other types of metallic support[4], or screws alone.[5]

In January of 1984 we first reported our early experience with the use of autograft and allograft femoral heads secured with screws.[6]

When to Graft the Rim. The need for a graft of the superior rim should be suspected preoperatively on the basis of both templating and the degree of disruption of Shenton's line. The final decision should be made at the time of surgery when the thickness of the medial wall can be assessed by means of a depth gauge; however, the decision should ideally be made before reaming commences because fixation of the graft may be more difficult after the acetabulum has been reamed.

It might be tempting to place the acetabular component at a higher level rather than to graft the rim but it should be remembered that the walls of the ilium converge sharply within ½ inch of the superior rim of the true acetabulum (Figure 5-3). Above this level, the bone stock is insufficient to provide both anterior and posterior coverage. Excessive abduction of the acetabular component insures coverage but risks instability. Very small cups need less coverage but require smaller head sizes, again compromising stability. With small cups the polyethylene liner is also thinner and with wear could lead to early implant failure.

A hip with mild superior migration can be reconstructed without a bone graft (Figures 5-4A and 5-4B). More significant migration will definitely need a graft (Figure 5-5). The decision is much more difficult in those patients with moderate migration (Figure 5-6A). Many of the more modern acetabular components are of lower profile than the previous components that were designed to be used with cement. Accordingly, it is sometimes possible now to use such components without a graft in situations that would have required a graft if the older deeper components were used. We will accept up to 8mm. of an uncovered superior edge of the acetabular component if there is complete anterior and posterior coverage (Figure 5-6B). Leaving more of the

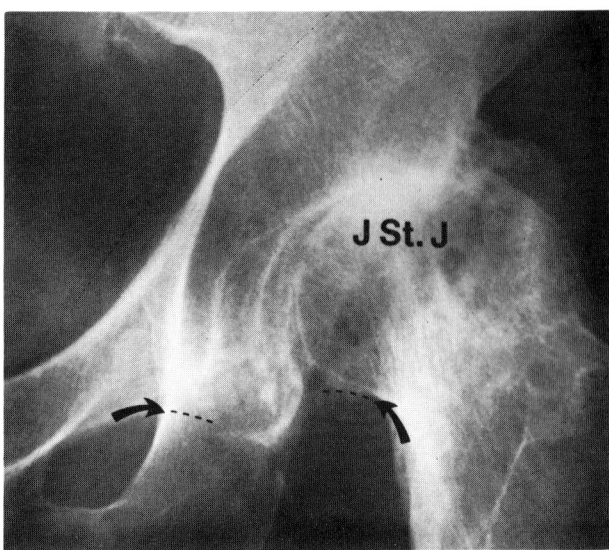

Figure 5-4A. A hip with mild dysplasia and minimal proximal migration does not need a graft.

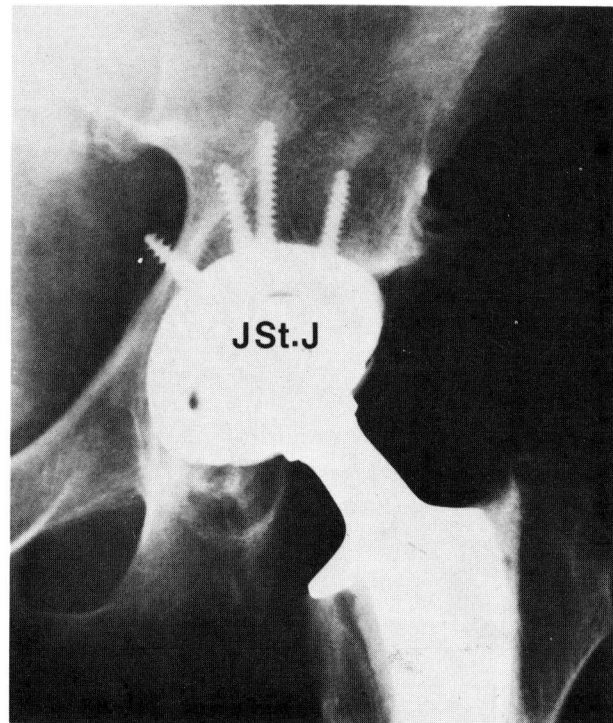

Figure 5-4B. The acetabular component is well covered by bone.

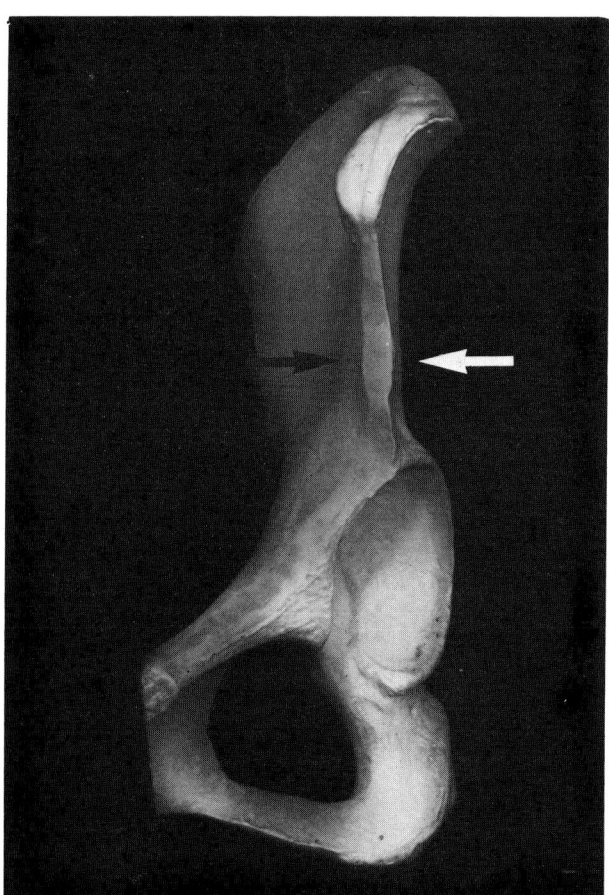

Figure 5-3. There is inadequate anterior-posterior bone to allow for stable proximal placement of the acetabular component.

superolateral edge uncovered increases the risk of socket breakout (Figures 5-7A and 5-7B).

Author's Preferred Treatment

Dealing with Small Superior Rim Defects That Do Not Require Grafting. If it is clear that a major graft will not be necessary, it is our preference to use the direct lateral approach.

With small rim deficiencies, proper placement of the acetabular component requires very careful reaming to

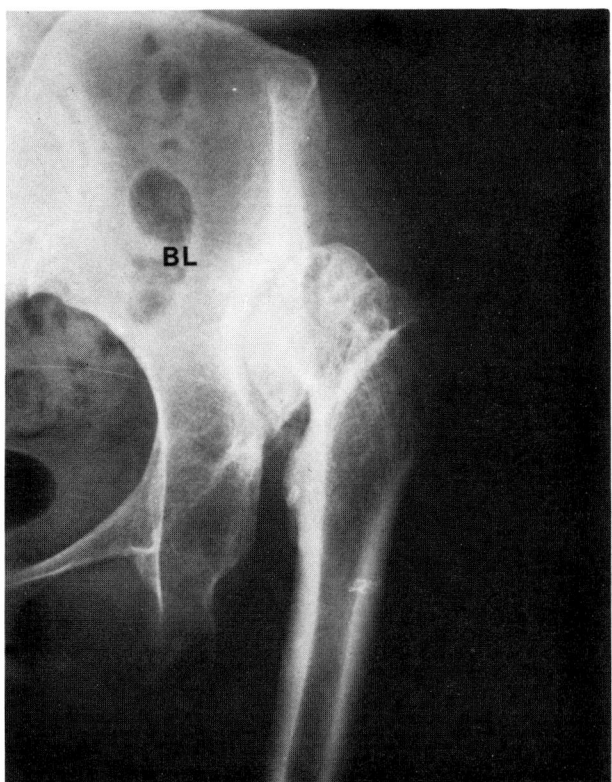

Figure 5-5. With such dramatic proximal migration, there will be no anterior-posterior stock to reconstruct the new acetabulum. An autograft will be necessary to carry out the reconstruction at the level of the true acetabulum.

avoid losing bone stock that might further compromise coverage of the acetabular component. If the surgeon begins with the templated reamer, oriented in the desired final position of the acetabular component, it is possible that superior rim bone could be inadvertently lost (Figure 5-8A). It is safer to begin with the smallest available reamer (usually 42 or 44mm.) and to first ream medially (Figure 5-8B). This reamer is then oriented into the position that will eventually be used for the final component. Progressively larger reamers are then used until further enlargement would remove bone from the rim (Figure 5-8B). Under certain circumstances, moderate thinning of the medial wall can be accepted to allow coverage of a bone ingrowth acetabular component used without cement. In general we prefer to use the largest component that will be well covered.

Technique for Superior Rim Defects That Require Grafting. Small superior rim defects can be grafted through either a posterior approach, or the direct lateral approach but our preference for most large rim defects is to use one of the transtrochanteric approaches.

If the patient's femoral head is available, it is helpful to make a mark on the head and on the acetabulum in the position of the weight-bearing axis (Figure 5-9C) before the head is divided from the neck, as congruity is often best with the graft in this position. The articulating surfaces should be cleaned of all soft tissues. It is not necessary to remove all cortical bone but we do prefer to shave the surface of the femoral head lightly with a reciprocating saw to remove any remaining cartilage and to roughen areas of eburnated bone (Figure 5-9A). The acetabulum should be

Figure 5-6A. The decision whether or not a graft will be necessary is harder to make preoperatively with moderate proximal migration and rim erosion.

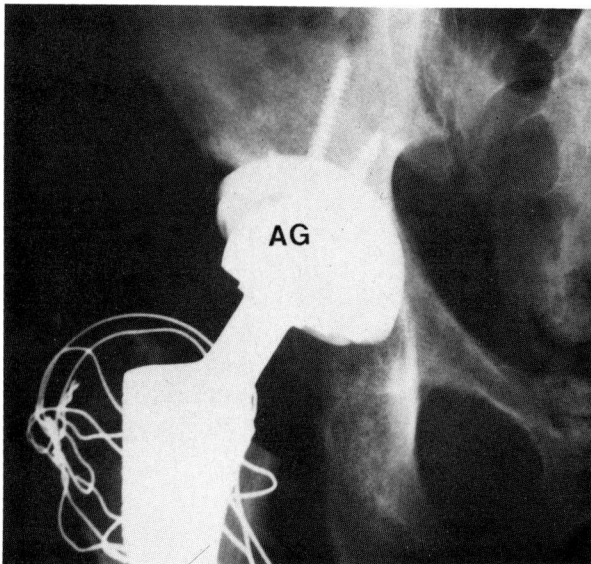

Figure 5-6B. We will accept up to 8mm. of uncovering of the superior edge of the acetabular component if there is complete anterior and posterior bony coverage. If an older, deep profile cemented component was used, it probably would have been necessary to graft the rim.

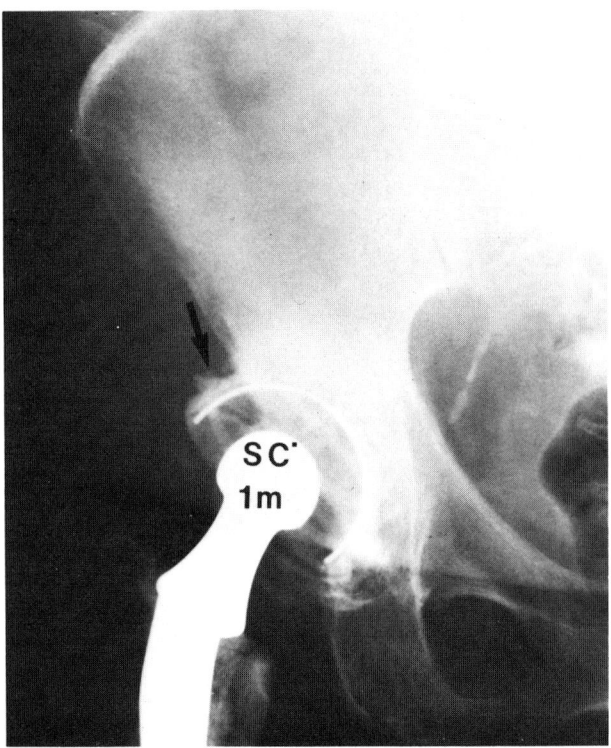

Figure 5-7A. At one month postoperatively, the lateral aspect of this acetabular component is unsupported by bone. Better coverage could have been achieved by reaming more medially and a graft probably would not have been needed but this acetabular component is at risk.

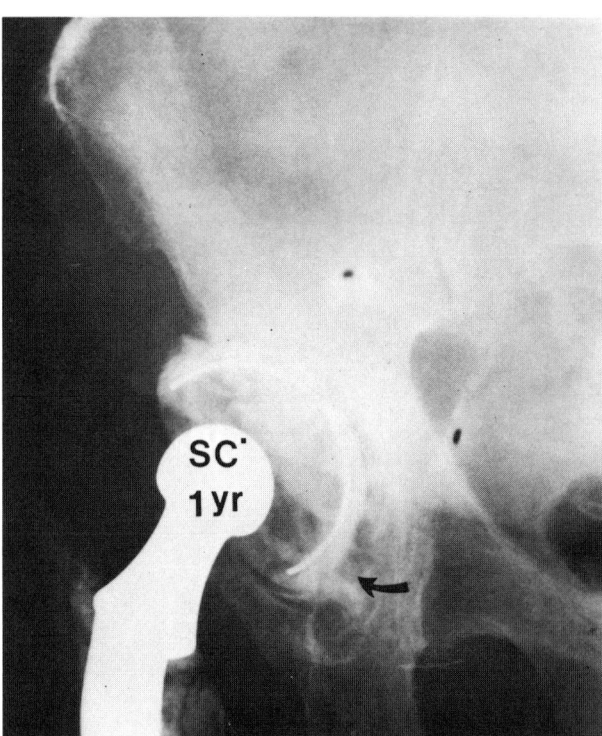

Figure 5-7B. At one year, superolateral migration is evident.

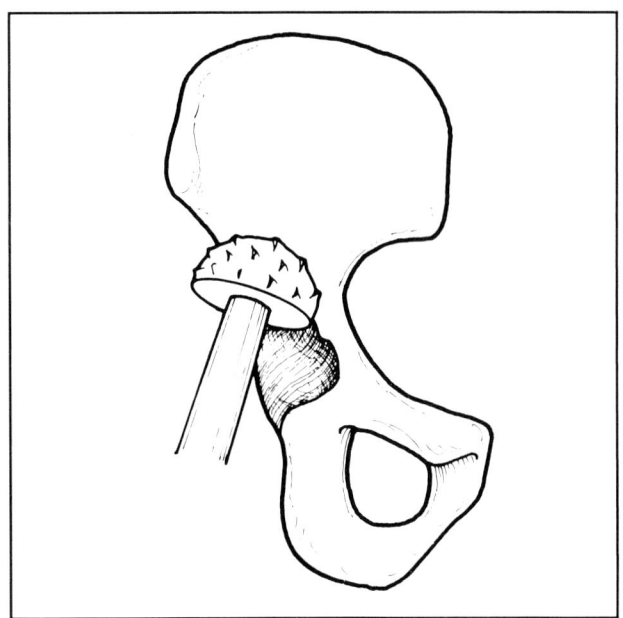

Figure 5-8A. If the surgeon begins with the reamer corresponding to the size of the templated component and orients it in the final desired position of the acetabular component, superior rim bone could be lost.

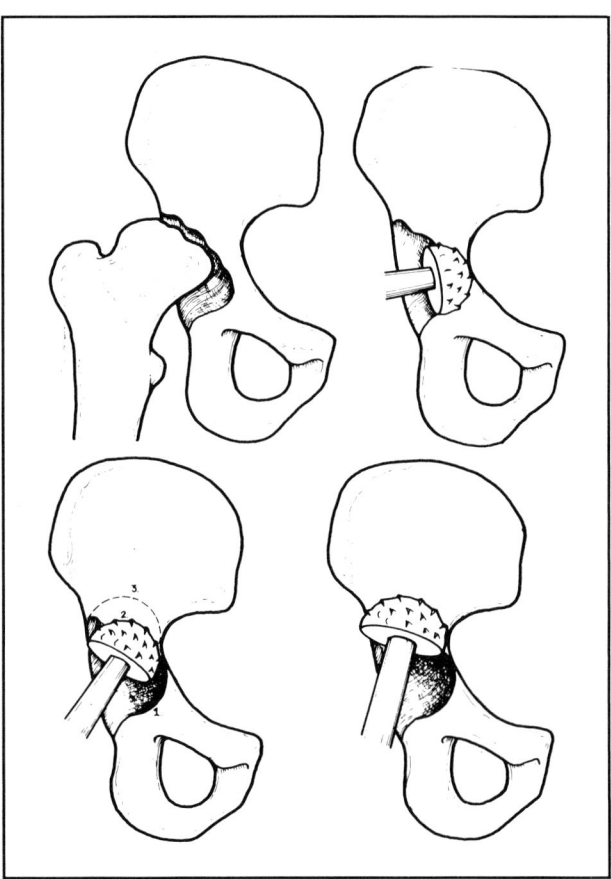

Figure 5-8B. It is safer to first ream medially with the smallest available reamer (usually 42 or 44mm.) and then to orient the reamer in the position that will eventually be used for the final component. Progressively larger reamers are used until further enlargement would remove bone from the rim.

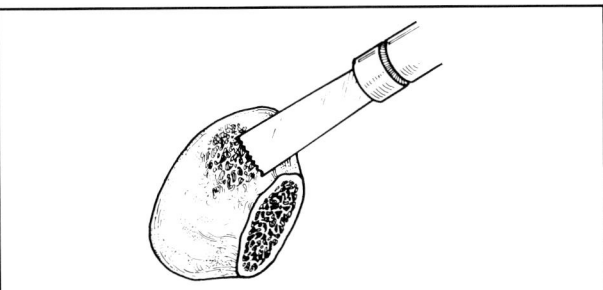

Figure 5-9A. It is not necessary to remove all cortical bone but it is preferable to shave off any remaining cartilage and to roughen areas of eburnated bone with a reciprocating saw.

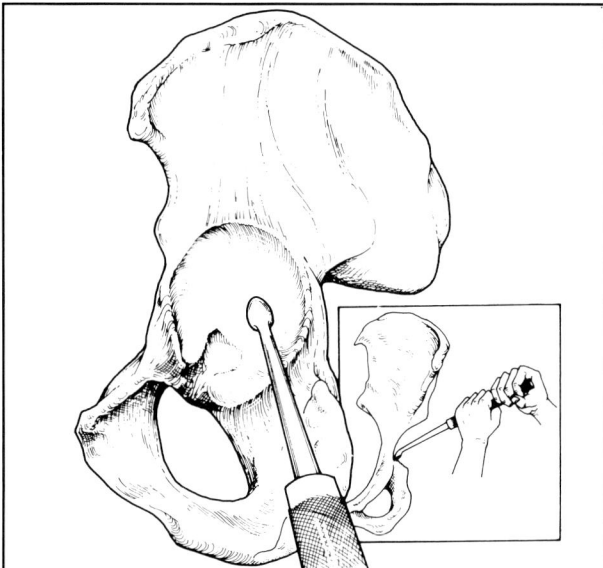

Figure 5-9B. Surfaces are cleared of all soft tissue. Any remaining cartilage may be removed with a large curette. Care is taken not to remove underlying bone.

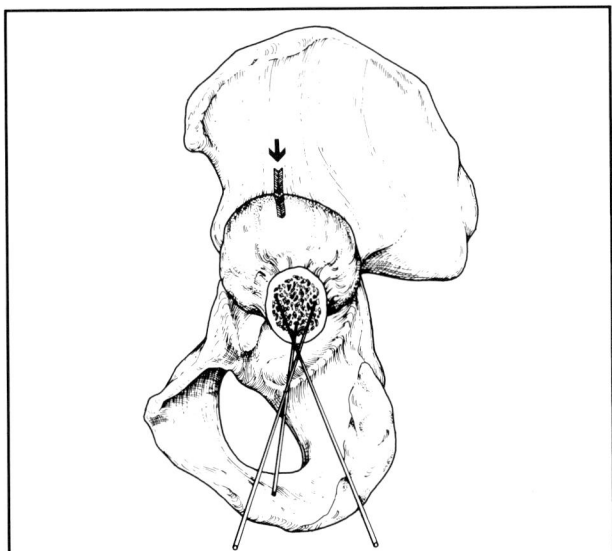

Figure 5-9C. The graft is secured in its most congruous orientation, which is usually in the position of weightbearing, determined by a mark made before the neck is divided. Three ³/₃₂nd K-wires are placed in the area that will subsequently be removed by the reamer.

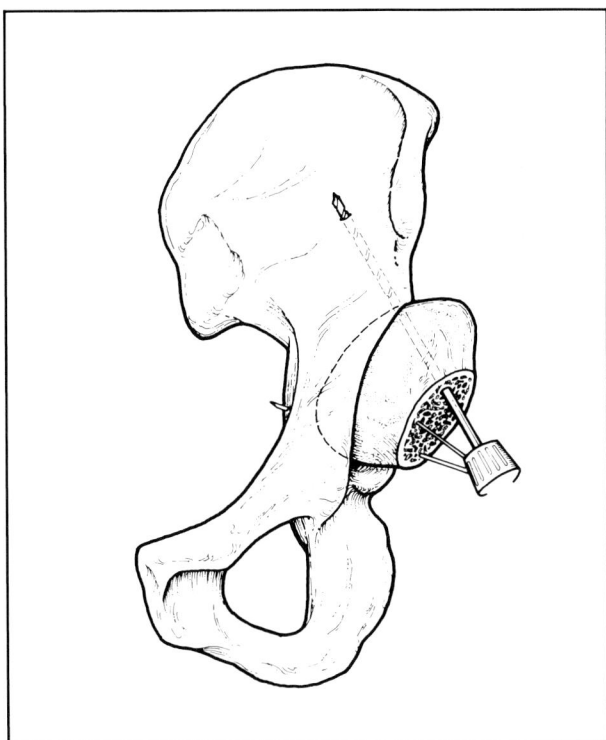

Figure 5-9D. Holes are drilled for screws superiorly, in the area that will not be reamed. It is important to orient these in the weight-bearing axis. A ⁹/₆₄th drill is appropriate for the 6.5mm. Vitallium screws that we prefer (Howmedica, Rutherford, NJ).

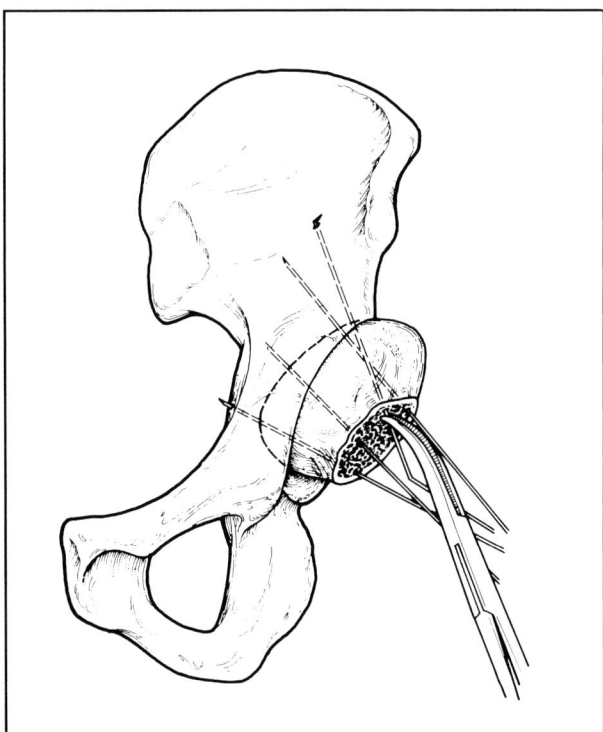

Figure 5-9E. A depth gauge is used to determine the appropriate length screw. Conventional depth gauges are usually not long enough and a simple but effective depth gauge can easily be made from a small smooth K-wire.

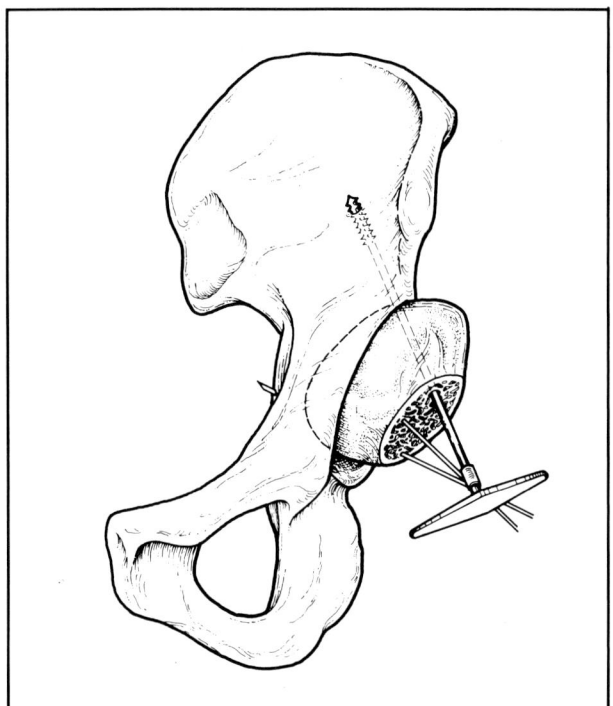

Figure 5-9F. The screw holes are tapped (6.5mm. tap).

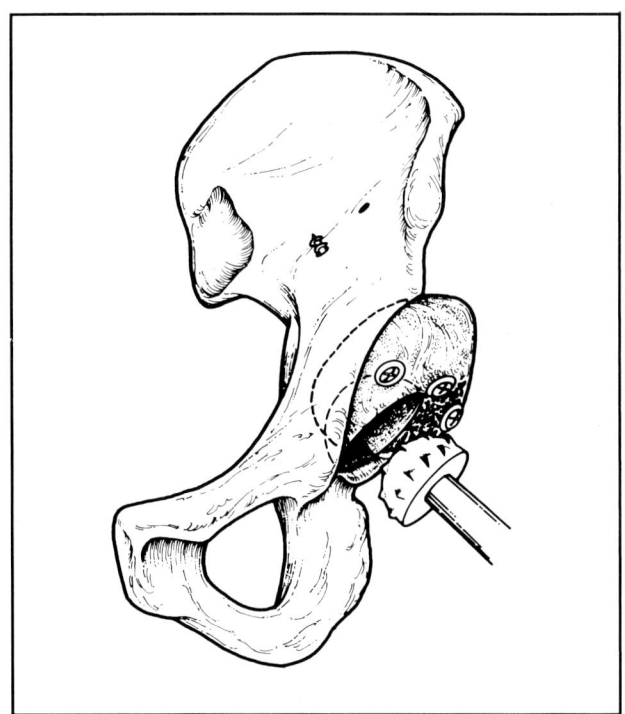

Figure 5-9H. Final acetabular preparation is carried out with standard reamers of appropriate size. The reamer should be spinning prior to making contact and initial pressure should be light in order to avoid the risk of sudden torque which could displace or fracture the graft.

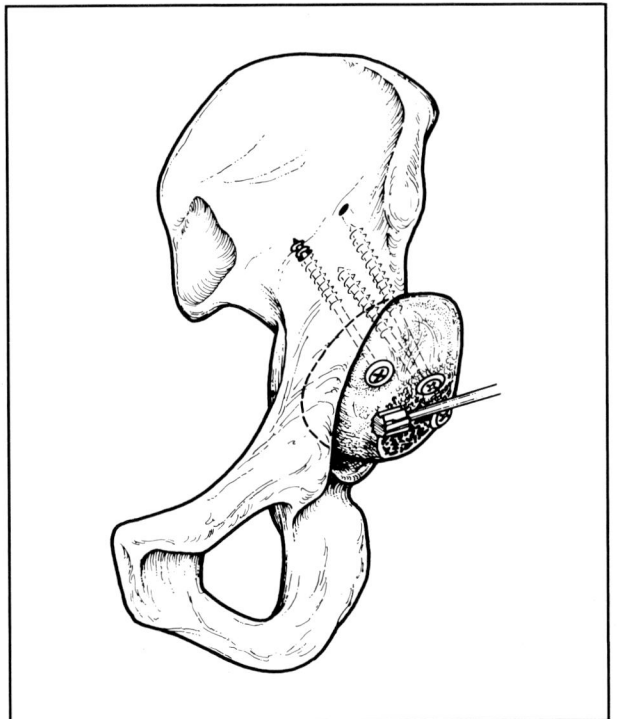

Figure 5-9G. Shaping of the new acetabulum is first started with a high-speed burr.

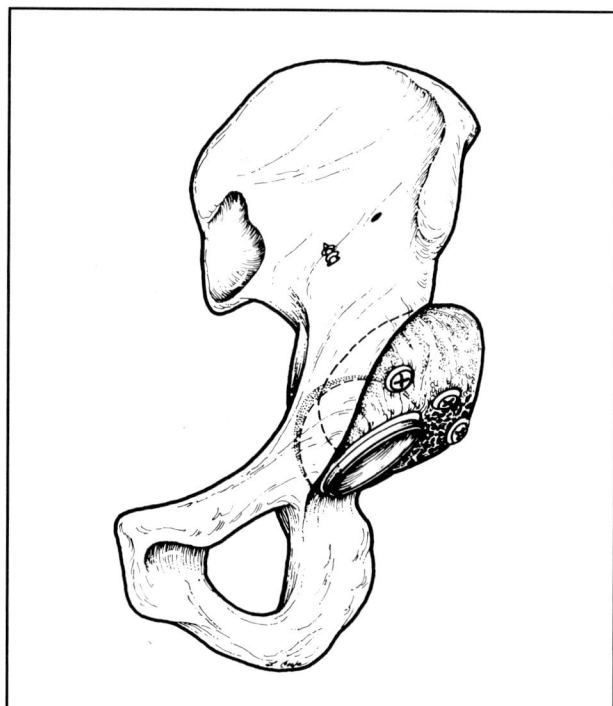

Figure 5-9I. Once the acetabulum has been reamed, the component can be placed in the optimal position of 40° to 45° of abduction and 30° to 35° of flexion and ideally should be completely covered by bone.

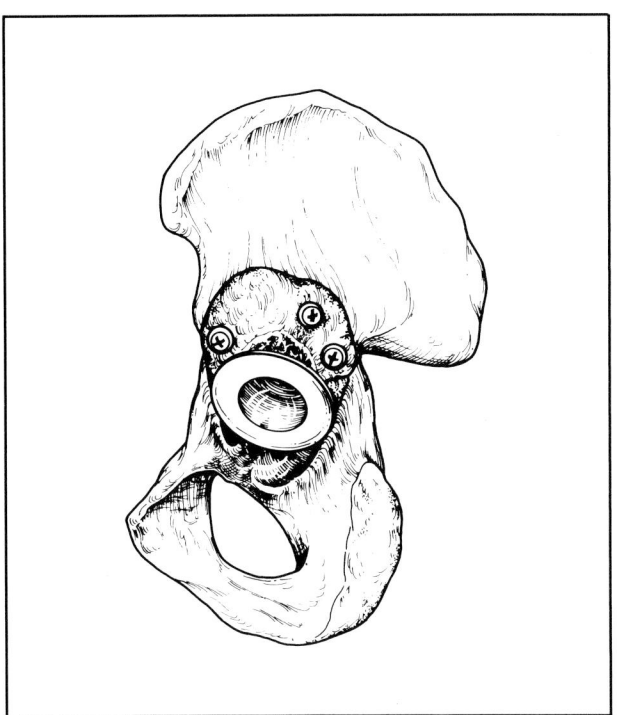

Figure 5-9J. The acetabular component should be well contained within the graft once the rim is reconstructed.

firmly curetted to create fresh surfaces (Figure 5-9B). If an allograft is used, it must be shaped with a reciprocating saw, or a high speed burr to maximize surface contact.

All major cysts are curetted and filled with morsellized bone that can be obtained from the femoral head in the region of the neck, from acetabular reamings or from the iliac crest. The head is then placed in the false acetabulum and is oriented in the position that provides the most congruous and stable fit. It is temporarily fixed using two or three #3/32 smooth K-wires (Figure 5-9C). An attempt should be made to place these wires inferiorly in the area that will eventually be reamed so that the superior portion of the graft will be available for insertion of cancellous bone screws. Great care should be taken to avoid directing wires, drills or screws toward the sciatic nerve and to avoid plunging through the inner wall of the ilium because neurovascular or urological structures within the pelvis could be damaged. Once the graft is secured by wires, drill holes are made for the appropriate screws (Figure 5-9D). A %4th drill is appropriate for the 6.5mm. Vitallium lag screws that are our preference (Howmedica, Rutherford, NJ). In determining the length of screws, a conventional depth gauge is seldom long enough. We therefore use a small K-wire with a bent tip (Figure 5-9E). The drill holes are then tapped (Figure 5-9F) and appropriate length screws are used.

It should be emphasized that the shear resistance of screws or bolts is limited and that stability of the graft must be determined solely by the superior bony buttress. The function of the screws is to hold the graft against the buttress and not to bear weight. For this reason, we now feel that lag

screws should be positioned as close to the line of the weight-bearing axis as possible and should be roughly parallel to one another. If there are any cancellous threads in the graft, the holes in the graft should be overdrilled to allow impaction of the graft against its bony buttress with weight bearing.

Although some authors have felt that bolts offer superior fixation to screws alone,[2] we feel that screws are more than adequate. If bolts are used, intrapelvic dissection is necessary in order to mount the nuts. If the obturator vessels are damaged, the resultant intrapelvic hemorrhage is extremely difficult to control. Because of the difficulty of attaching the nuts, the surgeon might also be tempted to use fewer bolts than would be ideal. Since the use of screws is relatively simple, we do not hesitate to use additional screws if required for stability.

Once the screws have been tightened securely, the K-wires are removed. It is usually necessary to remove excessive bone in the area of the new acetabulum, first using an oscillating saw. Initial shaping is done with a high-speed burr (Figure 5-9G) and then acetabular reamers are used for the final preparation of the acetabulum (Figure 5-9H). The reamer should be spinning prior to contact with the graft and initial pressure should be light to avoid undue torque which might compromise graft fixation. However, we have been impressed that fixation with two or three screws will almost universally prevent any motion of the graft while it is being reamed. As with the dysplastic acetabulum that does not require bone graft, it is important to begin with small reamers initially directed medially. Once the depth of the acetabulum has been maximized, the reamer is directed in the appropriate position of abduction and flexion. Superior reaming is then completed. If there is inadequate space for two or three screws at the periphery, we do not hesitate to add one or two countersunk screws within the reamed acetabulum. These screws should also be oriented as close as possible to the weight-bearing axis. Although washers are used whenever possible with peripheral screws, countersunk screws within the reamed acetabulum are used without washers.

After the rim has been reconstructed, the acetabular component should be placed in the optimal position of abduction (40° to 45°) and flexion (30° to 35°) and ideally should be entirely covered by bone (Figures 5-9I and 5-9J). We will, however, accept 8mm. of an uncovered superior rim as long as there is complete anterior and posterior coverage.

In the early part of our series, we used cement routinely. Because of the potential for bone lysis in association with cement and the encouraging early success of porous-coated acetabular components, we no longer use bone cement for the acetabular component. In using sintered acetabular components we have accepted less than 20% contact with host bone and more than 80% contact with autograft or allograft bone. If cement is used, it is advisable to use a preliminary small bead of cement at the interface between the graft and the host bone in order to block intrusion of cement when the final cement bolus is pressurized.

Clinical Examples

Case 1

The patient seen in Figure 5-10A was 64 when she presented with hip pain secondary to hip dysplasia and degenerative arthritis. Her femoral head is in a false acetabulum. If the acetabulum were reconstructed at the level of the false acetabulum, there would not be enough anterior and posterior bone stock to contain the component. If the true acetabulum was used without a graft, more than one half of the acetabular component would be uncovered. Her femoral head was used as an autograft, utilizing the technique previously outlined (Figure 5-9). We routinely used cement in 1981 when this patient was operated on but would now use an uncemented acetabular component. Gait training began on the third postoperative day, her hospital stay was eight days and she was kept on partial weightbearing with crutches for eight weeks. Radiographs at five years and five months show slight medial migration of the washers that we have interpreted as demonstrating that the graft has revascularized and is remodeling in the most lateral area that is not stressed (Figure 5-10B and 5-10C). At follow up of six years and two months, she rates 100 on the Harris scale.

Case 2

The patient seen in Figure 5-11A was 60 when he presented in 1976 with degenerative arthritis secondary to

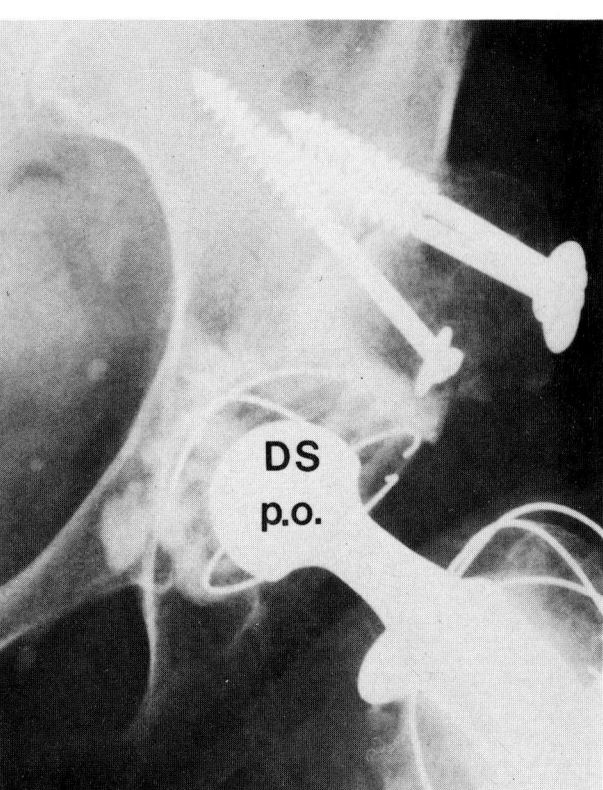

Figure 5-10B. The immediate postoperative appearance of the autograft femoral head secured in the false acetabulum. The superior rim is restored. The inferolateral portion of the graft has been trimmed away to minimize impingement of the greater trochanter.

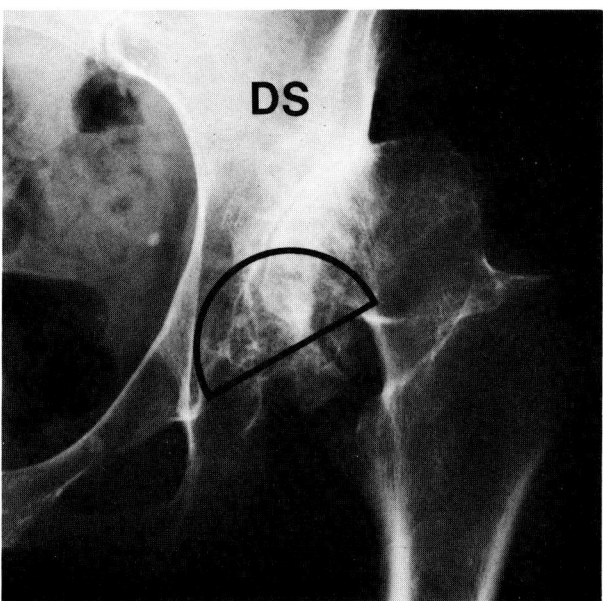

Figure 5-10A. Shenton's line is dramatically broken. If the acetabulum was reconstructed at the level of the false acetabulum, there would not be enough anterior and posterior bone stock to contain the component. If the true acetabulum was used without a graft, more than one half of the acetabular component would be uncovered.

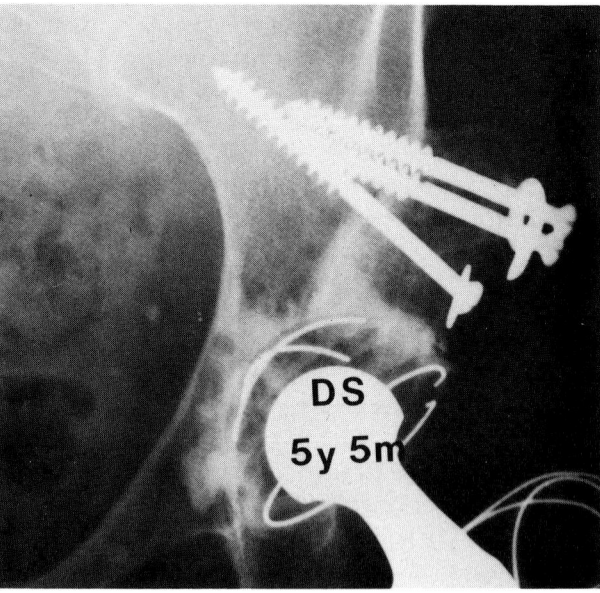

Figure 5-10C. There has been little change at five years, five months. The washers have migrated medially a bit. We have interpreted this as demonstrating revascularization of the graft and remodeling of the bone at the unstressed periphery. There may be a radiolucent line starting to form inferiorly in the area where the acetabular component contacts the ungrafted bone but there is none in the area of the graft. The patient rates 100, six years after her procedure.

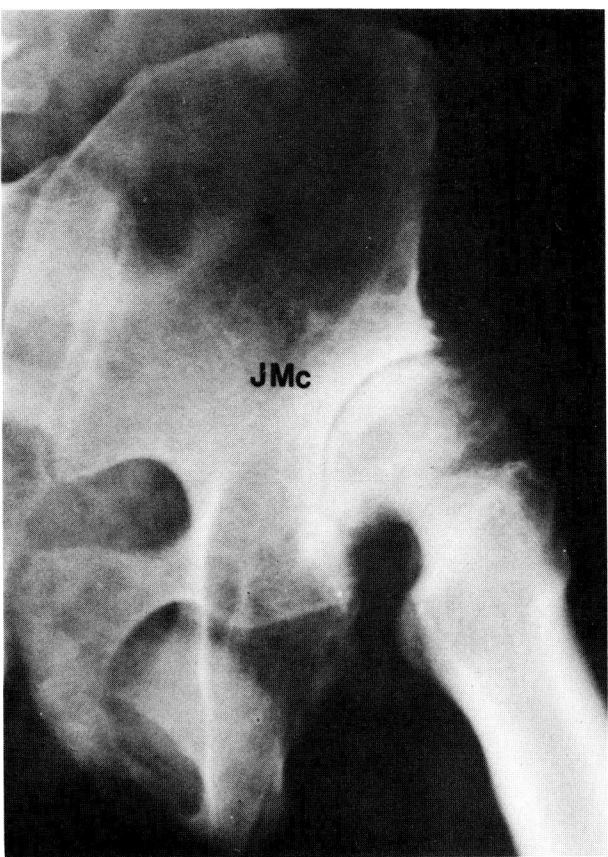

Figure 5-11A. Degenerative arthritis in a 60 year old man with congenital dysplasia. The head is in a false acetabulum.

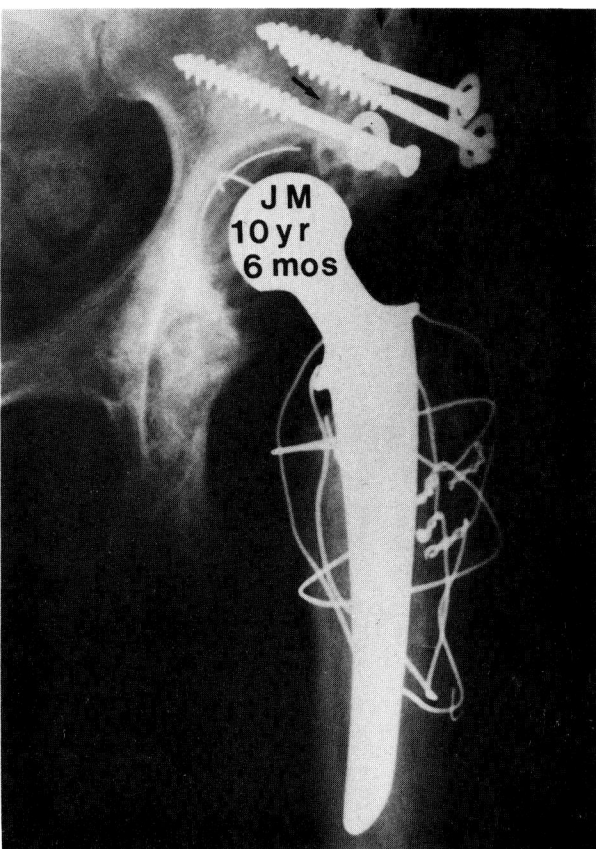

Figure 5-11B. The femoral head was used as an autograft and at ten and one half years the graft continues to appear sound (outlined by arrows). The washers have moved medially. Note the absence of radiolucent lines. The patient rates 92.

congenital dysplasia. His femoral head is almost entirely in a false acetabulum. Autograft reconstruction of the superior rim was carried out using his femoral head. Cement was used. Ten and a half years since his surgery, he now rates 92 on the Harris scale. His graft continues to look sound by x-ray. The washers have moved medially. The bone-cement interface remains benign (Figure 5-11B).

Case 3

The patient seen in Figure 5-12A was 62 when he presented with pain secondary to degenerative arthritis. The femoral head had subluxed laterally and had eroded the superior rim of the acetabulum. Preoperative templating suggested that a portion of the acetabular component would remain uncovered if a graft was not used (Figure 5-12A). Although this case is borderline and perhaps could have been done without a graft, the patient's femoral head was used as an autograft in conjunction with an uncemented PCA acetabular component (Howmedica, Rutherford, NJ). The acetabular component has contact with viable bone over two thirds of its surface (Figure 5-12B). Because the need for only a small graft was anticipated, the direct lateral approach was used. The hospital stay was eight days and the patient was protected with crutches for seven weeks. Followup is short at two years, five months but he rates 100 and his acetabular graft appears to have united (Figure 5-12C).

Case 4

The patient seen in Figure 5-13A was 75-years-old when he presented with a resection arthroplasty following a septic, failed Moore prosthesis (Figure 5-13A). The original organism was *Pseudomonas*. The sedimentation rate had been normal and the patient demonstrated no signs of infection for approximately one year at the time of reconstruction. A femoral head and neck allograft obtained from a formal harvest was used in a manner similar to that described for the autografts except that the head required more extensive preparation to be congruent with the acetabular defect (Figure 5-13B). Autogenous bone was taken from the iliac crest and from acetabular reamings. Tobramycin impregnated cement was used. He was protected for eight weeks with axillary crutches, and then used a cane for outside walking for balance purposes only. There was no evidence of residual infection at the time of his death from unrelated causes four years, eight months since his operations. He rated 92 on the Harris scale. At his last radiograph at three years, one month, his graft continued to appear satisfactory by x-ray. The washers had migrated medially (Figure 5-13C).

Superior and Posterior Rim Defects (Figure 5-14). Combined superior and posterior rim defects occur

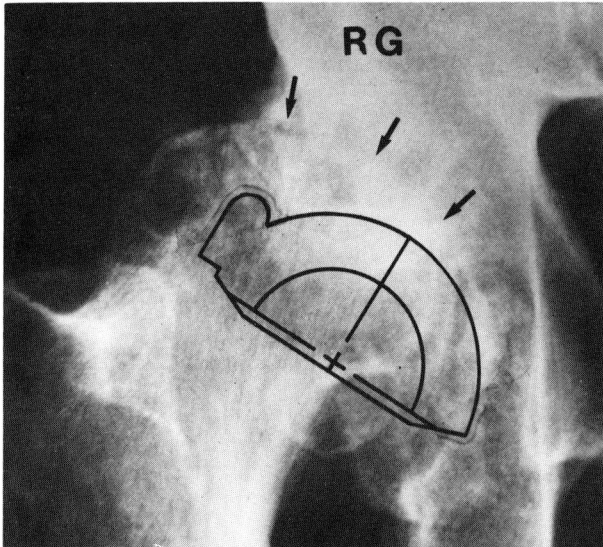

Figure 5-12A. This 62 year old man presented with pain secondary to degenerative arthritis. Preoperative templating suggests deficiency of the superior rim if the true acetabulum was used. This case is borderline and perhaps could have been done without a graft.

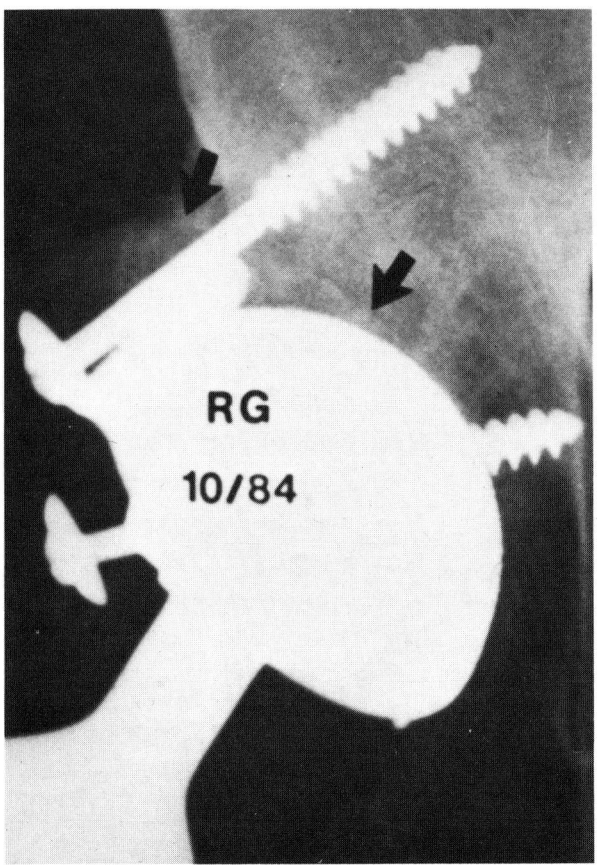

Figure 5-12B. The femoral head autograft is secured by two screws. One is superior and anterior and the other is posterior to the acetabular component. Ideally, the inferior screw should have been oriented in the axis of weightbearing. Two thirds of the surface of this uncemented component contacts living host bone and one third rests on allograft.

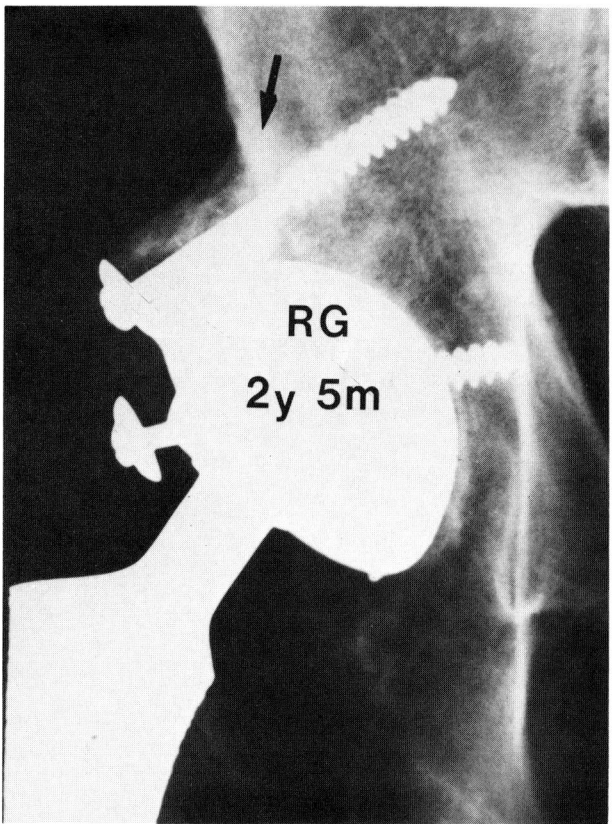

Figure 5-12C. At two years, five months the graft appears to have united. The patient rates 100.

much less frequently than do simple superior rim defects. In our series, only two patients had an isolated combination of a superior and posterior rim defects (2.6%). However, superior and posterior rim defects, in combination with other acetabular defects, occurred in twelve other patients (16%).

This defect almost always is the results from failed previous surgery. It may rarely be seen in congenital dislocation or with significant dysplasia.

Review of Literature. It has long been suspected that the forces on the posterior rim are excessive with such activities as getting out of a low chair or climbing stairs. This has been verified by recent studies by Harris and Hodge using an instrumented prosthesis.[7] Harris and Gerber have shown that acetabular prosthesis breakout is likely to occur if the posterior rim is left deficient.[8] Other authors have described methods of using autograft or allograft femoral heads and screws to reconstruct the posterior rim in a similar fashion to their reconstruction of the superior rim.[4,10] Borden has used femoral heads to reconstruct the posterior rim and has secured these grafts with contoured acetabular reconstruction plates extending from the ischium to the ilium.[9]

Author's Preferred Treatment. The posterior approach can be used for grafting isolated superoposterior rim problems in many cases. However, we prefer the greater access afforded by one of the transtrochanteric approaches.

In the first of the two patients in our series, we used an autograft which included the femoral head and neck. In the

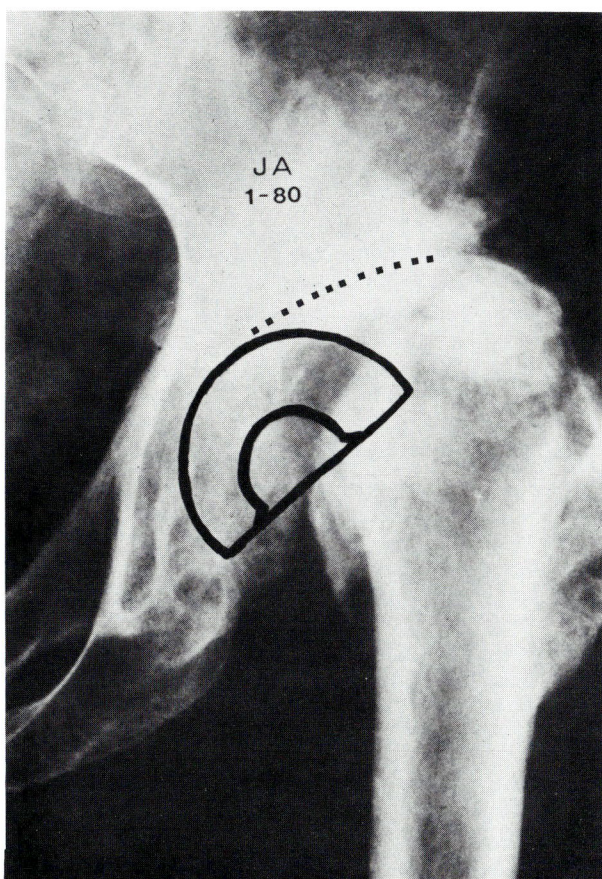

Figure 5-13A. This 75 year old man had a resection arthroplasty following a pseudomonas infection associated with a Moore prosthesis. A preoperative template shows how much of the acetabular component would have been uncovered if a graft had not been used.

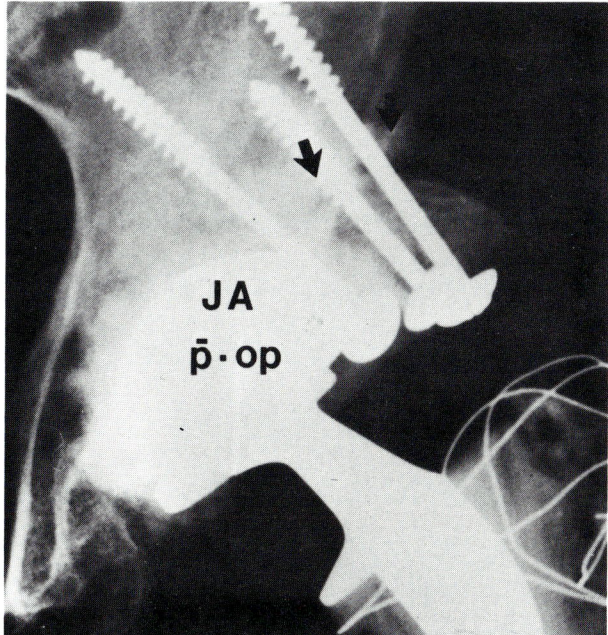

Figure 5-13B. The immediate postoperative x-ray shows a peripheral gap between the allograft and the patient's false acetabulum. There is morsellized autograft within this gap.

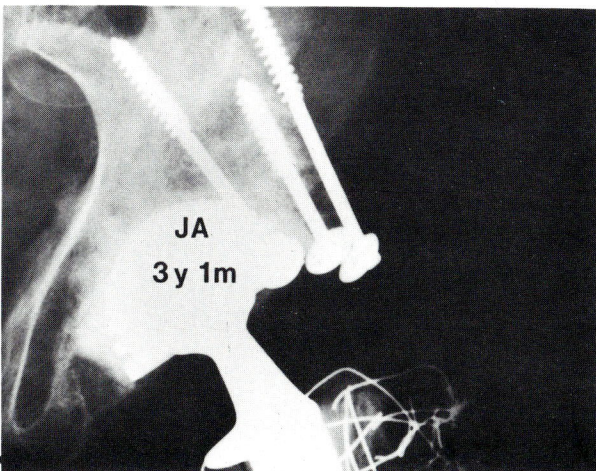

Figure 5-13C. The graft appears to be doing well at three years, one month. The peripheral gap has filled. There are no radiolucent lines between the cement and the graft. A faint line may be forming inferiorly where the cement is in contact with the patient's bone. The patient rated 92 and used a cane only for balance.

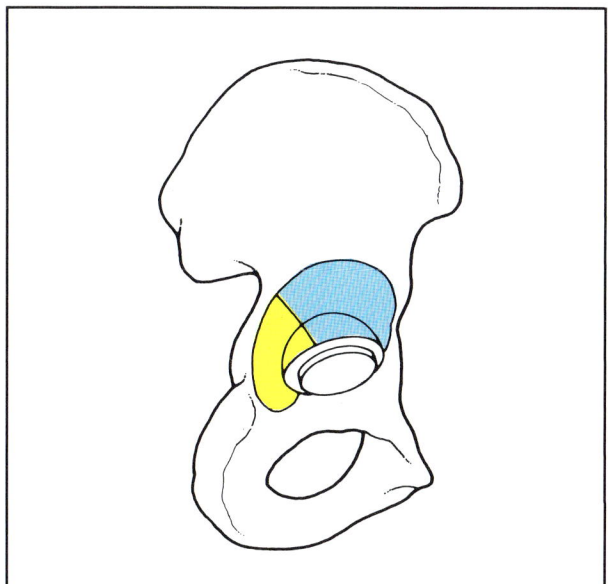

Figure 5-14. Superior and Posterior Rim Defects.

second case, the head, neck and intertrochanteric area of an allograft femur were all used. The techniques for graft and host preparation and graft fixation are as described in the previous section. Although we have not used Borden's technique of acetabular reconstruction plates,[9] this method would seem to be very appropriate if the graft was not secure by screws alone or if there was a true posterior column defect.

Clinical Examples

Case 1

The patient seen in Figure 5-15A was 52 when he presented in 1979 with a resection arthroplasty one year follow-

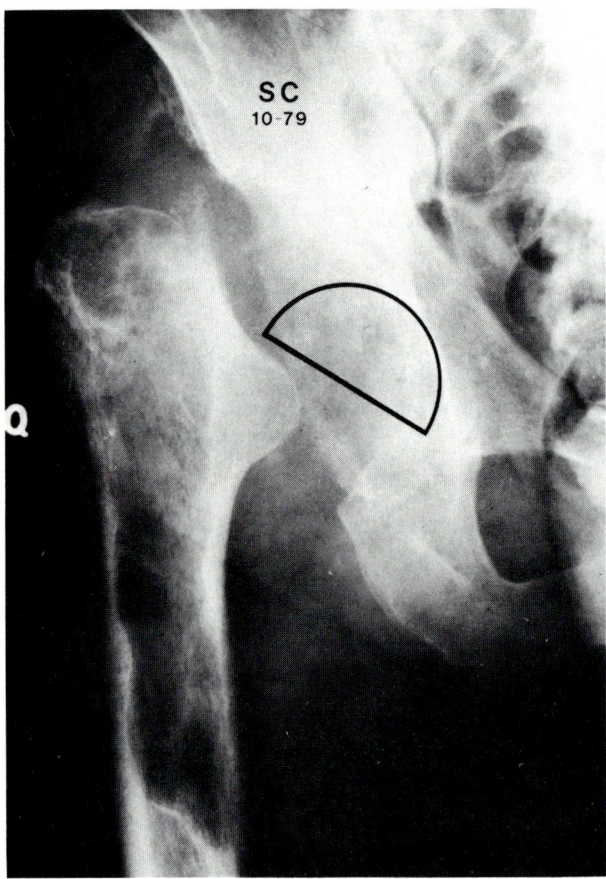

Figure 5-15A. This 52 year old man had a resection arthroplasty following hip sepsis with a hematogenous beta streptococcus. One year after a resection arthroplasty, there is deficiency of the superior and posterior rim.

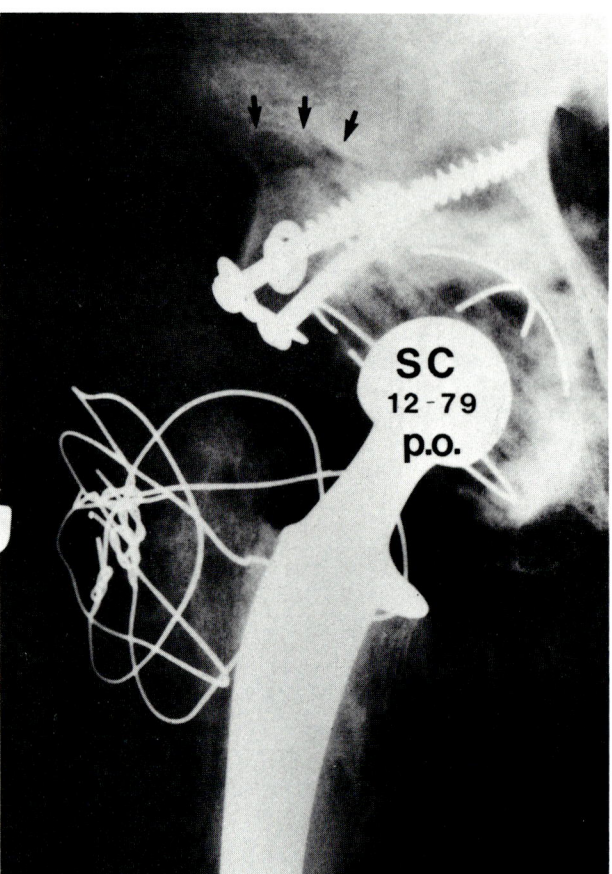

Figure 5-15C. Immediate postoperative appearance of the superior and posterior rim reconstruction. The gap at the periphery of the allograft was packed with morsellized autogenous bone.

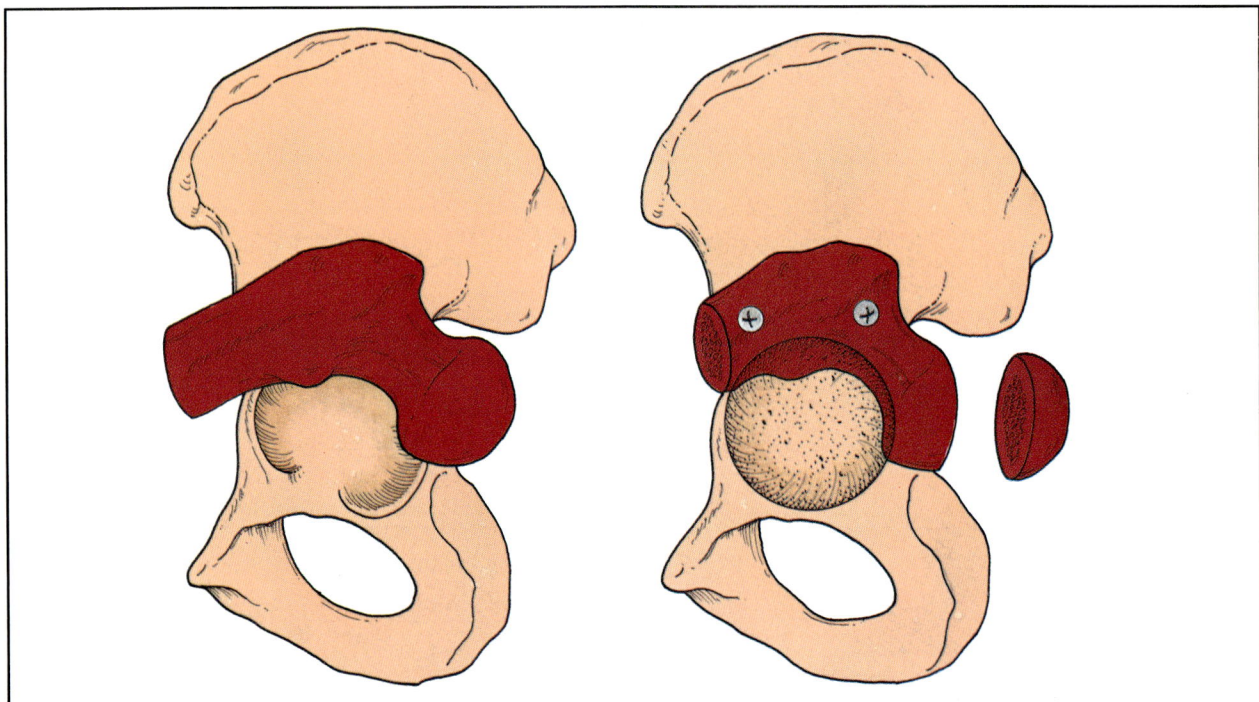

Figure 5-15B. A proximal femur including the head, neck, and intertrochanteric area provided superior and posterior coverage.

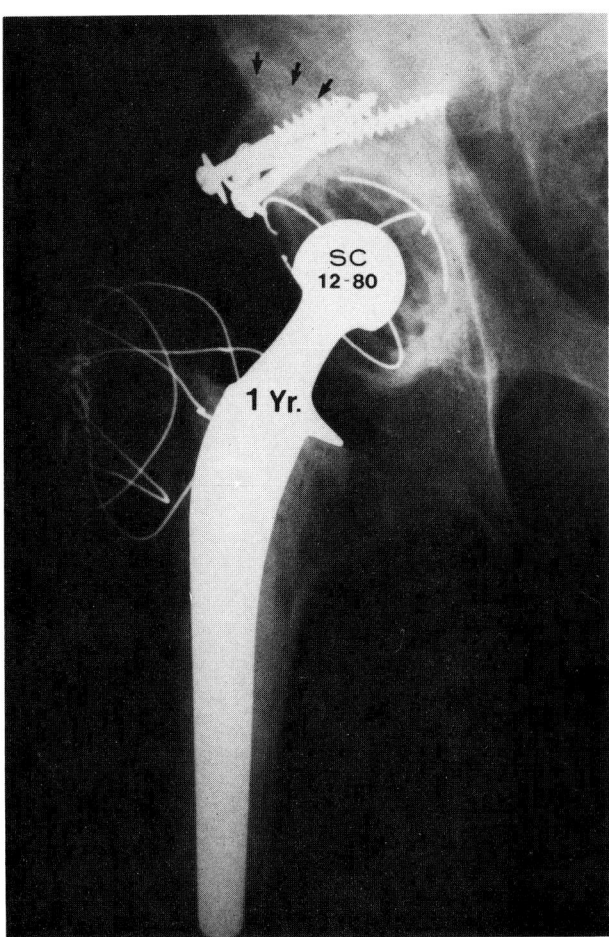

Figure 5-15D. The peripheral gap has filled in by one year.

ing hip sepsis. The organism was a beta-hemolytic streptococcus.

At the time of revision, the sedimentation rate was normal and there was no sign of infection. A proximal femur, including the head, neck and intertrochanteric area, was obtained from a formal harvest and provided superior and posterior coverage (Figures 5-15B and 5-15C). The graft was contoured with a high-speed burr to fit the false acetabulum and fixation was achieved by means of the methods previously described. Tobramycin impregnated cement was used. The hospital stay was eight days and the patient was protected with crutches for eight weeks. At one year, the peripheral gap between the graft and the acetabulum had filled in (Figure 5-15D). Seven and a half years since his surgery, he now works as a farmer and rates 100. His most recent x-rays (Figure 5-15E) look very satisfactory despite transverse orientation of the screws.

Case 2

The patient seen in Figure 5-16A was 54 when she presented with arthritis secondary to a dysplastic hip. Although her preoperative x-ray suggested only a superior rim defect, there was a surprisingly large deficiency of the posterior rim as well. Her femoral head and neck were used to reconstruct the superior and the posterior rim (Figure 5-16B). No morsellized bone was used at the autograft-host interface and this was radiographically evident at four

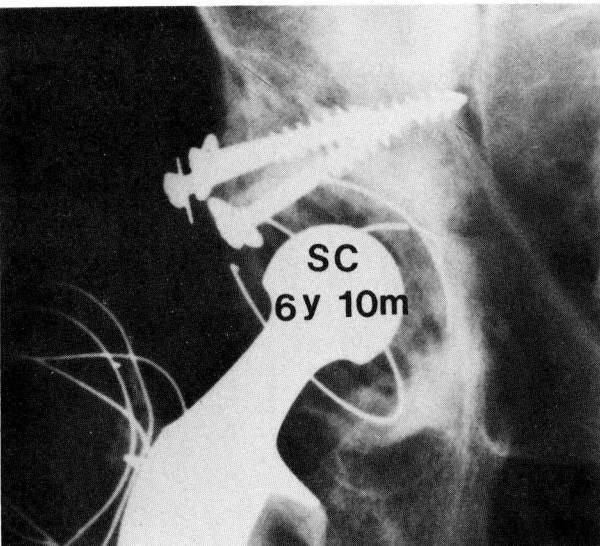

Figure 5-15E. X-rays taken at six years, ten months show that the interface is no longer visible. The component remains stable and no radiolucent lines are present. The washers have migrated medially. Ideally, the screws should have been oriented more closely to the weight-bearing axis. At seven and one half years, the patient rates 100 and works as a farmer.

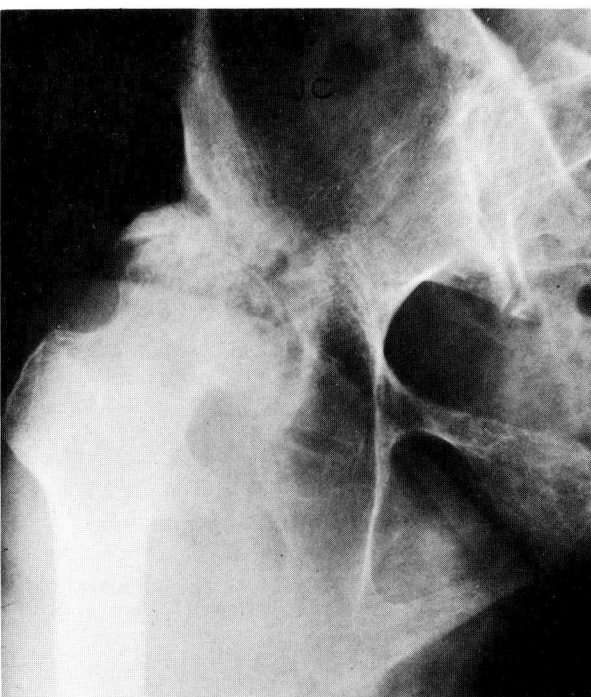

Figure 5-16A. This 54 year old woman had degenerative arthritis secondary to congenital dysplasia. This preoperative x-ray shows the head in a false acetabulum. The superior rim would be deficient if the true acetabulum was used without a graft. The posterior rim was more deficient than would seem apparent from this x-ray.

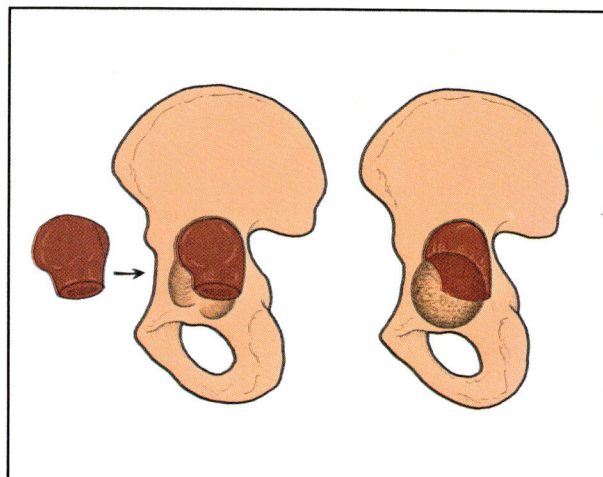

Figure 5-16B. The patient's femoral head and neck were used to reconstruct the superior and posterior rim.

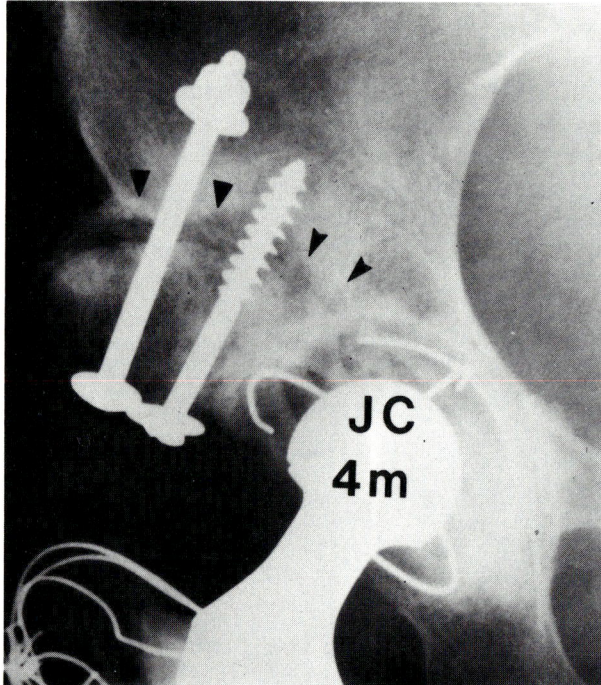

Figure 5-16C. Four months postoperatively, the autograft-host interface is evident. Unfortunately morsellized bone was not used to fill the gap. We would now use a second screw rather than the bolt.

months (Figure 5-16C). She is now eight years and eleven months since her surgery and rates 98 on the Harris scale. Her only disappointment is the fact that as a result of an asymptomatic but completely dislocated contralateral hip, the operated side is long by comparison. Her graft appears satisfactory on her most recent x-ray (Figure 5-16D).

Intra-acetabular Defects (Figure 5-17)

Isolated intra-acetabular defects are rare. They are usually associated with other defects of the rim or the medial wall. In our series we had only three patients (4%) with pure intra-acetabular defects. However, in the whole series, there were 19 additional patients who had intra-acetabular defects in association with other acetabular defects, making a total of 22 patients (29%) who had significant intra-acetabular deficiency

Intra-acetabular defects are almost always secondary to failed cemented hip replacements. The most common cause of small intra-acetabular defects is lysis about a cement keying hole. Large intra-acetabular defects usually result from superior migration of a loose cemented acetabular component with associated bone lysis.

Review of Literature. Reports in the literature concerning intra-acetabular grafts are sparse but Tranck as well as Harris and Jasty have used femoral heads; Scott and Murray have advocated the use of morsellized bone in conjunction with bipolar prosthesis for treatment of this defect.[11-14]

Authors' Preferred Treatment. The direct lateral approach is adequate for small intra-acetabular defects, but we prefer one of the transtrochanteric approaches for large defects.

Small intra-acetabular defects, with an otherwise intact superior intra-acetabular surface, can be filled with morsellized bone, used in conjunction with an uncemented acetabular component. Large defects, with inadequate bone to stabilize an acetabular component, require a solid graft contoured to fit the defect.

Significant superior intra-acetabular migration in the presence of an intact rim, tempts one to accept the proximal

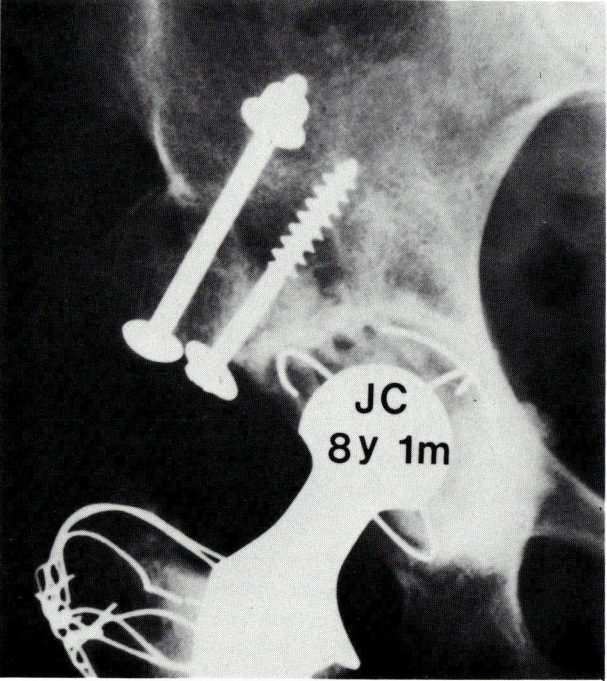

Figure 5-16D. At eight years, one month, the gap between the graft and the false acetabulum has filled in. There is no radiolucency. The patient rates 98.

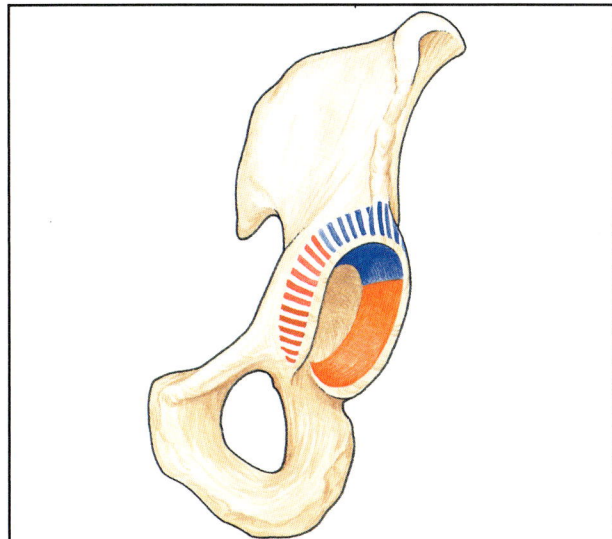

Figure 5-17. Intra-acetabular defects.

position of the acetabulum for component support; however, this situation creates two problems. First, the center of rotation moves proximally and the abductors become lax as their origins and insertions move closer. This problem can be resolved by distal trochanteric transplantation and/or by use of a longer femoral neck. However, the second problem, which is impingement of the femoral component on the anterior or posterior rim can cause dislocation. Minor impingement can be corrected by resection of the rim but with significant proximal migration, it may be necessary to resect a significant portion of the anterior or posterior columns to prevent impingement. Modest proximal migration of the acetabular roof can be managed by a protrusio-type of acetabular component such as the PCA (Howmedica, Rutherford, NJ), but major proximal migration is better treated by a solid graft placed against a thin layer of morsellized bone so that the center of rotation of the hip can be brought inferiorly. The solid bone graft is held in place with screws at the periphery of the reamed acetabulum or by countersunk screws within the acetabulum.

Clinical Examples

Case 1

The patient whose preoperative x-ray is seen in Figure 5-18A, was 69-years-old when he presented with a loose surface replacement acetabular component. At the time of surgery, in addition to a significant superior intra-acetabular defect that was apparent on the preoperative AP x-ray, he was found to have a very large ischial defect that was more than 3cm. in diameter. The ischial defect was grafted with a separate, smaller femoral head. This head and the defect were reamed with corresponding female and male cup arthroplasty reamers. Morsellized autograft and allograft bone was used to graft the small defects of the dome, and then a large femoral head was used to bring the center of

rotation inferiorly (Figures 5-18B and 5-18C). The basic technique of holding these grafts was similar to that described before except for the fact that they were temporarily held with transverse smooth K-wires through the rim while the definitive screws were inserted from below. At the time of this patient's operation (1984), we elected to cement the acetabular component because there was minimal contact of the porous surface with living bone (Figure 5-18D). We would now use an uncemented component with screws. The femoral component is uncemented.

This man is now three years, four months since surgery. His graft appeared to be doing well at three and a half years (Figure 5-18E). He plays tennis three hours a day, seven days a week (against advice) and rates 96.

Case 2

The patient whose x-rays are seen in Figure 5-19A is a 51-year-old hospital maintenance worker who had a failed surface replacement prosthesis.

The rim of the acetabulum was entirely intact. If the proximal position of the acetabular dome had been accepted for the new component, it would have been necessary to trim away so much anterior bone to provide clearance for the femoral component that an anterior column defect might have been created (Figure 5-19B). Morsellized autograft from the femoral head and from the iliac crest was mixed with morsellized cancellous allograft and was firmly impacted into the superior defect. An allograft medial femoral condyle was used to provide a massive solid graft that was large enough to fill the anterior, superior and posterior intra-acetabular defect when inserted transversely (Figure 5-19C). This graft was also impacted against the

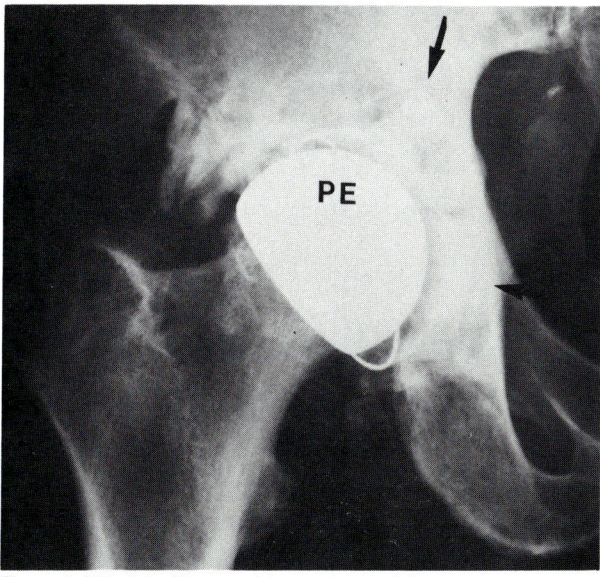

Figure 5-18A. This 69 year old man had a failed surface replacement. The immediate pre-revision x-rays have been lost but this x-ray taken one year previously shows a significant superior intra-acetabular defect as well as a posterior (ischial) defect. The rim was intact as was the medial wall.

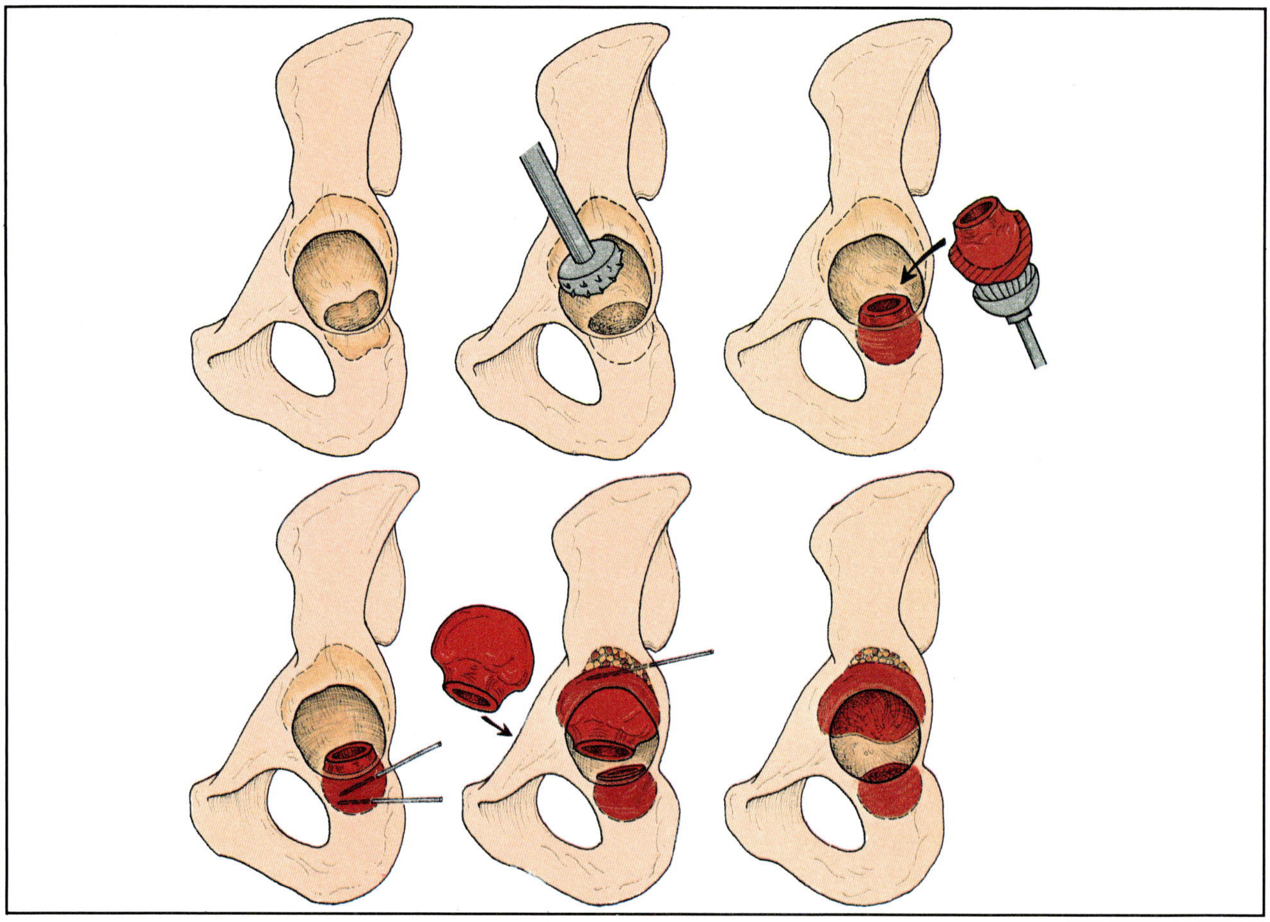

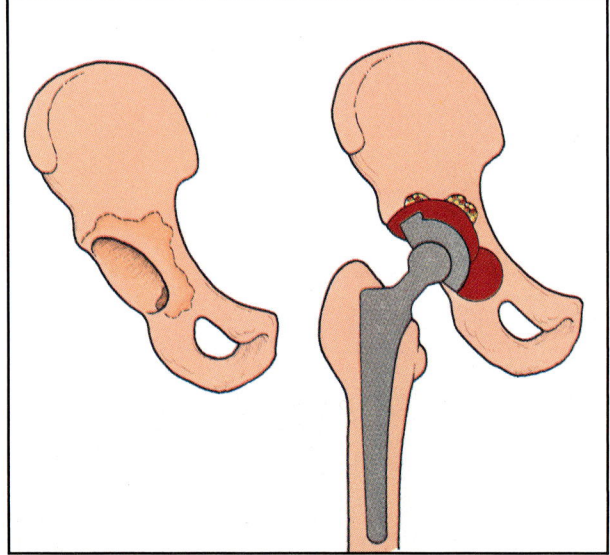

Figure 5-18B. The ischial intra-acetabular defect was filled with a small femoral head. Small irregularities in the superior intra-acetabular defect were filled with morsellized bone and the major defect was reconstructed by means of a large femoral head.

Figure 5-18C. The tracing on the left demonstrates the defect that was evident on the AP x-ray view. The ischial defect was filled with a small femoral head. The small superior intra-acetabular defects were reconstructed with morsellized bone and a separate larger head was used for the major superior defect.

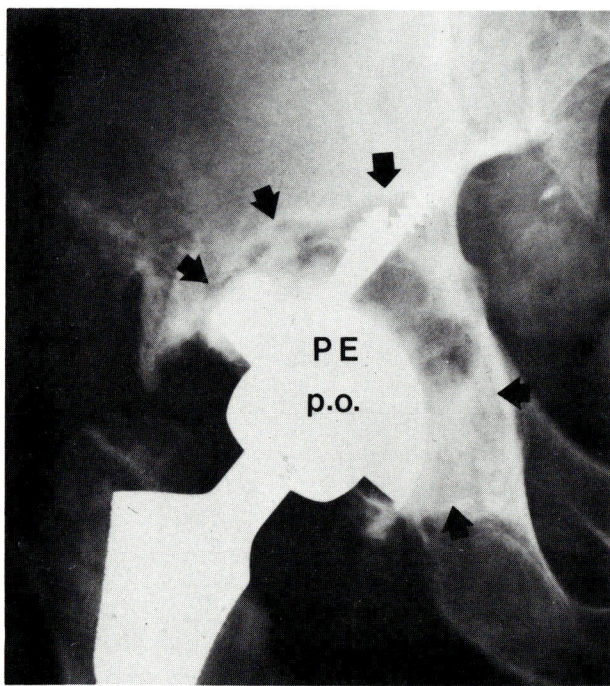

Figure 5-18D. The superior intra-acetabular defect is outlined by the arrows. The two inferior arrows show the periphery of the small femoral head in the ischial defect.

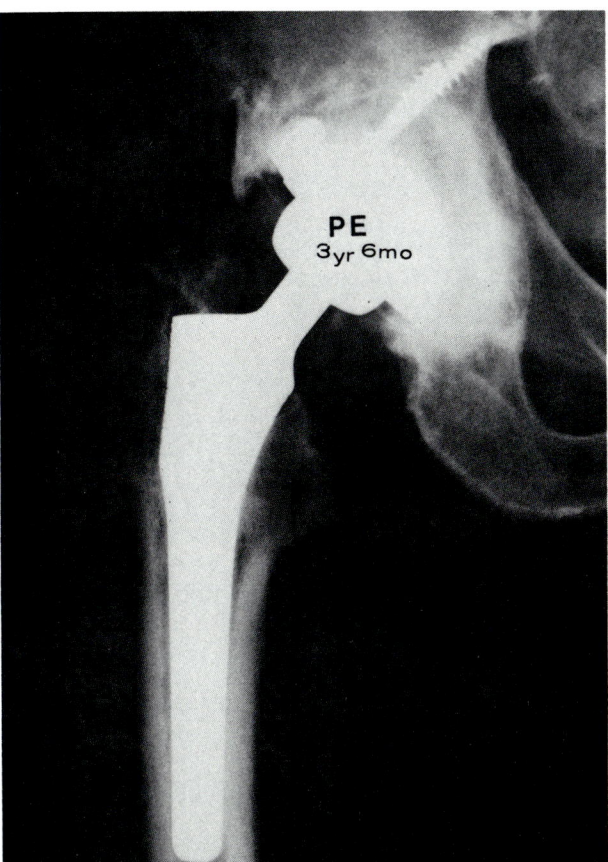

Figure 5-18E. At three and one half years, the morsellized bone between the superior femoral head, graft and the intra-acetabular defect appears to have incorporated. The patient plays tennis three hours every day and rates 96.

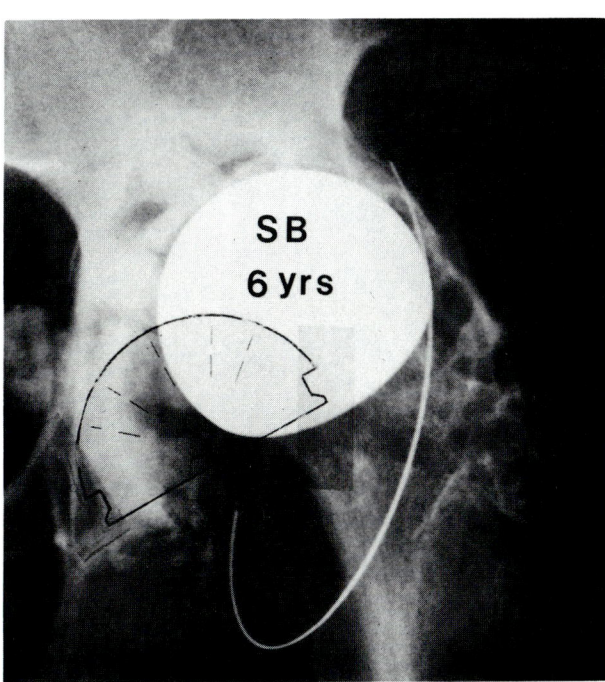

Figure 5-19A. This 51 year old man had a surface replacement arthroplasty six years previously. There were very large anterior, superior, and posterior intra-acetabular defects. The rim was intact and the medial wall had only a small perforation.

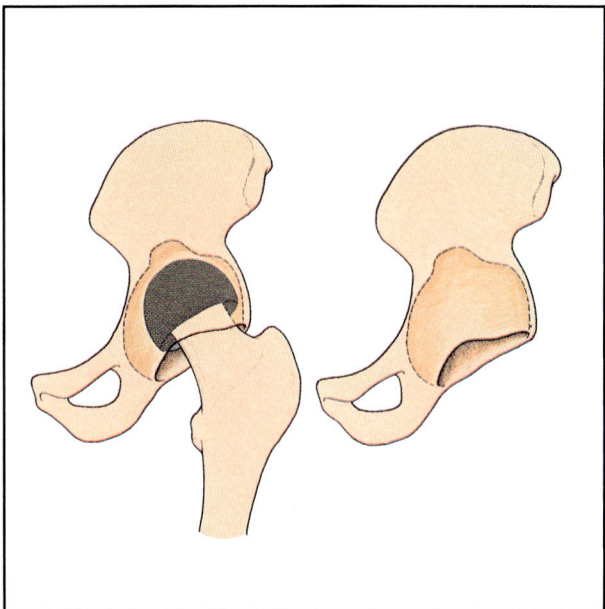

Figure 5-19B. A tracing made from the x-ray shows the significant anterior, superior, and posterior intra-acetabular defect. If the superior position of the acetabular roof was accepted, it would have been necessary to resect a significant amount of the rim.

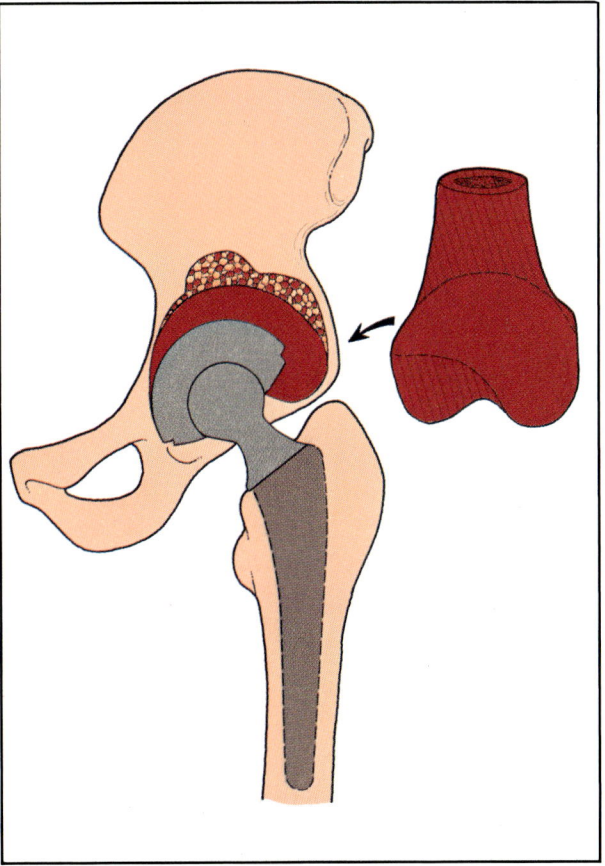

Figure 5-19C. A mixture of morsellized autograft and allograft was used to fill the irregularities of the superior and posterior intra-acetabular defect and then a graft from the distal femur was used to reconstruct the major anterior, superior, and posterior intra-acetabular defect.

morsellized bone. The graft was mechanically stable but additional fixation was provided by means of two peripheral lag screws and by means of the screws of the Harris-Galante uncemented acetabular component (Zimmer, Warsaw, IN). Although only one fifth of the acetabular component was in contact with living bone, it was used without cement. This patient is very motivated and left the hospital on the fifth postoperative day on two axillary crutches. At six weeks he began to use a cane and at nine weeks he returned to work as a maintenance worker and has walked without support since then (Figures 5-19D and 5-19E). At six months his x-rays appear satisfactory (Figure 5-19F). He has formed some heterotopic bone but at short followup of ten months rates 98.

Case 3

The patient whose x-rays are seen in Figure 5-20A was 46 when he presented with loose acetabular and femoral components. He had undergone multiple previous operations following a fracture dislocation, 18 years previously. These included three cup arthroplasties, a Moore prosthesis, and finally a total hip replacement. His femoral reconstruction will be discussed in the section on femoral grafts (Figure 5-9).

The rim was intact and the intra-acetabular defect was more modest than that seen in Case 2. Morsellized autograft bone was used medially and in the small superior intra-acetabular defects. An uncemented PCA protrusio cup (Howmedica, Rutherford, NJ) was used to move the center of rotation distally and laterally. With minimal trimming of the anterior rim, impingement was prevented (Figure

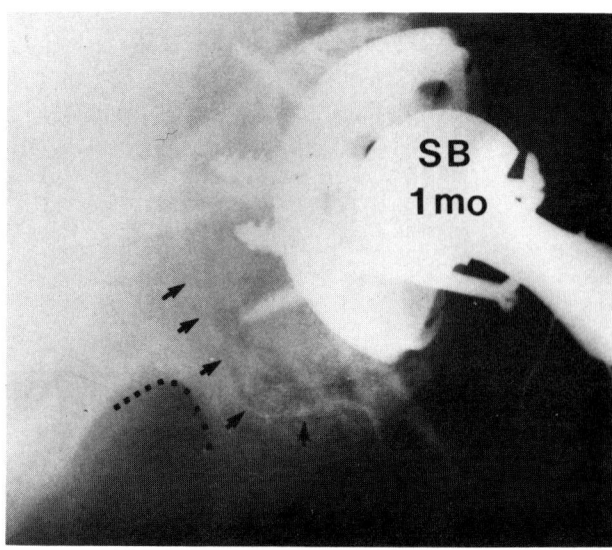

Figure 5-19E. The lateral view demonstrates the significant reconstruction of the posterior intra-acetabular defect.

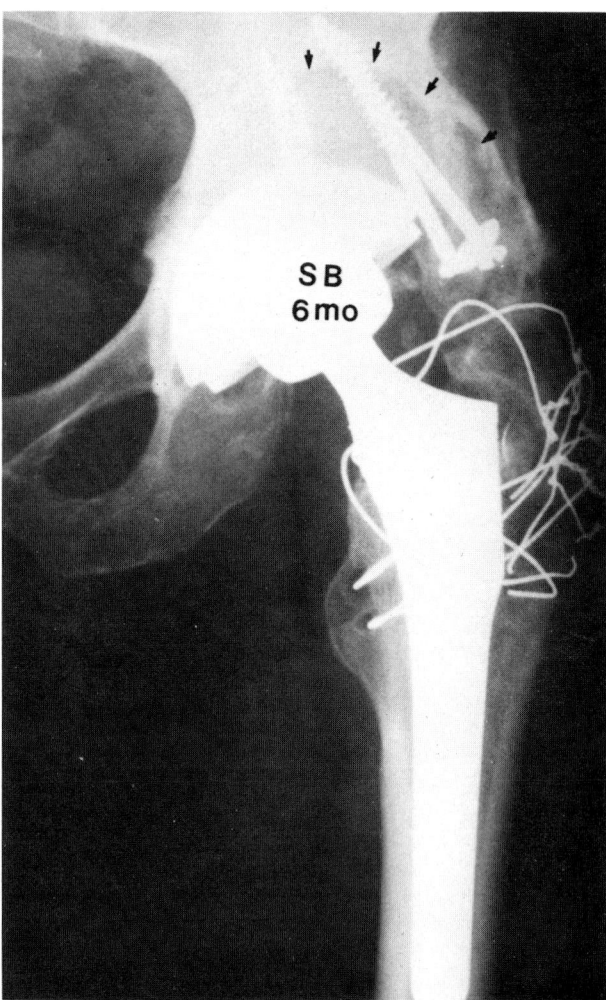

Figure 5-19F. The graft appears to be doing well at six months. The morsellized bone between the acetabular roof and the allograft distal femur appears to have incorporated. Some heterotopic bone has formed laterally and the patient only flexes 100°. Nevertheless, at short followup of ten months he rates 98.

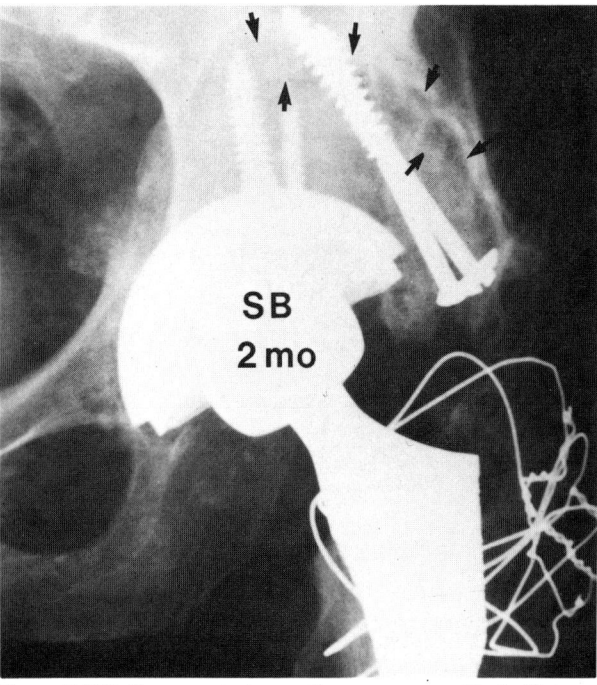

Figure 5-19D. The area between the arrows was filled with morsellized bone. A distal femur was used to reconstruct the major superior and posterior intra-acetabular defects.

5-20B). This man has returned to heavy work as an automobile mechanic and at short term followup of one and a half years rates 98 on the Harris scale. His acetabular reconstruction looks satisfactory and the small superior intra-acetabular grafts appear to have incorporated (Figure 5-20C).

Protrusio Acetabulum (Figure 5-21)

Unlike other defects, protrusio acetabulum frequently occurs as an isolated problem. In our series, five hips (6%) presented with protrusio alone but there was one other patient with the combination of protrusio and a medial wall defect to make a total of six patients (8%) with protrusio problems in our total series.

The etiology of protrusio acetabulum was congenital (Otto pelvis) in three, failed Moore prosthesis in two, and rheumatoid arthritis in one.

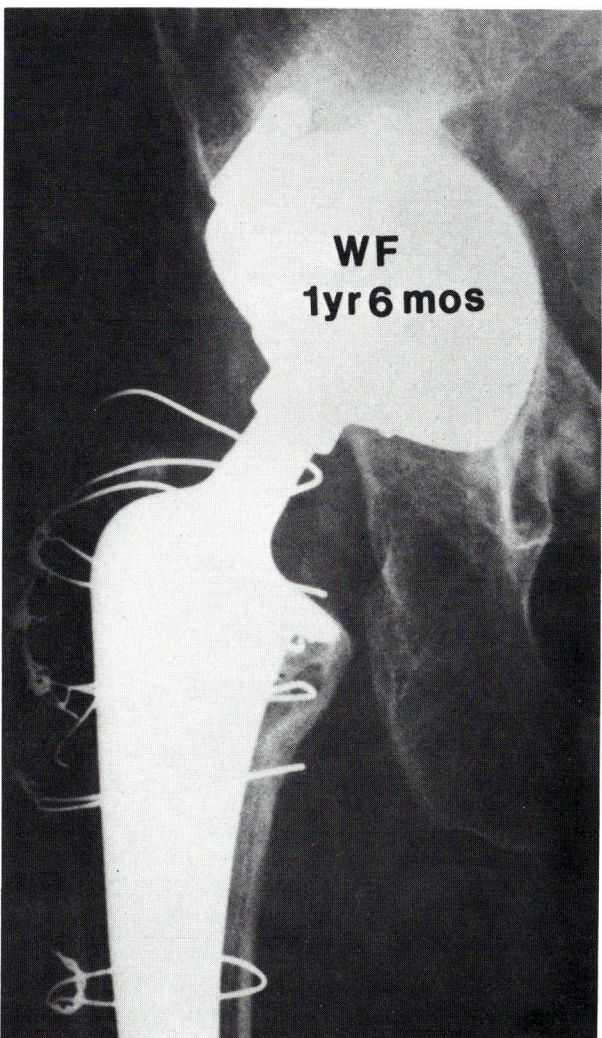

Figure 5-20C. At one and one half years, the morsellized bone appears to have incorporated. The patient works as an automobile mechanic and rates 98.

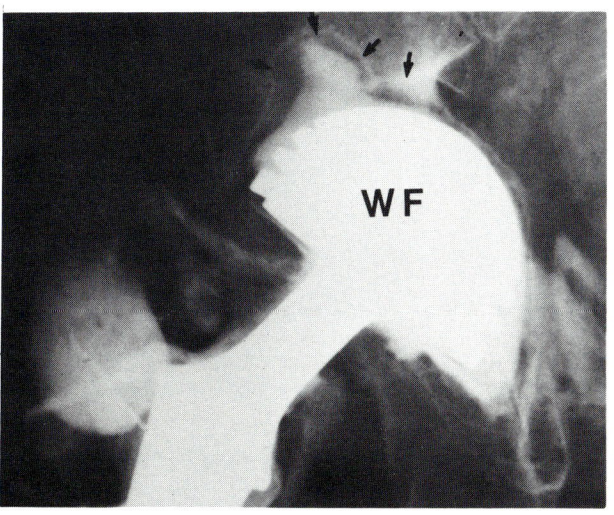

Figure 5-20A. This 49 year old man had a failed total hip replacement. The rim is intact and the superior intra-acetabular defect is more modest than in Case 1. The medial wall was thin but intact.

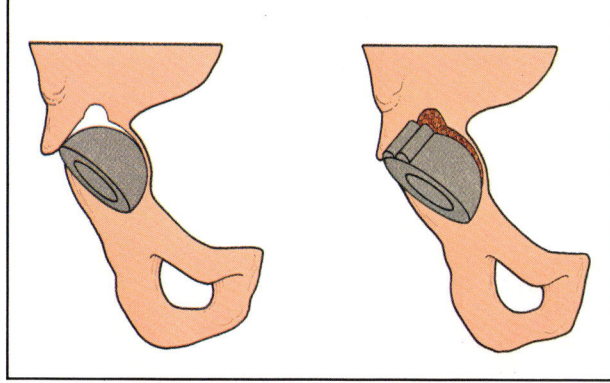

Figure 5-20B. The smaller superior intra-acetabular defects were filled with morsellized bone. Additional morsellized bone was placed medially. An uncemented PCA protrusio cup (Howmedica, Rutherford, NJ) was used to move the center of rotation more distally and laterally.

Review of Literature. Protrusio acetabulum in association with total hip replacement has been recognized as a problem for some time. In 1975, Hastings and Parker pointed out the forces involved on the medial wall and reported their experience with autogenous grafts used both with and without additional mechanical support.[15] In that same year, Salvati et al. reported on intra-pelvic protrusion of cemented acetabular components used for protusio and recommended bone grafting.[16] Ranawat et al. reported a high incidence of radiolucent lines when nonmetal backed polyethylene acetabular components were used with cement alone and recommended mesh, titanium shells or bone grafts.[17] Sotelo-Garza and Charnley reported good results with nonmetal backed polyethylene cups used with cement, but also described their experience with bone grafts in four patients.[18] In revision surgery, Bierbaum advocated leaving the old acetabular component and cement if this complex was stable and using it as a base for a new cemented acetabular prosthesis.[5] Other authors have rec-

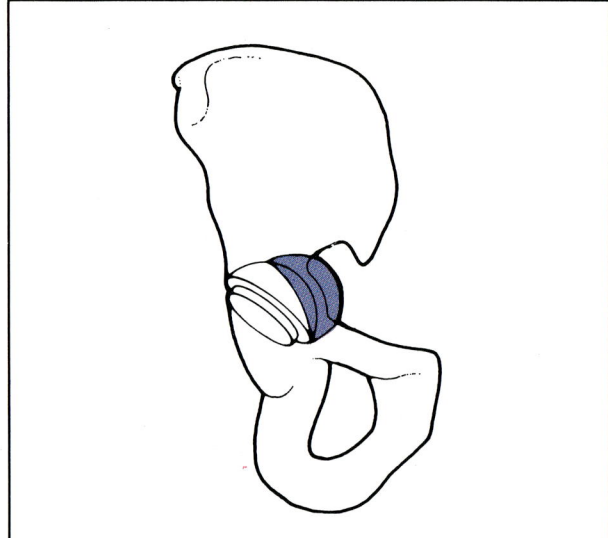

Figure 5-21. Protrusio acetabulum.

ommended the use of femoral heads alone, or femoral heads used in conjunction with protrusio rings and/or mesh.[19,22]

Author's Preferred Treatment. The direct lateral approach provides adequate exposure for isolated protrusio acetabulum defects.

We feel bone grafts in conjunction with metal-backed components provide the best solution to protrusio acetabulum in primary or revision total hip replacement. Mesh adds little strength not provided by a metal backed component. Protrusio shells do not offer any advantage in the treatment of protrusio acetabulum and in fact probably cause medial acetabular stress shielding and should not be used. Shallow protrusio defects can be managed by conventional or by protrusio style uncemented acetabular components. Larger defects can be dealt with by means of morsellized autogenous bone in conjunction with noncemented acetabular devices. Very large defects may need solid bulk grafts. Although we used cement in conjunction with solid bone grafts in the early part of our series, we now feel that cement is not necessary in the treatment of protrusio acetabulum.

Clinical Examples

Case 1

The patient seen in Figure 5-22A was 67 when she presented in 1980 with a failed Moore prosthesis. An allograft femoral head was first reamed with a female cup reamer of the same size as the outer diameter of the Moore prosthesis. The acetabulum was then curetted to remove all soft tissue. The graft was placed in the acetabulum temporarily to make sure that the fit was accurate and then was removed. The periphery of the patient's acetabulum was lightly over-reamed until the reamer was covered by the acetabular rim. Excessive bone from the inferior portion of

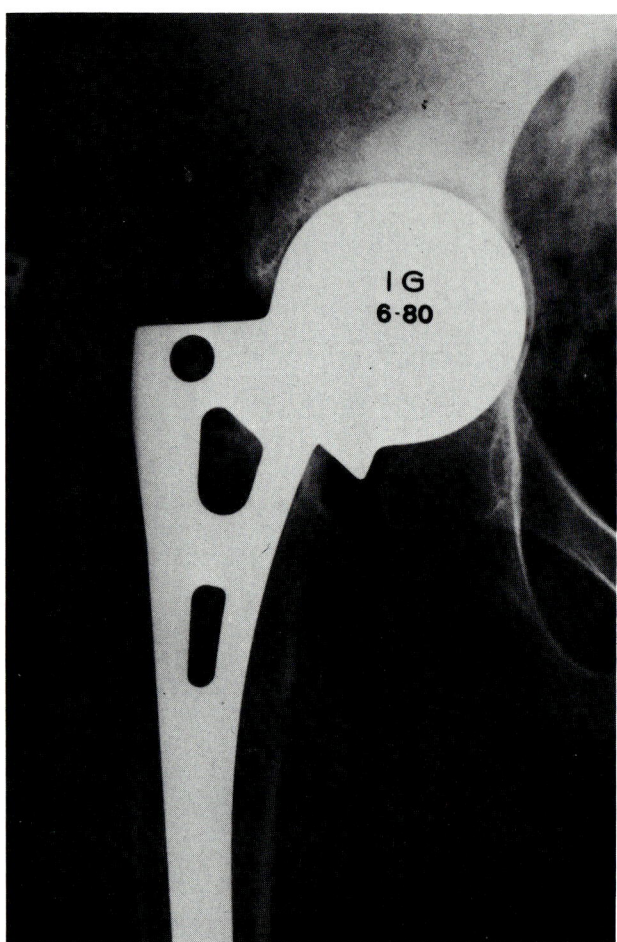

Figure 5-22A. This 67 year old female had a painful hip secondary to protrusion of a failed Moore prosthesis that was also loose in the femoral shaft.

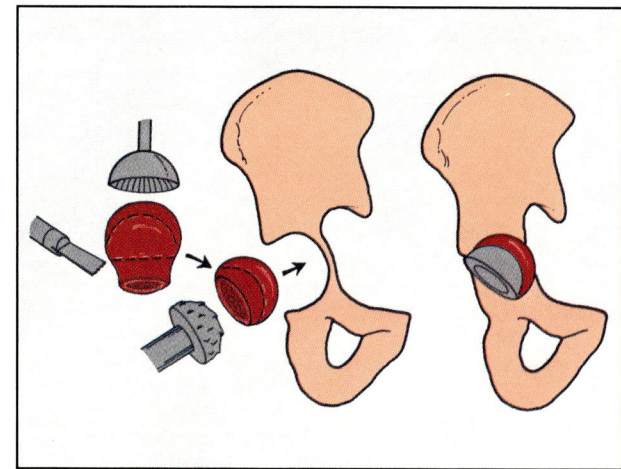

Figure 5-22B. A femoral head allograft was first reamed with a female cup reamer of the same diameter as the Moore prosthesis. The excess bone was removed with a reciprocating saw. The rim and the outer portion of the allograft were reamed with the same male reamer. The acetabulum was cleaned of soft tissues by means of a currette and the graft impacted into its depth. A bead of cement was used at the periphery of the graft to prevent intrusion of the final bolus of pressurized cement. We would now use an uncemented acetabular component.

the head and neck was removed with a reciprocating saw and then the graft was held with bone clamps and was reamed with the same reamer that had been used for the rim of the acetabulum (Figure 5-22B). The reamed allograft was then impacted into the depths of the acetabulum and a bead of cement was placed around its periphery to prevent intrusion of pressurized cement. The final cementing was done with a pressurization system. One month following surgery, the graft-host interface was clearly visible (Figure 5-22C). By 18 months, the interface between the graft and the pelvis was less evident and a radiolucent line began to form laterally (Figure 5-22D). At five years the host-graft interface has disappeared and the lateral radiolucency has extended more medially suggesting that the graft has incorporated and is now participating in the usual membrane formation associated with cement (Figure 5-22E). We would now use an uncemented acetabular component in this situation. This patient did well initially but in recent years the femoral component has shown radiological evidence of loosening and she now complains of thigh pain. At followup of seven years she rates 82.

Case 2

The patient seen in Figure 5-23A is a 59 year old woman who presented with severe rheumatoid arthritis. A femoral

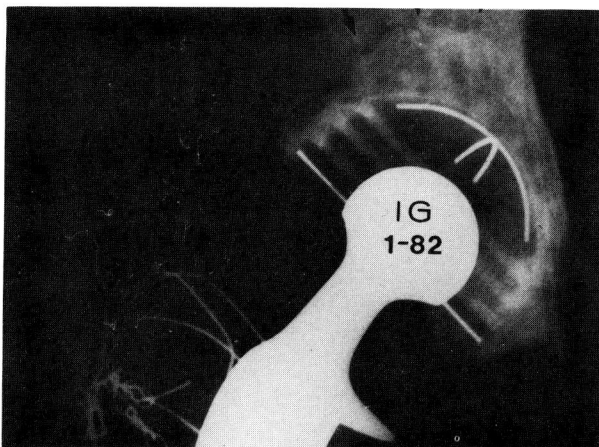

Figure 5-22D. Within 18 months of surgery, the graft-host interface has filled in considerably. A zone I radiolucency has appeared.

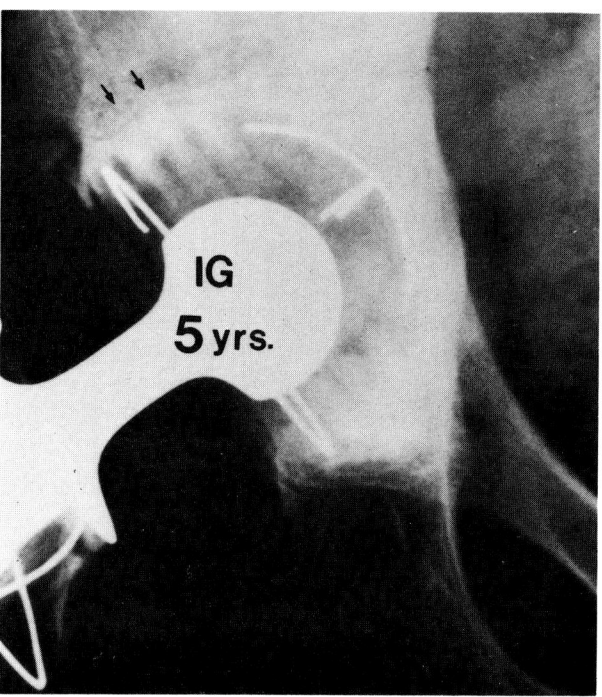

Figure 5-22E. At five years, the interface between the graft and the pelvis has disappeared and the lateral radiolucency has extended, suggesting that the graft has revascularized and is now participating in the usual membrane formation associated with cement. Although the acetabular graft seems to be doing well, the femoral component shows radiological evidence of loosening and at seven years the patient is having some thigh pain. She rates 82.

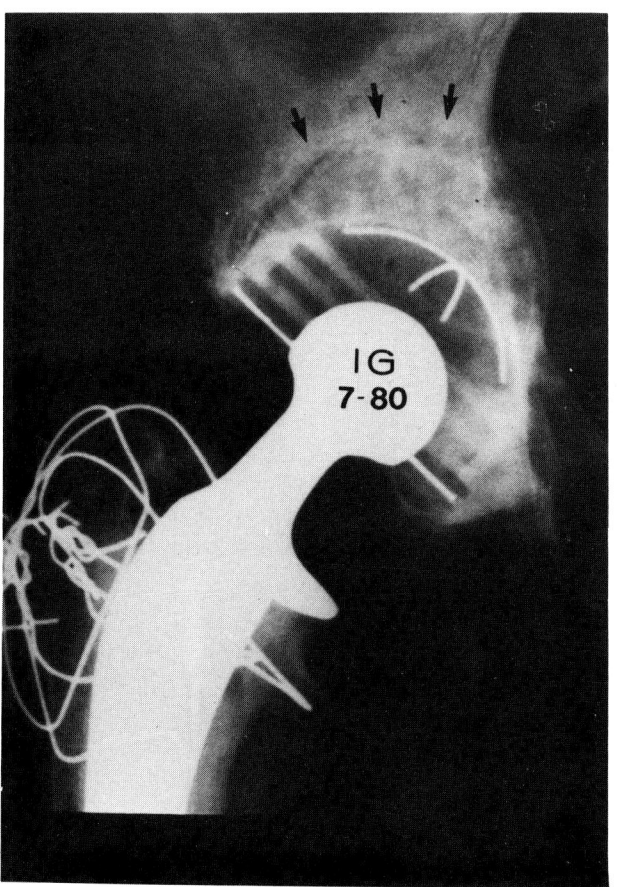

Figure 5-22C. One month following surgery the graft-host interface is clearly visible.

head autograft was used with cement using the same technique as described for Case 1 except for the fact that the femoral head was denuded of soft tissue but not reamed (Figure 5-23B). Although this patient is doing well at six and a half years and rates 92, a significant radiolucent line has developed between the cement and the graft (Figure 5-23C), suggesting that the graft has revascularized and now has entered into the usual loosening process. We now would deal with the same problem by means of an uncemented acetabular device used with morsellized bone from the patient's femoral head.

Case 3

The patient seen in Figure 5-24A is a 40-year-old woman with congenital protrusio acetabulum. Despite a relatively wide joint space following an unsuccessful cheilectomy, she had limited motion and rated 42 preoperatively on the Harris scale. An uncemented acetabular component was used with a solid autograft that was fashioned from her femoral head. Approximately 60% of the sintered surface was in contact with viable acetabular bone (Figure 5-24B).

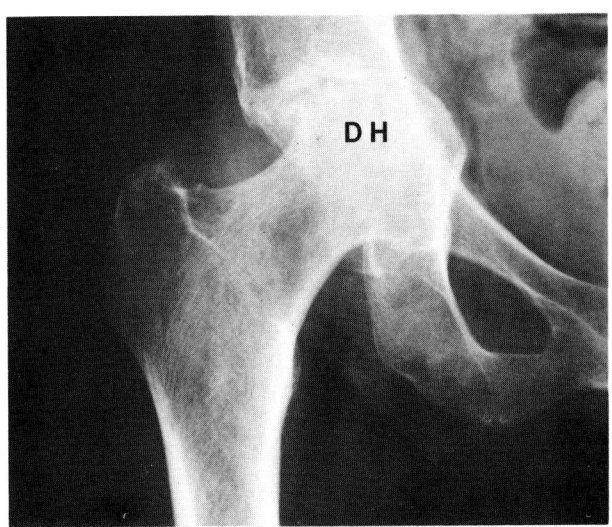

Figure 5-23A. This 59 year old woman had protrusio acetabulum secondary to rheumatoid arthritis.

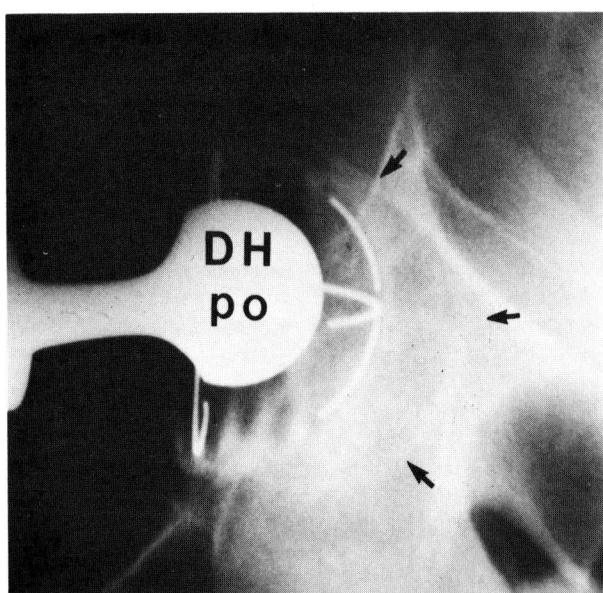

Figure 5-23B. The patient's femoral head was denuded of soft tissue and used as a solid graft. The acetabular component was cemented and immediately postoperatively, the bone cement interface looked benign.

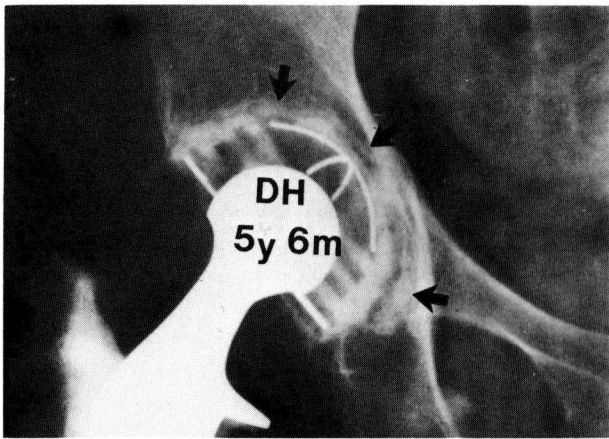

Figure 5-23C. At five and one half years, the patient rates 92 but an ominous radiolucent line has formed between the bone graft and the cement suggesting that the graft has revascularized and loosening may occur. We would now use morsellized bone from the patient's femoral head in conjunction with an uncemented acetabular component.

At short followup of two years, ten months, her graft continues to look very satisfactory (Figure 5-24C). She rates 98.

Case 4

The patient seen in Figure 5-25A was 69 when she had a right primary total hip replacement for congenital protrusio acetabulum. Morsellized autograft bone was used in conjunction with a conventional uncemented PCA component (Figure 5-25B). She is doing well at followup of two and a half years and the morsellized bone appears to have incorporated (Figure 5-25C). A protrusio-type cup without grafting probably would have proven satisfactory for such a mild defect.

Perforation of the Acetabular Medial Wall (Figure 5-26)

In our series, isolated perforations of the medial wall were rare and were seen in only two patients (2.9%). However, in combination with other defects they were quite commom and occurred in 14 additional patients. There were therefore 16 patients (23%) with perforation of the medial wall of the acetabulum.

Perforation of the medial wall most commonly results from a previous failed total hip replacement. In our series, 14 patients had medial wall perforation as a result of failed arthroplasty. Two patients had medial wall defects secondary to trauma.

Review of Literature. McCollum et al. reported their experience with cemented prostheses, used in association with solid bone grafts, Vitallium mesh and Eichler rings to deal with medial acetabular perforations.[19] Mendes et al. felt that strips of cancellous bone, covered with mesh and used with cement, provided a successful reconstruction.[23]

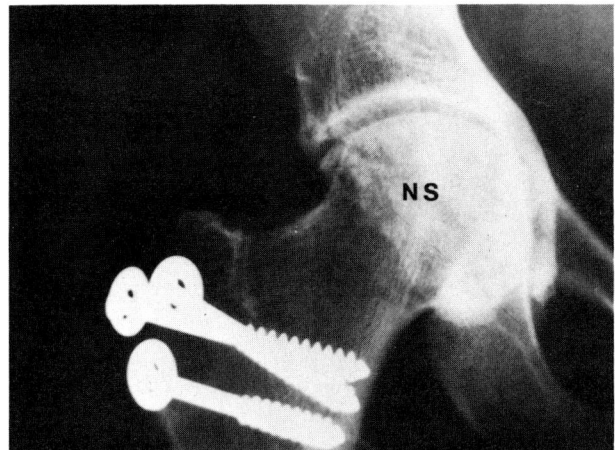

Figure 5-24A. Despite the relatively wide joint space, this 40 year old woman had pain and very limited motion. She rated 42.

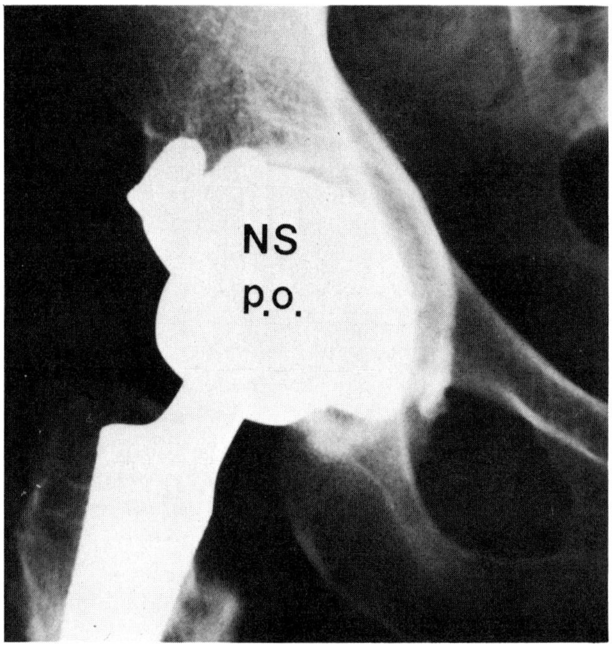

wall but when these are combined with other defects we prefer one of the transtrochanteric approaches.

Our original experience with medial wall perforations was in association with cemented total hip replacements. Because of the need to contain liquid cement, we felt that it was necessary to use solid grafts that completely occluded the defect. We have used full thickness iliac crest grafts placed intrapelvically and lagged with outside screws to occlude a perforation (Figure 5-30) but the risk of excessive bleeding has led us to abandon this technique. Hat-shaped grafts can be used within the depths of the acetabulum but may force the acetabular component laterally, requiring an additional superior rim graft for coverage (Figure 5-37). Since we now rarely use cement on the acetabular side, our preference is now to use strips of cortical and cancellous bone to fill the perforation and then to use an uncemented

Figure 5-24B. A solid autograft from the patient's femoral head was shaped to fit the defect and an uncemented PCA low profile acetabular component (Howmedica, Rutherford, NJ) was used.

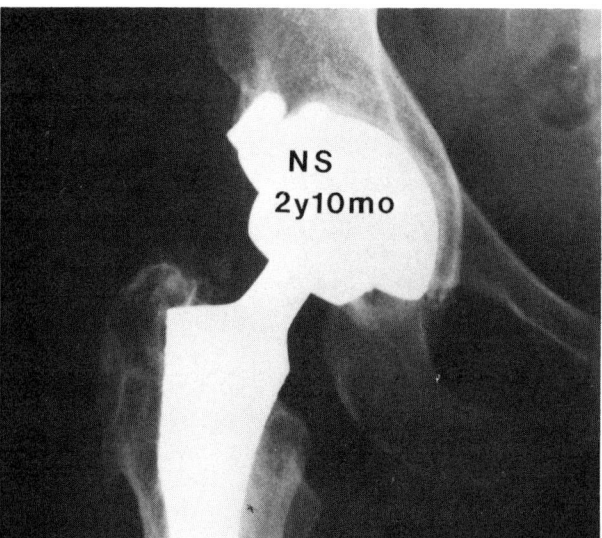

Figure 5-24C. At two years, ten months the graft-host interface is not visible and the patient rates 98. Although this graft appears to be doing well, we would now use morsellized bone to fill the defect because it is much easier technically and appears to incorporate very quickly.

Cameron has advocated cancellous strips and a Charnley cement restrictor for small perforations; a larger free block of cortico-cancellous bone with bone chips, flexible wire mesh and cement for larger perforations; and finally chips of bone and a bipolar prosthesis for large medial wall defects.[24]

Scott and Murray have advocated the use of large bipolar prostheses used in association with morsellized bone against the defect.[13,14] Morley and Schmidt described their technique of sculpting a femoral head to plug the defect and felt that resection arthroplasty may be the only alternative in certain patients with marked lysis.[21]

Author's Preferred Treatment. The direct lateral approach is adequate for isolated perforations of the medial

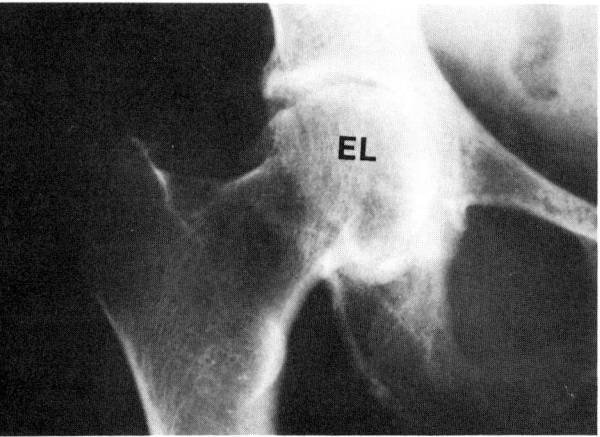

Figure 5-25A. This 69 year old woman presented with degenerative arthritis secondary to mild congenital protrusio acetabulum.

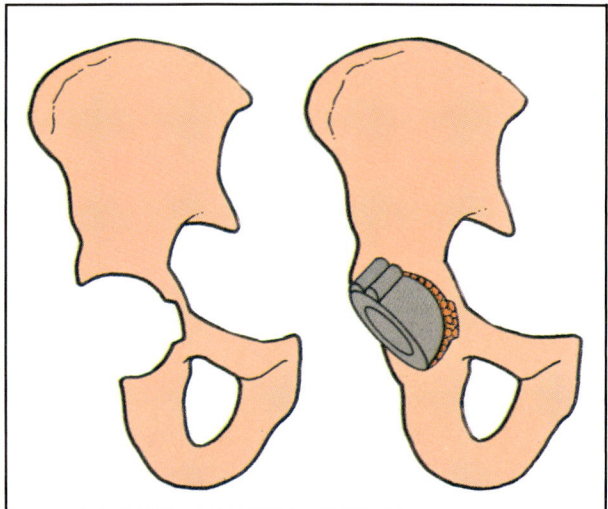

Figure 5-25B. Morsellized autograft from the patient's head was used with an uncemented low profile PCA acetabular component (Howmedica, Rutherford, NJ).

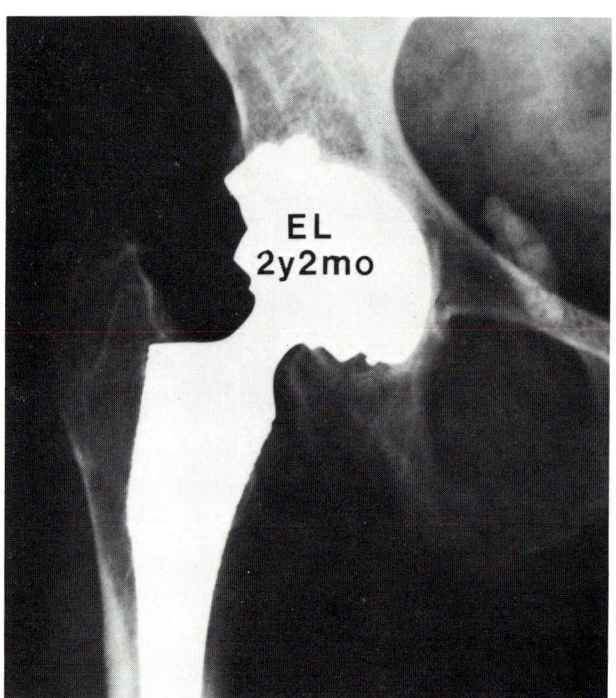

Figure 5-25C. The autograft appears to have incorporated well at two years, two months. A protrusio-type cup used without morsellized bone probably would have proved satisfactory for such a mild defect.

porous coated acetabular component that is large enough to span the defect. Stability is achieved by contact with the anterior and posterior columns and with the dome of the acetabulum. Intrapelvic pressure holds the cortical strips against the acetabular component that acts as a mold. Incorporation of the grafts appears to occur very quickly because of the rich blood supply of the iliacus. This technique is technically less demanding than the use of solid bone grafts and does not compromise the volume of the acetabulum.

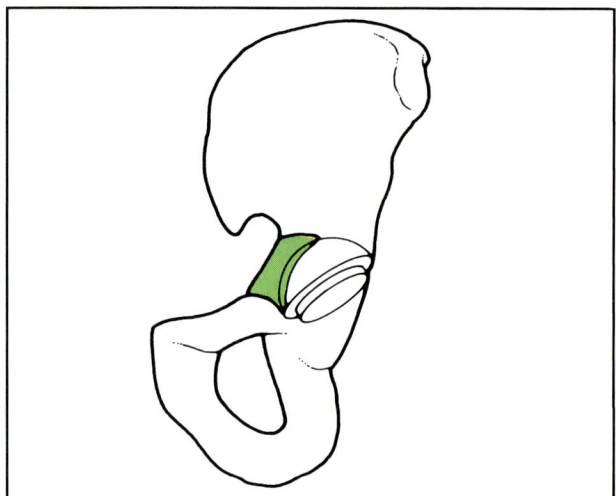

Figure 5-26. Perforation of the medial wall of the acetabulum.

Clinical Examples

Case 1

The patient seen in Figure 5-27A was 36 when she presented in 1982 with traumatic arthritis following an intrapelvic fracture-dislocation of her hip. The medial perforation was grafted with her femoral head which was shaped somewhat like a cap with the brim preventing the crown from protruding further intrapelvically (Figure 5-27B). Cement was used.

At followup of five years, she rates 85 but has some discomfort in her hip with excessive activity, such as skiing. A radiolucent line has formed between the cement and the inferior and superior acetabular margins (Figure 5-27C), but there is no radiolucency between the autograft and the cement, which suggests that the graft has not yet completely revascularized. We would now treat this defect by means of cortical and cancellous strips and an uncemented Harris-Galante acetabular component (Zimmer, Warsaw, IN).

Case 2

The patient seen in Figure 5-28A was 32 when she presented with a loose acetabular component, eight years after a cemented total hip replacement. The medial perforation was approximately 3cm. in diameter, and there were minor defects in the superior intra-acetabular region. Cortical and cancellous autogenous strips were used to fill the medial perforation and morsellized bone was used in the irregularities of the superior acetabular region (Figures 5-28B and 5-28C). The femoral component was not loose and was left in place. Because of the short neck and neutral anteversion of the femoral component, very accurate positioning of the uncemented acetabular component was necessary to prevent dislocation.

It is now two years since her procedure and the cortical and cancellous strips appear to have incorporated (Figure 5-28D). She rates 100, works full-time as a nurse, and holds an additional part-time job as well.

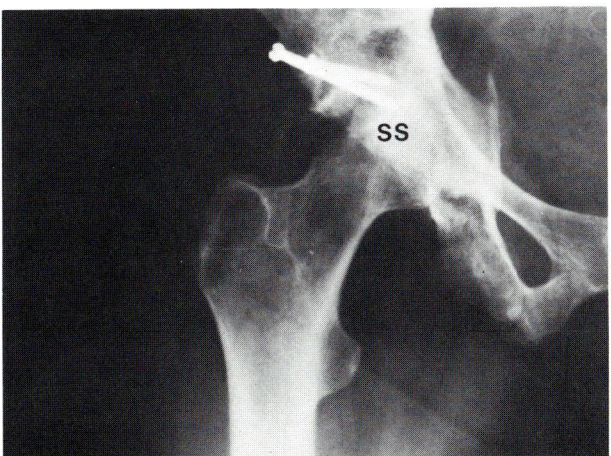

Figure 5-27A. This 36 year old woman had traumatic arthritis with a medial acetabular defect that measured 2cm. in diameter.

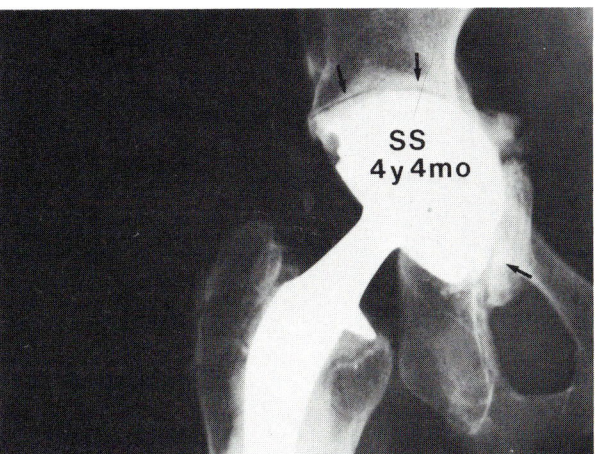

Figure 5-27C. At four years, four months, the graft appears to be incorporating but a radiolucent line has formed superiorly and inferiorly where the cement is in contact with living bone. The patient is beginning to have pain with excessive activity and rates 85. We would now deal with this defect by means of cortical and cancellous strips and an uncemented acetabular component.

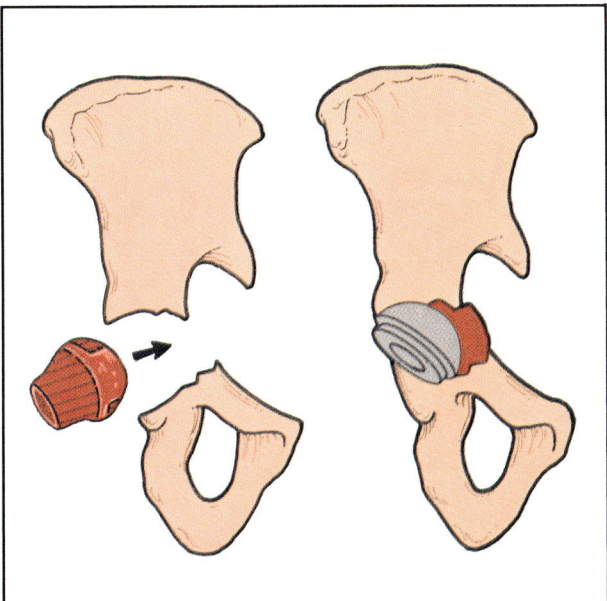

Figure 5-27B. The patient's femoral head was shaped like a hat. The brim prevented the crown from dislocating within the acetabulum.

Combined Acetabular Defects

Protrusio and Perforation of the Medial Wall (Fig. 5-29)

This combination of defects occurred in only one patient in our series (1.4%). The etiology in this patient was trauma although this combination could theoretically occur in other patients with failed total hip replacements.

Author's Preferred Treatment. The direct lateral approach is adequate to deal with both the protrusio and the medial wall defects. As with isolated medial perforations, we initially felt that it was important to occlude the defect completely in order to contain cement. Because we now use

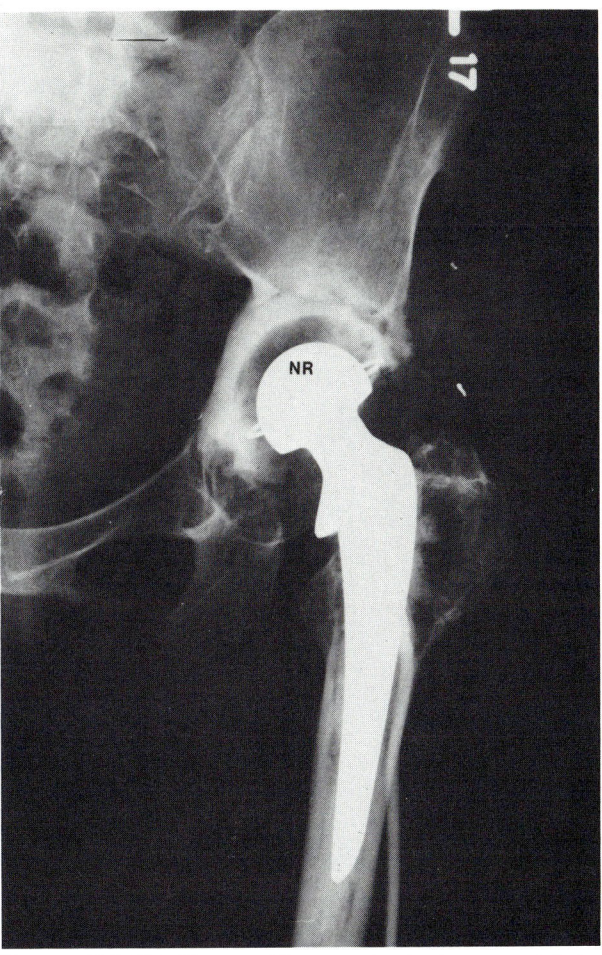

Figure 5-28A. This 32 year old woman had a loose acetabular component eight years after a cemented total hip replacement. The medial perforation measured almost 3cm. in diameter. The femoral component was not loose despite moderate calcar resorption.

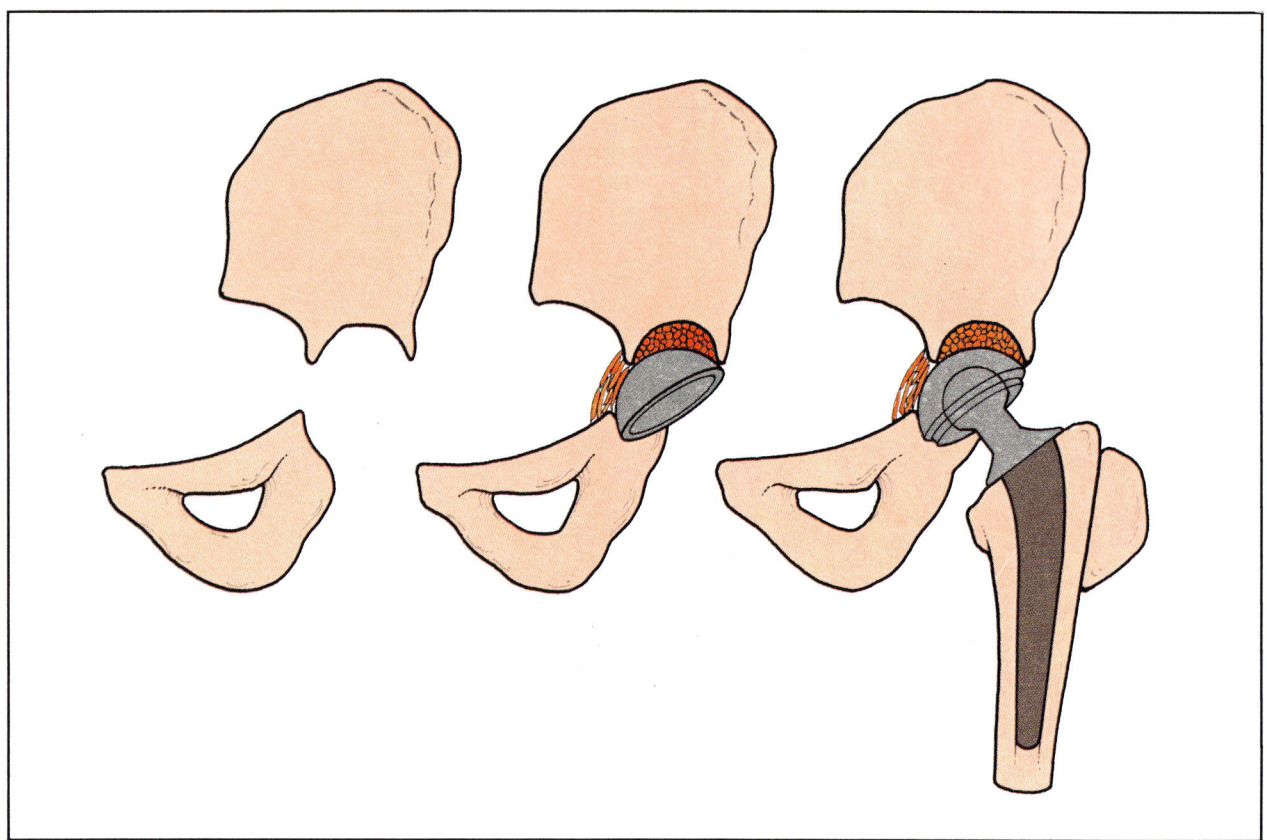

Figure 5-28B. Morsellized bone was used to fill the superior intra-acetabular irregularities, and cortical and cancellous strips from the iliac crest were used to reconstruct the medial perforation.

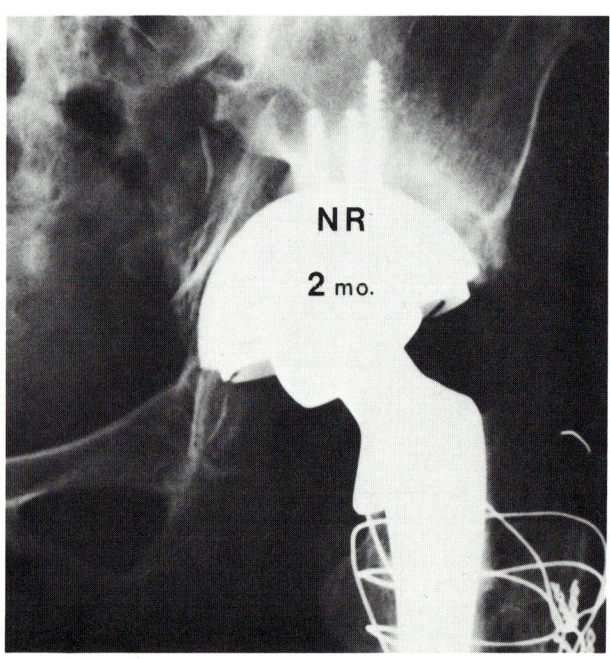

Figure 5-28C. An uncemented Harris Galante acetabular component (Zimmer, Warsaw, IN) was used. At two months the graft had begun to incorporate and the patient began to use a cane. The femoral component had a short neck and was in neutral anteversion, making acetabular positioning very critical to avoid dislocation. The greater trochanter was transplanted distally to provide increased stability.

uncemented sintered acetabular components in virtually all cases, the perforation can be managed more easily by means of cortical and cancellous autograft strips and the protrusio problem by morsellized or solid grafts. The acetabular component must extend well beyond the margins of the perforation.

Clinical Example

Case 1

The patient seen in Figures 5-30A and 5-30B was 62-years-old when she presented in 1980 with a significant perforation of the medial wall in association with protrusio acetabulum secondary to a central fracture-dislocation of her hip. We elected to occlude the medial defect by means of a full-thickness iliac crest graft placed intrapelvically and lagged with screws from the outside (Figure 5-30C). This required a separate incision over the iliac crest. The large defect in the iliac crest was repaired with mandibular mesh (Figure 5-30D) (Howmedico, Rutherford, New Jersey). Intra-operative and postoperative bleeding was excessive and she required over 20 units of blood, probably because of injury to the obturator vessels. At five years, the graft appears to have incorporated (Figure 5-30E) and there is no sign of loosening but the protrusio problem was not addressed and at followup of six and a half years the patient

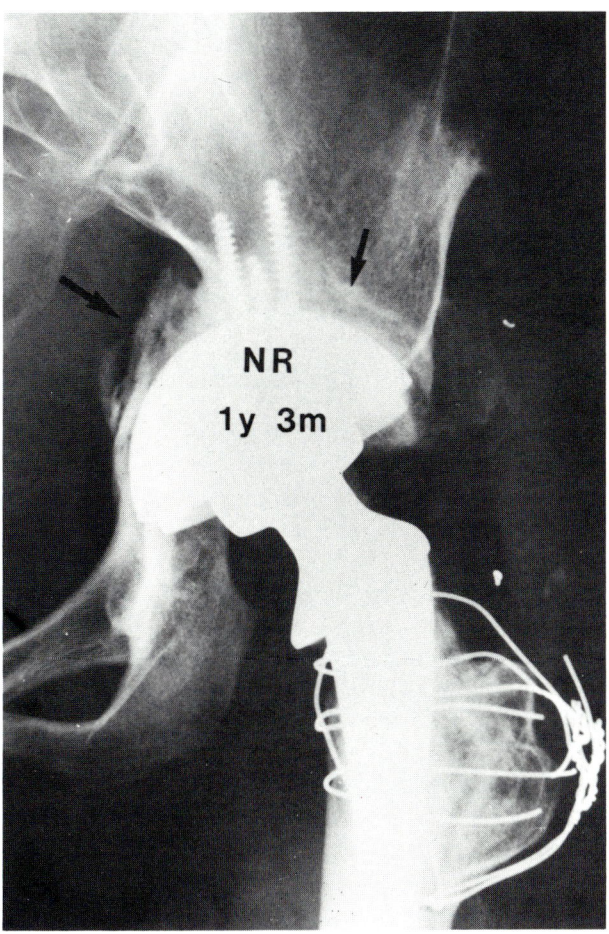

Figure 5-28D. At one year and three months the grafts look very satisfactory. The patient works as a nurse without restrictions and rates 100.

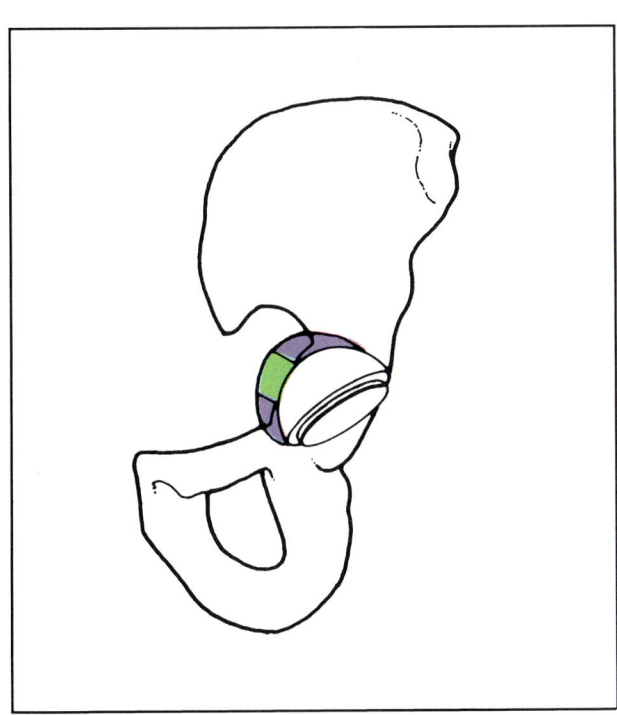

Figure 5-29. Protrusio and perforation of the medial wall.

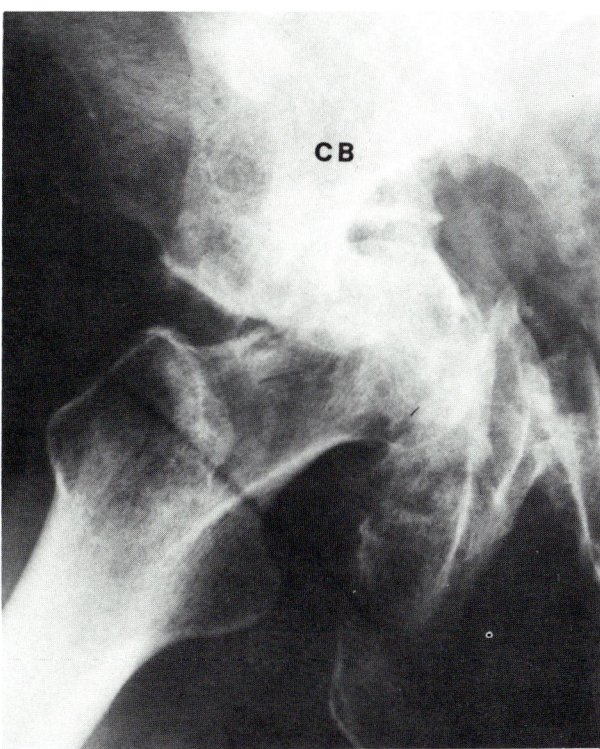

Figure 5-30A. This 62 year old woman had a central fracture dislocation of her hip when she was struck by an automobile four years prior to admission. She has protrusio acetabulum and a perforation of the medial wall.

complains of groin pain, particularly with straight leg raising. We feel that this is because the center of rotation of the acetabulum is too medial, causing irritation of the iliopsoas as it passes over the prominent anterior rim of the acetabulum. The patient uses a cane for outside walking and rates only 75.

If we were to deal with the same problem today, we would fill the medial perforation with autogenous strips, reposition the denuded femoral head in the depths of the acetabulum in order to move the center of rotation laterally and would use an uncemented acetabular component fixed with screws.

Superior Rim and Superior Intra-acetabular Defects (Figure 5-31)

This combination of defects occurred in seven patients in our series (10%). The etiology in every case was failed total hip replacement associated with bone lysis.

Author's Preferred Treatment. One of the transtrochanteric approaches is preferable. It is our feeling that all rim defects should be dealt with by means of solid grafts. Because this particular defect occurs most commonly in association with failed total hip replacement, autogenous femoral head bone is almost never available and allograft bone must be used. In the majority of cases we have used allograft femoral heads but do not hesitate to use other

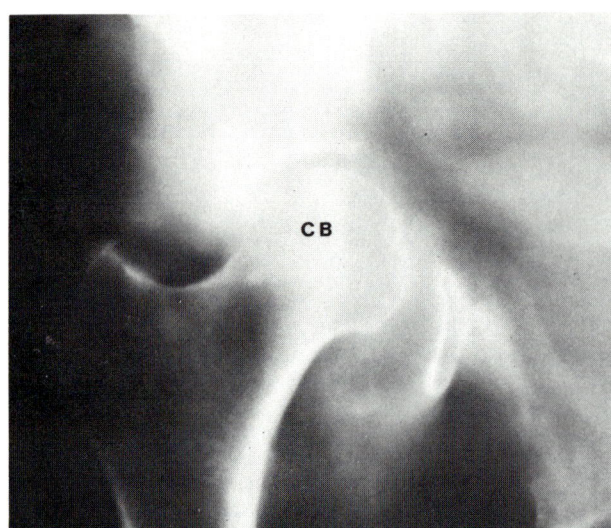

Figure 5-30B. The magnitude of the medial defect is shown by this tomogram.

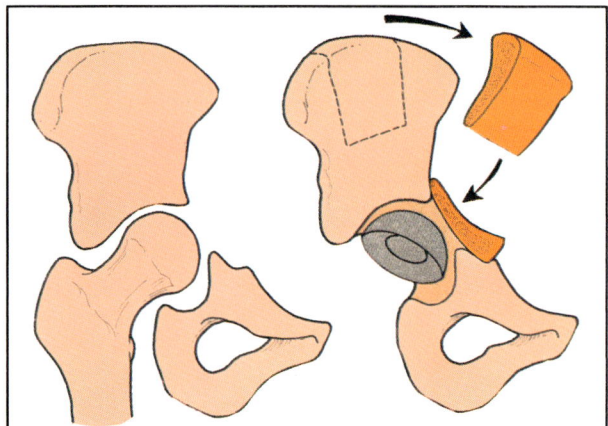

Figure 5-30C. A full thickness iliac crest graft was placed intra-pelvically and lagged by screws from the outside.

sources of larger solid allograft bone.

The intra-acetabular defects may be dealt with by morsellized bone if they are small, but with large defects in the weight-bearing area, solid grafts are desirable since they move the center of rotation distally.

Although our initial experience was with the use of cement, it is now our feeling that these defects can almost always be dealt with by means of cementless acetabular components.

Clinical Examples

Case 1

The patient seen in Figure 5-32A was 60 when he presented in 1982 with loose acetabular and femoral components, 12 years after his initial arthroplasty for degenerative arthritis. There were significant superior rim and superior intra-acetabular defects, with an intact medial wall. Morsellized cancellous autogenous and allograft bone was used in conjunction with a large femoral head to reconstruct both the intra-acetabular and rim defect (Figure 5-32B). Although cement was used in this case, we would now use an uncemented component.

The original fit of the femoral head against the superior rim was poor (Figure 5-32C). At four years, eight months, this area of poor contact seems to be filling in (Figure 5-32D). There is no radiolucency between the graft and the cement. The patient rates 95, nine years, four months after his surgery.

Case 2

The patient seen in Figure 5-33A was 68 when he presented with a failed total hip replacement that was loose on both the acetabular and femoral sides, eleven and a half years after his initial arthroplasty for degenerative arthritis.

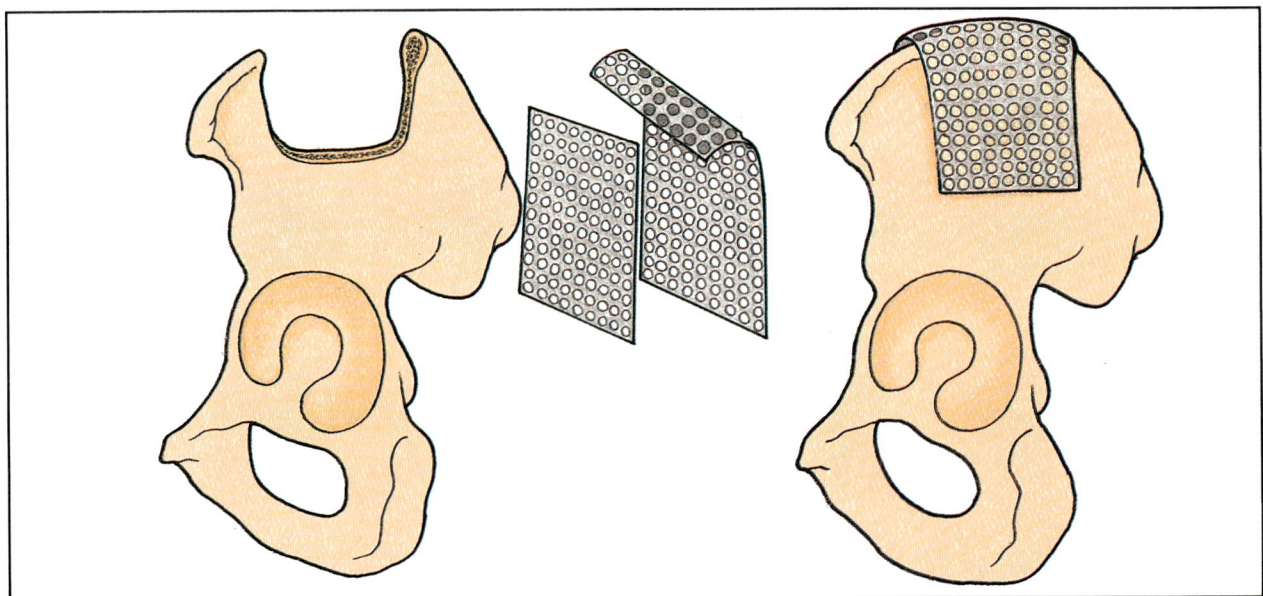

Figure 5-30D. Chrome cobalt mandibular mesh (Howmedica, Rutherford, NJ) was used to occlude the defect and to avoid herniation.

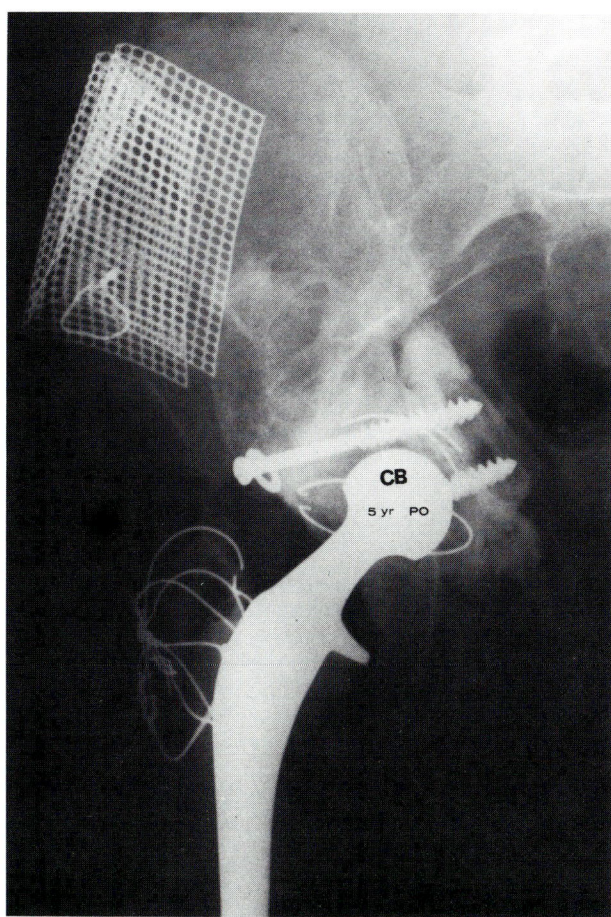

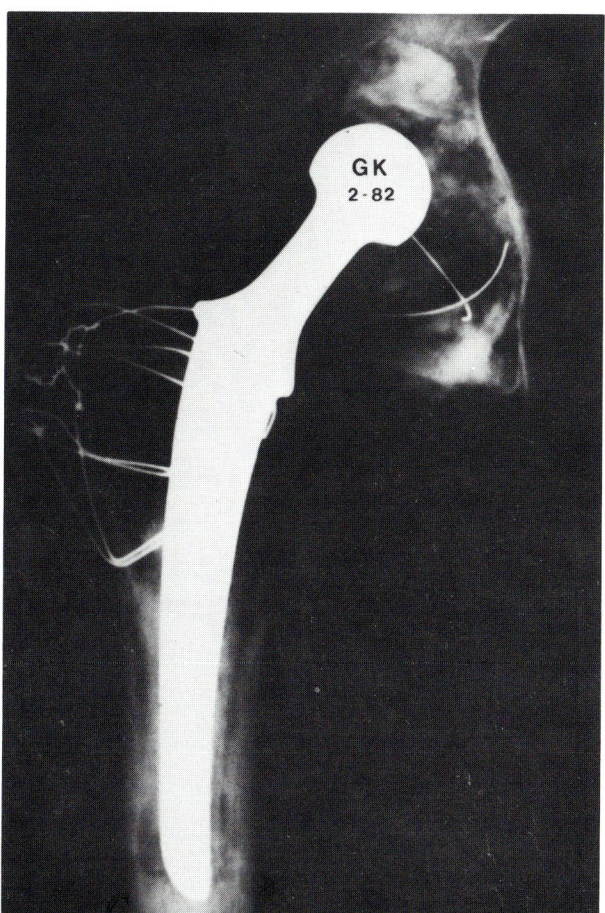

Figure 5-30E. At five years, the graft appears to have united and there is no radiolucency. At follow up of six and one half years, the patient complains of pain in the groin, probably from irritation of the psoas tendon because the protrusio defect was not corrected. She uses a cane for outside walking and rates only 75.

Figure 5-32A. This 60 year old man had a loose acetabular component twelve years after his initial total hip replacement. There is a defect of the superior rim and superior intra-acetabular area.

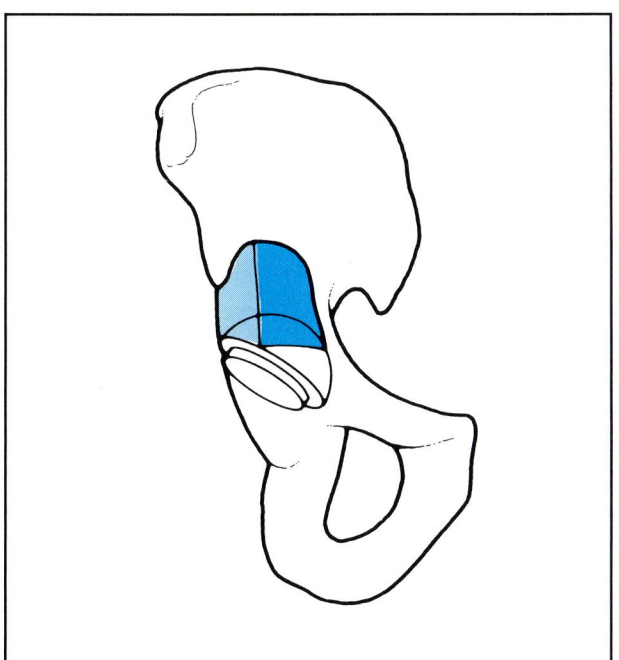

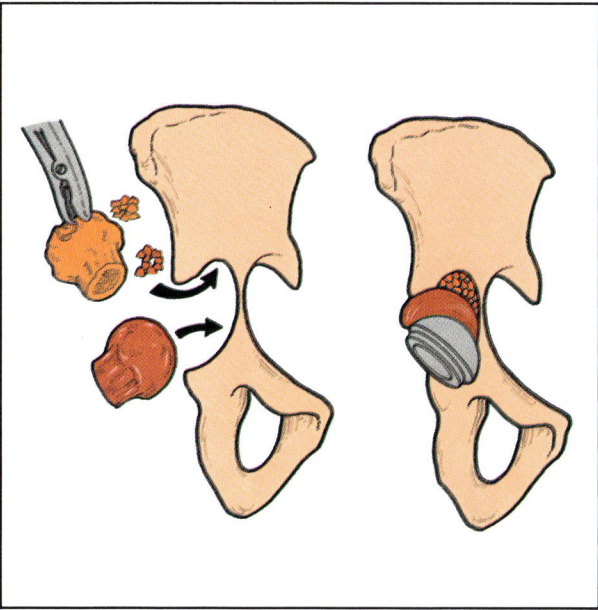

Figure 5-32B. The smaller superior intra-acetabular defects were filled with morsellized bone from an allograft femoral head, mixed with morsellized autogenous iliac crest graft. The superior rim and the major superior intra-acetabular defects were reconstructed with a single large femoral head.

Figure 5-31. Superior rim and superior intra-acetabular defects.

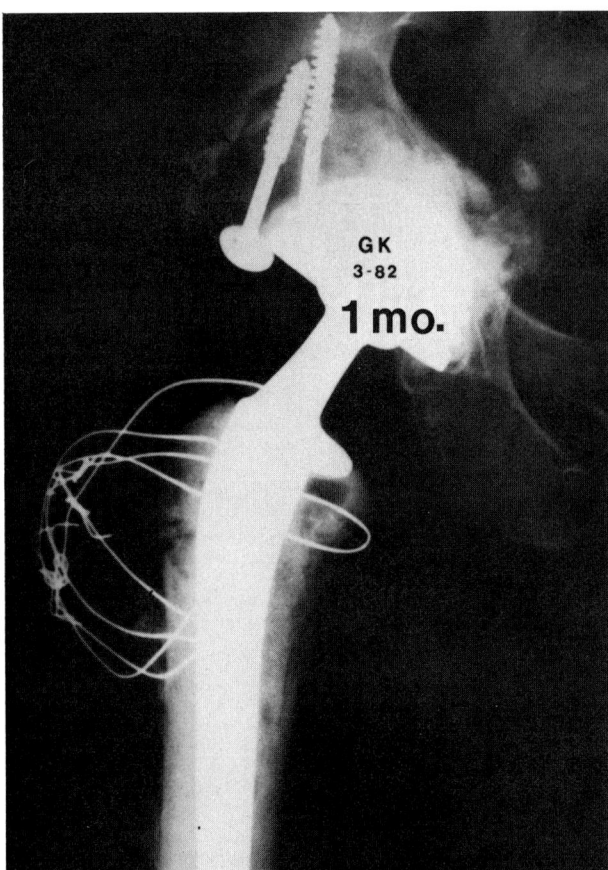

Figure 5-32C. Although the superior intra-acetabular defect was packed with bone, the significant gap between the graft and the pelvis laterally (arrows) was not recognized at surgery and was not packed.

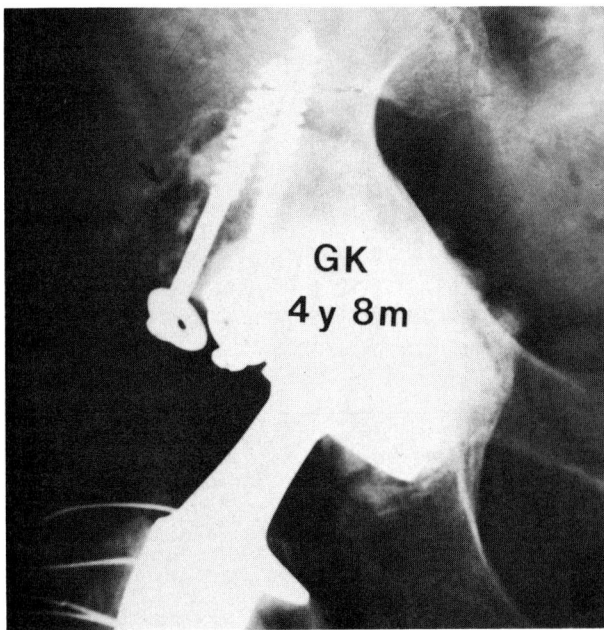

Figure 5-32D. At four years and eight months, the small superior intra-acetabular defect which was packed with bone has partially incorporated. The superolateral defect is filling in. The washers have migrated medially in the area at the periphery of the graft that is not stressed. The patient rates 95.

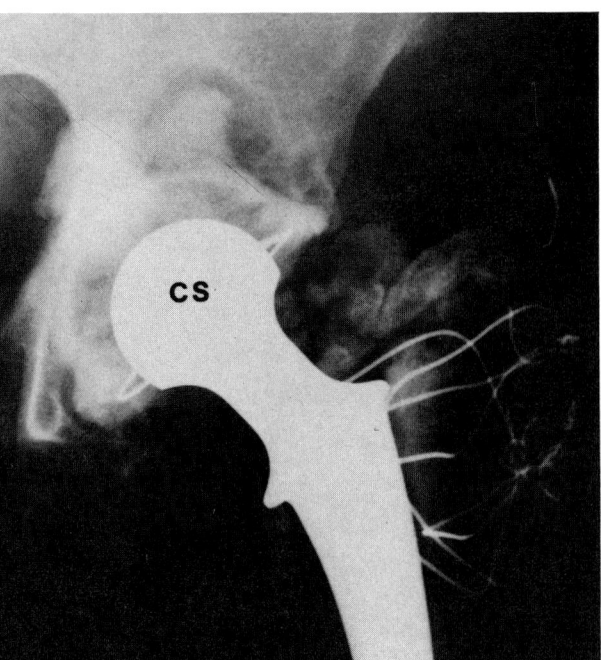

Figure 5-33A. This 68 year old man had a loose femoral and acetabular component. Note the significant lysis about the superior intra-acetabular keying hole and about the cement in the area of the rim.

He had a modest superior rim defect and a significant superior intra-acetabular defect secondary to lysis about a keying hole. The small intra-acetabular defects were filled with morsellized autogenous and allograft bone. A large femoral head was used to provide support in the superior intra-acetabular area and the superior rim in order to bring the center of rotation down to the anatomical position. An uncemented acetabular component was used and the superior screws of the acetabular component helped to fix the femoral head graft as well. The loose femoral component was replaced by an uncemented porous coated device (Figure 5-33B). At short-term followup of one year, five months, the patient rates 100 and his grafts appear satisfactory (Figure 5-33C).

Case 3

The patient seen in Figure 5-34A was 58 when she presented with a failed total hip replacement. Her original diagnosis was congenital dysplasia with degenerative arthritis. Her first total hip was performed in 1976 and was revised to a cemented long stem prosthesis in 1978 because of a fractured stem.

She had significant superior rim and superior intra-acetabular defects. An allograft femoral head was shaped like a mushroom to restore both intra-acetabular and superior rim bone stock. Morsellized autogenous bone was placed in the depths of the intra-acetabular defect before the graft was impacted (Figure 5-34B). The graft was inherently stable, but two cancellous screws were used for additional fixation. An uncemented acetabular component was used (Figure 5-34C).

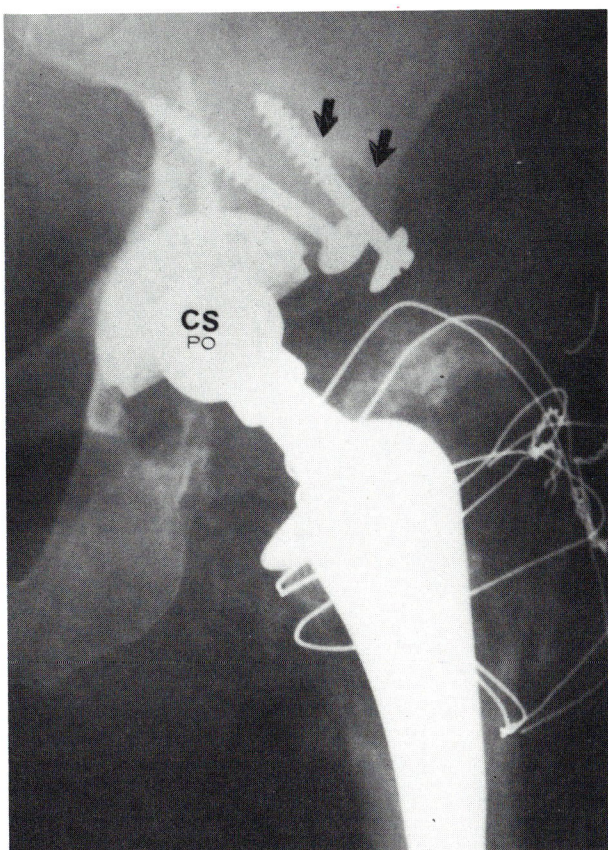

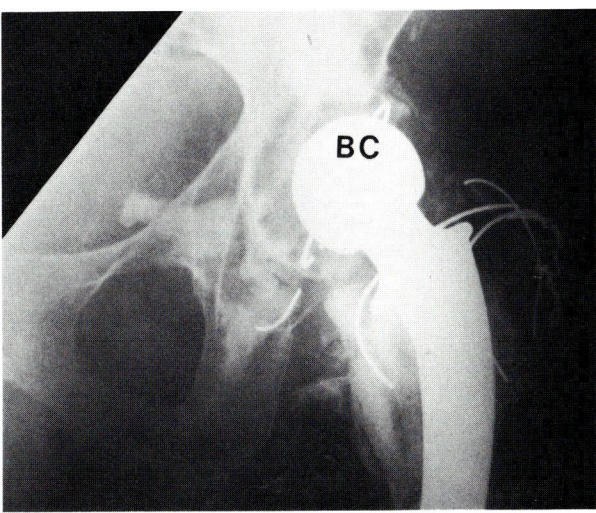

Figure 5-34A. This 58 year old woman presented with a superior rim and superior intra-acetabular defect.

Figure 5-33B. The small superior intra-acetabular defects were filled with a mixture of morsellized autograft and allograft bone. A large allograft head was used to reconstruct the major intra-acetabular and superior rim defect. Both components are uncemented.

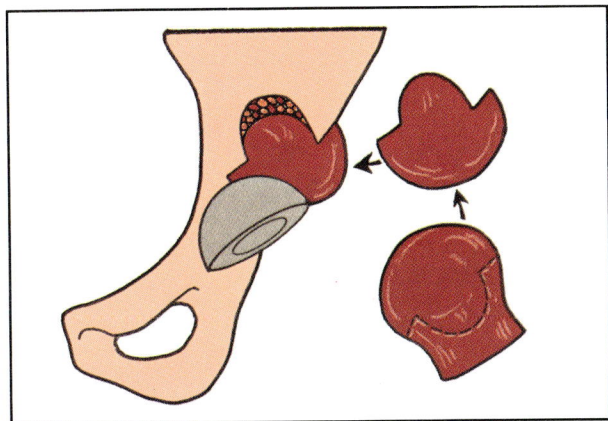

Figure 5-34B. The superior intra-acetabular defect was first packed with a mixture of allograft and autograft bone. A femoral head allograft was shaped like a mushroom and was used to reconstruct the superior rim and the superior intra-acetabular defect.

At two months, she was started on a cane. At seven months, the superior rim portion of the graft has probably fractured (Figure 5-34D). The orientation of the screws in the line of weightbearing has allowed the graft (and acetabular component) to migrate to a position of stability and fixation of the acetabular component does not seem to be compromised. If the screws were more transverse, the rim of the graft might not have fractured but union also might not occur. This patient has mild thigh pain, probably unrelated to her acetabular component. She does not take analgesics but still uses a cane and rates 80.

Superior Rim, Superior Intra-acetabular Defects, and Perforation of the Medial Wall (Figure 5-35)

This particular combination occurred in only three cases in our series (4%). The etiology in all was failed total hip

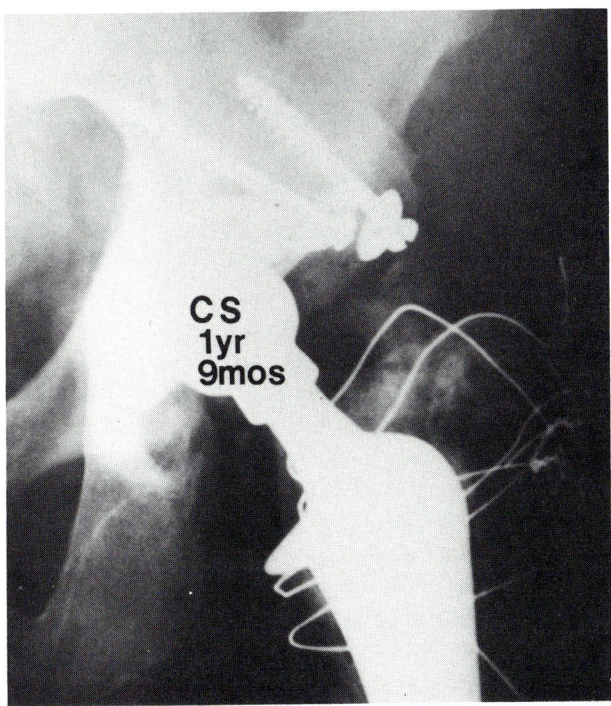

Figure 5-33C. At follow-up of one year and nine months, the grafts appear to be doing well. The patient rates 100.

replacement. Two patients had a failed mold arthroplasty prior to their total hip replacements.

Authors' Preferred Treatment. Such major defects require extensive exposure; we prefer one of the transtrochanteric approaches. Our initial experience was with cement used in conjunction with solid grafts to contain the cement. We still use solid grafts to provide superior rim support and to reconstruct very large intra-acetabular defects but now prefer autogenous iliac cortical and cancellous bone strips for the perforation in conjunction with uncemented acetabular prostheses.

Clinical Examples

Case 1

The patient seen in Figure 5-36A was 68 when she presented in 1981 with a failed total hip replacement. Her original diagnosis was bilateral congenitally dislocated hips. She had undergone multiple previous operations including an open reduction, a shelf procedure, three mold arthroplasties and two total hip replacements. She was a small woman who weighed less than one hundred pounds and there was very little acetabular stock to work with at the time of her final revision.

Unfortunately, laceration of the femoral artery vein and

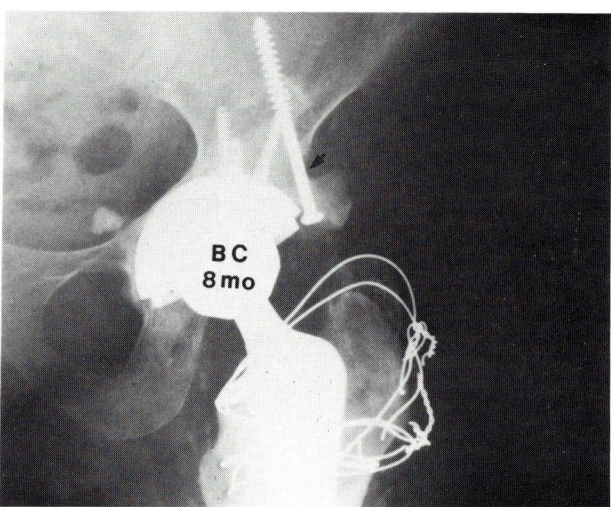

Figure 5-34D. At eight months, the superior rim portion of the femoral head graft has probably fractured because of superior migration of the intra-acetabular portion to a position of stability. However, fixation of the acetabular component does not seem to be compromised. The patient has mild thigh pain which is probably not related to her acetabular component. She does not take analgesics but still uses a cane and rates 80.

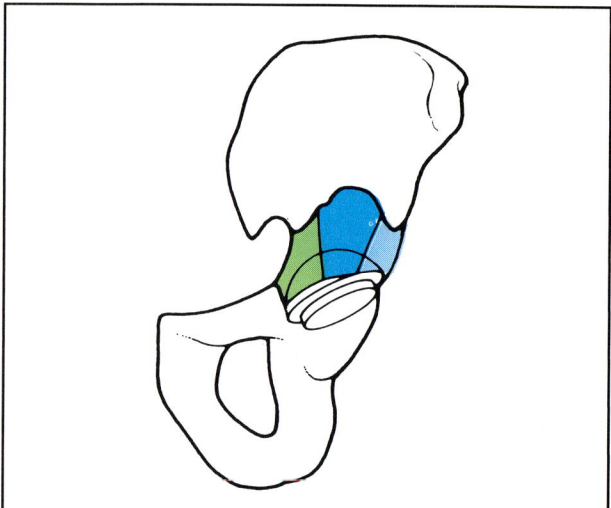

Figure 5-35. Intra-acetabular, superior rim, and medial wall defects.

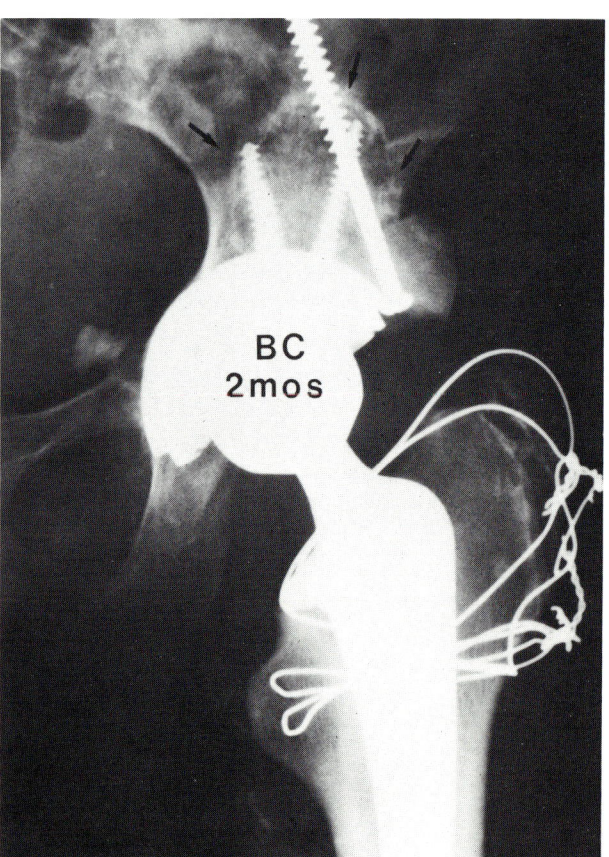

Figure 5-34C. An uncemented Harris Galante acetabular component was used (Zimmer, Warsaw, IN). At two months, the patient was started on a cane.

nerve occurred intra-operatively and required reconstruction of the artery. With multiple previous operations through an anterior Smith-Petersen incision, the iliopsoas had long been destroyed and these neurovascular structures were encountered directly over the anterior portion of the capsule. The orthopedic procedure was terminated, the artery was repaired and the vein ligated. Normal circulation to the extremity was restored but the patient has a permanent femoral palsy. Three months later, because of continued disabling hip pain the patient insisted that the hip be reconstructed.

A large femoral head was oriented so that it would reconstruct the superior rim, the intra-acetabular area and

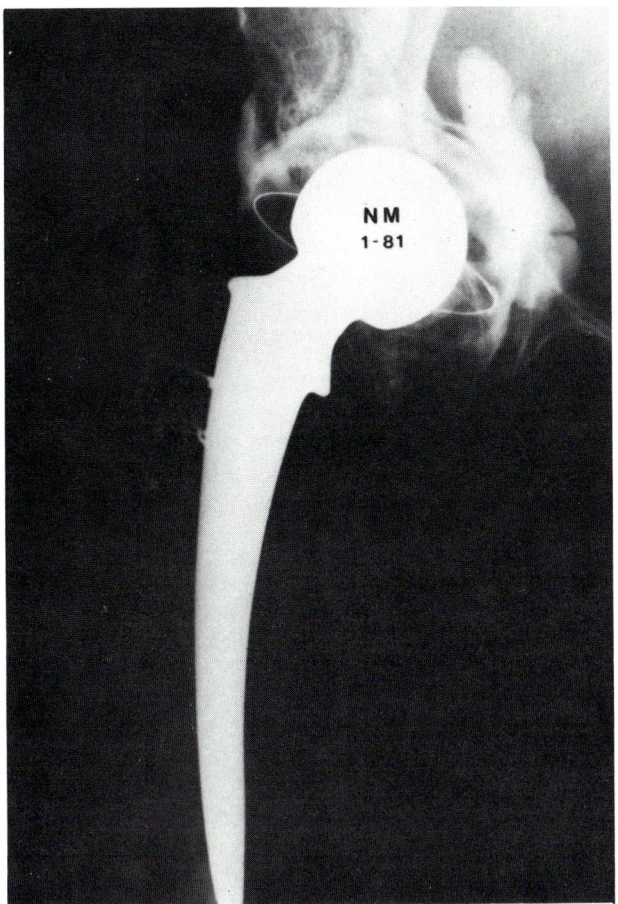

Figure 5-36A. This 68 year old woman had undergone multiple previous operations and presented with this complex superior rim and superior intra-acetabular defect as well as perforation of the medial wall. Despite dramatic stress shielding of her femur, the femoral component was not loose.

the medial perforation (Figure 5-36B). Morsellized allograft bone was first placed in the defect against the iliacus and this was held in place by the solid femoral head allograft. Cement was used. She dislocated once six weeks postoperatively and required open reduction. An early post-operative x-ray (Figure 5-36C) shows an inferomedial radiolucent area at the bone-cement interface.

At follow-up of six years, two months, the graft appears to be doing well and the inferomedial radiolucent line is unchanged (Figure 5-36D). The patient is pleased with her function but has a significant abductor lurch and requires a cane for walking. She has a completely paralyzed quadriceps related to her devastating neurovascular complication and rates only 72.

We would still deal with the rim and superior acetabular defect by means of a solid graft but would now use autograft cortical and cancellous strips for the medial perforation in conjunction with an uncemented acetabular component.

Case 2

The patient seen in Figure 5-37A was 45 when he presented in 1982 with a failed total hip replacement with

loosening of both components. He had undergone two previous cup arthroplasties prior to his initial total hip replacement. Although it is not completely obvious on the preoperative x-ray, there was a significant medial perforation which measured 2.5cm. in diameter. One large femoral head was shaped like a straw hat to fill the medial defect. The brim of the hat stabilized the graft but pushed the acetabular component laterally. A second large femoral head was used to reconstruct the superior intra-acetabular area and the lateral rim. This second head helped to move the center of rotation inferiorly. Morsellized allograft bone was used to fill the smaller defects in the dome of the acetabulum (Figure 5-37B). Cement was used.

The patient is now five years, four months since his surgery, works ten hours a day on his feet as a machinist and functions extremely well with a Harris rating of 100. X-rays at four and a half years look satisfactory (Figure 5-37C). There are no radiolucent lines.

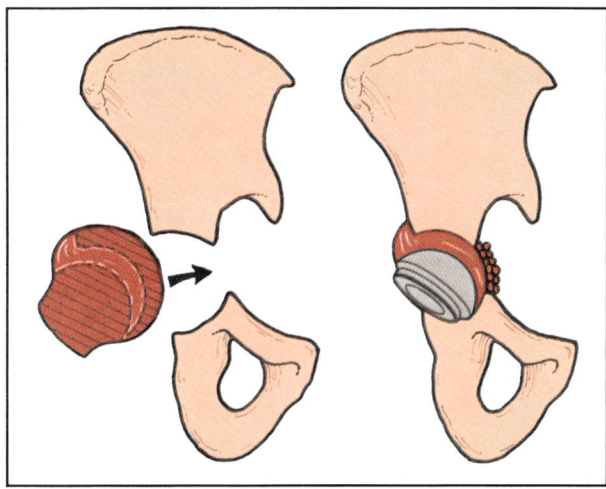

Figure 5-36B. Morsellized allograft was first placed in the perforation. A single femoral head was then used to reconstruct all the defects.

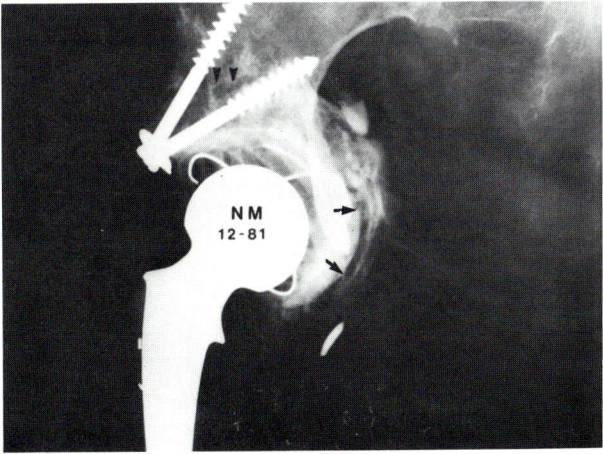

Figure 5-36C. In the immediate post-operative period, graft and component orientation are satisfactory but there is a cement-bone radiolucency visible inferomedially (Zone III).

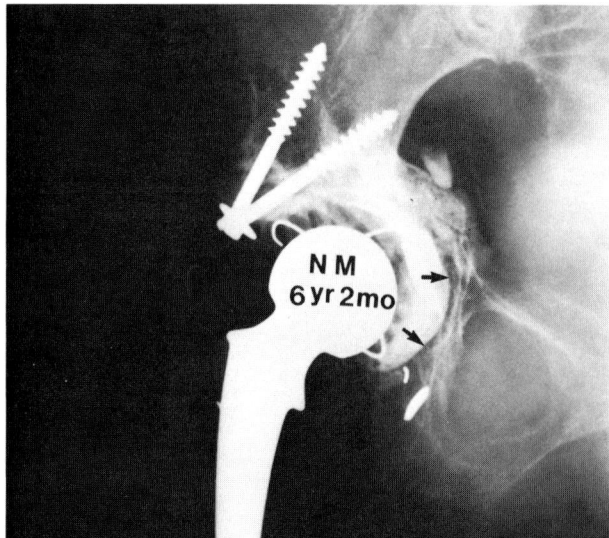

Figure 5-36D. At six years and two months, the graft appears to have incorporated. The inferomedial radiolucent zone is unchanged from early post-operative x-rays. The patient still requires a cane because of abductor weakness and a paralyzed quadriceps. She rates 72.

At present, we would still deal with the superior intra-acetabular defect and the rim defect by means of an allograft femoral head but would reconstruct the medial defect with autogenous strips of cortical and cancellous bone in association with an uncemented acetabular component.

Case 3

The patient whose x-rays are seen in Figure 5-38A was 38 when he presented with pain secondary to a loose acetabular component. He had the initial diagnosis of ankylosing spondylitis. At age 19 he had his first operation which was probably a Judet prosthesis. This was changed to a Moore prosthesis one year later. At age 31 he had his first total hip replacement. Two years later he began to have pain and x-rays demonstrated loosening of the acetabular component. The femoral component was not loose. He had a modest superior rim defect but the superior intra-acetabular defect was significant and the medial perforation was large enough to allow the acetabular component and cement to dislocate intrapelvically. Cortical and cancellous strips were used to fill the medial perforation, a mixture of morsellized autogenous and allograft bone was placed in the intra-acetabular defect; and, a single very large allograft femoral head was used to reconstruct all three defects (Figure 5-38B). Cement was used. X-rays at four years looked very satisfactory (Figure 5-38C). The patient did very well for five years, walked without support and rated 88.

At five and a half years he fell and had pain but did not return for followup. X-rays at six years, two months (Figure 5-38D) showed that the acetabular component was loose. The patient rated 69. At revision, the acetabular component was grossly loose but the architecture of the acetabulum remained intact and an uncemented PCA protrusio

acetabular component (Howmedica, Rutherford, NJ) was used. No further grafts were necessary (Figure 5-38E).

The patient dislocated one week postoperatively. A closed reduction was performed and the acetabular component did not loose fixation. The patient, now seven months since his final revision, has no pain and does not use support. He has a mild abductor lurch because of previous surgical damage to the abductor muscles and rates 86.

We would now still use autogenous strips for the medial perforation and morsellized bone for the superior intra-acetabular defect but might have used a very large uncemented Harris-Galante acetabular component (Zimmer, Warsaw, IN) instead of the large femoral head. If the hip was unstable because of shortening, a femoral head graft could still have been used to bring the center of rotation distally; however, there was a major error in the original reconstruction in that the two screws were oriented transversely and probably prevented proper impaction and remodeling of the graft.

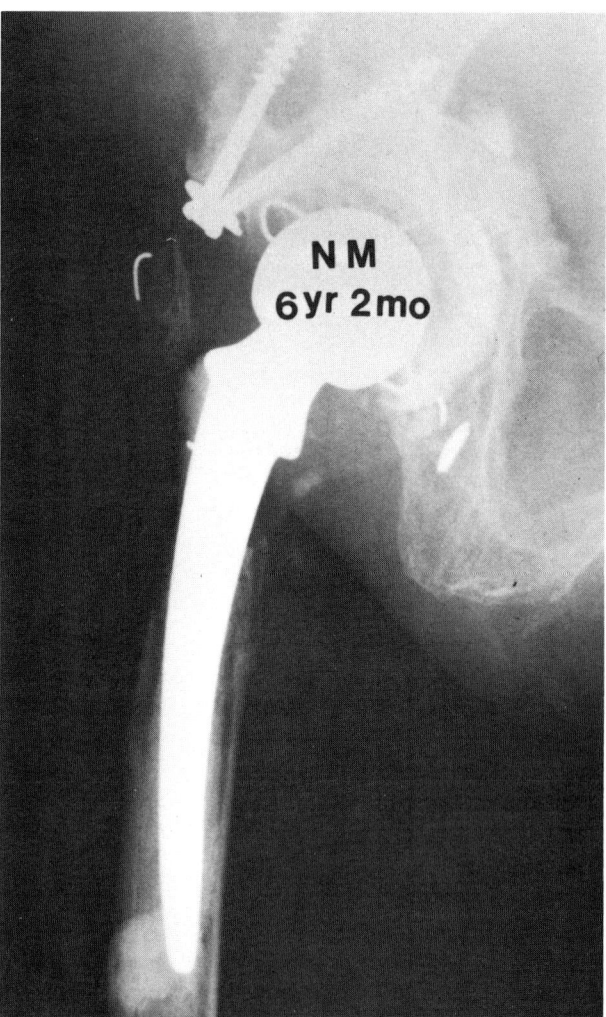

Figure 5-36E. Note the dramatic stress shielding of the proximal femur. However, the component is not loose and the patient does not have pain. Proximal migration of the greater trochanter probably contributes to her abductor lurch.

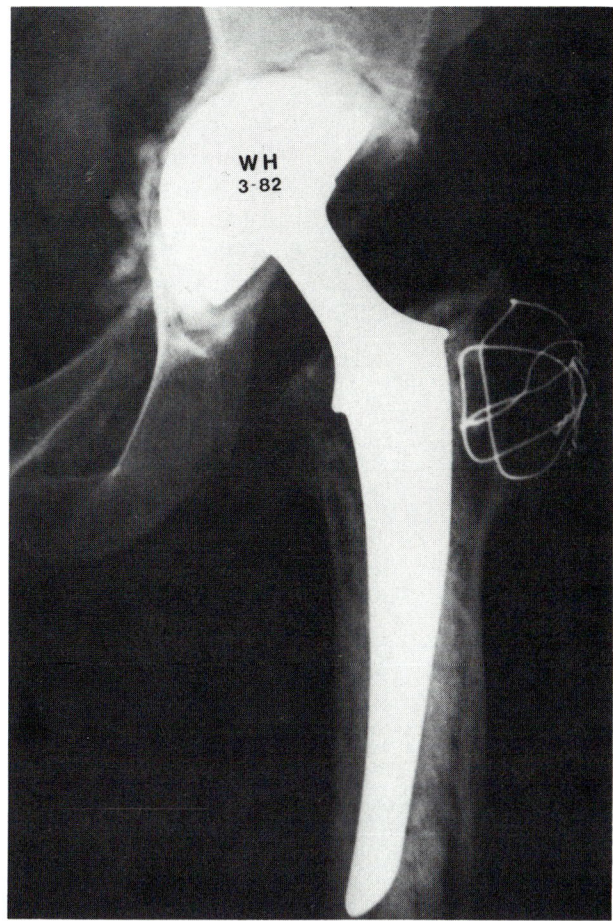

Figure 5-37A. This 45 year old man had undergone two cup arthroplasties prior to this failed total hip replacement. The medial perforation was 2.5cm. in diameter.

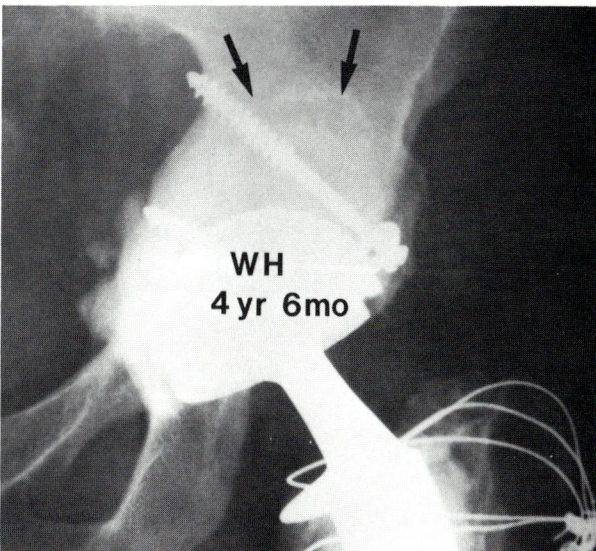

Figure 5-37C. X-rays at four years and six months appear satisfactory. The morsellized bone in the superior intra-acetabular area appears to have incorporated. There are no radiolucent lines. At follow-up of four years and ten months, the patient rates 100.

Case 4

The patient seen in Figure 5-39A was 53 at the time she presented with a loose acetabular component, 12 years after her primary total hip replacement for hip dysplasia. There was significant lysis of the acetabulum. The defect in this particular patient was much larger than could be accommodated by one femoral head and we elected to use a distal femoral condyle as shown in Figures 5-39B and 5-39C.

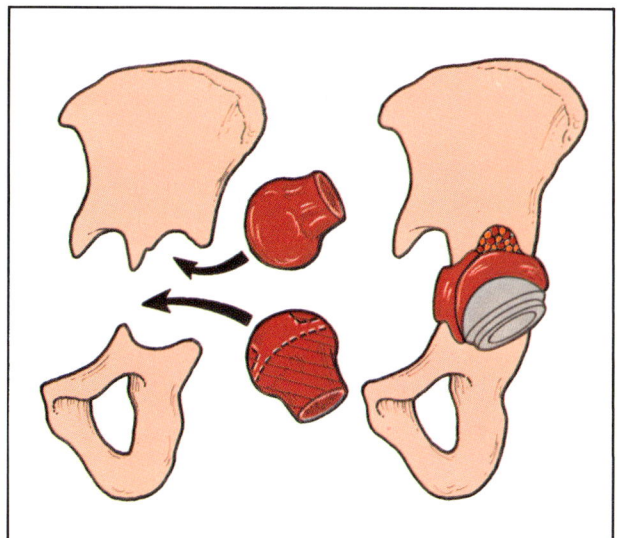

Figure 5-37B. One allograft femoral head was shaped like a hat and was used to occlude the medial perforation. Morsellized allograft bone was used for the smaller superior intra-acetabular defect. A second allograft femoral head was used to move the center of rotation inferiorly, and because the acetabular component was pushed laterally by the head used to reconstruct the medial perforation, this graft also provided superior rim support.

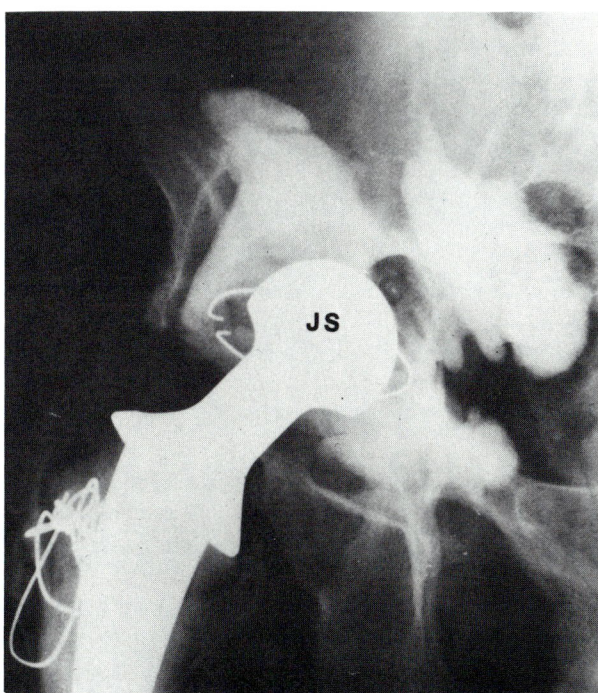

Figure 5-38A. This 38 year old man with ankylosing spondylitis had pain secondary to a loose acetabular component which had been inserted seven years previously.

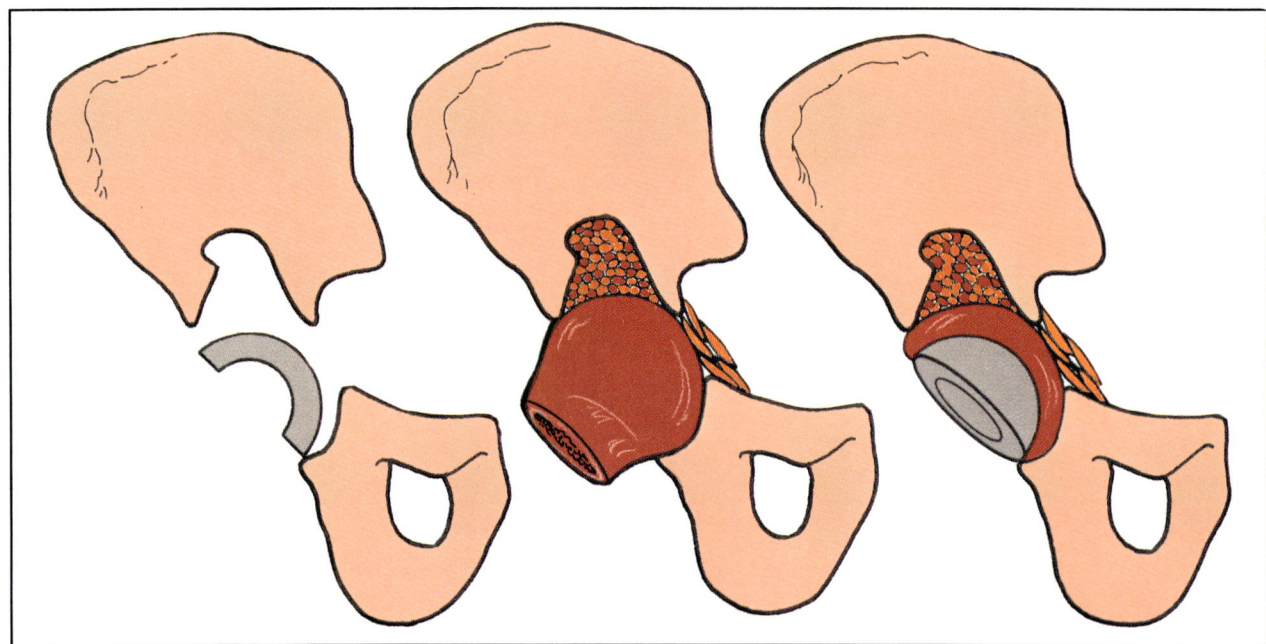

Figure 5-38B. The superior rim defect was modest but the superior intra-acetabular and the medial defects were large enough to allow the acetabular component and the cement to sublux intrapelvically. Autogenous strips were placed in the medial defect and morsellized bone was placed in the superior intra-acetabular defect. One very large femoral head was used to reconstruct all defects.

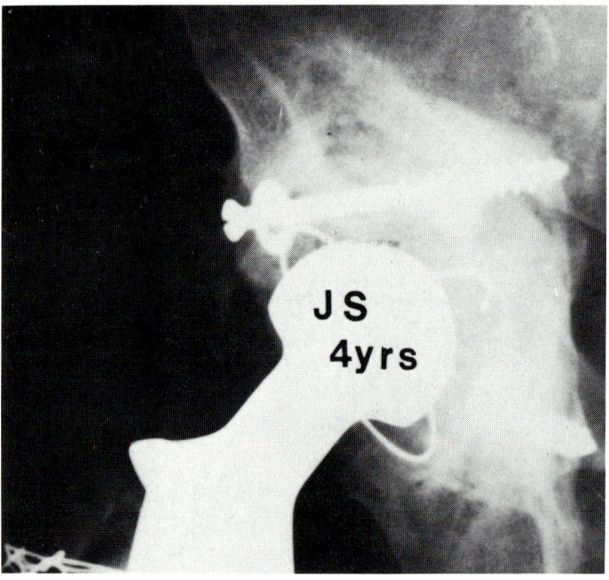

Figure 5-38C. The grafts appeared to be doing well at four years and the patient rated 88.

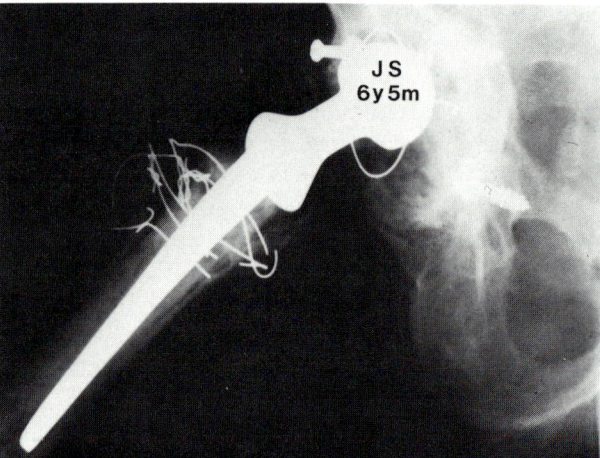

Figure 5-38D. X-rays at six years and two months showed that the acetabular component was loose. There was a major technical error in the original reconstruction in that the two screws were oriented transversely and potentially could have kept the graft from impacting and/or remodeling. Note that the superior screw has fractured.

This graft was large enough to fill the intra-acetabular defect, the lateral rim defect and the significant medial wall perforation. Prior to putting in the solid graft, morsellized autogenous and allograft bone was used superiorly to fill the irregular intra-acetabular defects, and cancellous and cortical strips from the iliac crest were used to fill the medial defect. Although there was stress shielding and lysis of the proximal femur, the femoral component was not loose by x-ray or clinical examination and was left in place (Figure 5-39D).

This patient did well and was discharged from the hospital on the sixth postoperative day, moved from two crutches to a cane at six weeks and was off of all support by three months. At short followup of twelve months, she rates 94 and the graft appears to be doing well by x-ray (Figure 5-39E). She has no hip pain but has a limited exercise tolerance because of an unrelated lumbar disc problem with pain in the typical sciatic distribution.

Superior Intra-acetabular Defects and Perforation of the Medial Wall (Figure 5-40). This particular

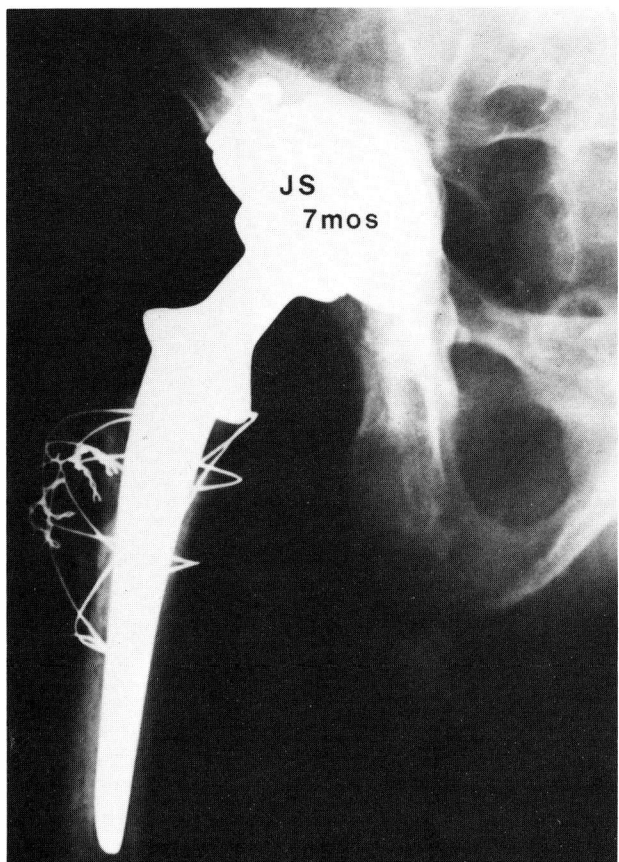

Figure 5-38E. At revision, the architecture of the acetabulum was close to being normal and an uncemented PCA protrusio component (Howmedica, Rutherford, NJ) was used. No further grafting was necessary.

combination is rare and occurred in only three patients (4%). The etiology in all cases was failed total hip replacement with lysis associated with a loose cemented acetabular component (Figure 5-40).

Authors' Preferred Treatment. The direct lateral approach is satisfactory for reconstruction of the medial perforation and for small superior intra-acetabular defects; but if the superior intra-acetabular defect is large, we prefer one of the transtrochanteric approaches.

Since the rim is intact, it is not necessary to use a solid graft to reconstruct this area. As with other significant superior intra-acetabular defects, however, it may be necessary to use a large solid graft to bring the center of rotation distally. Small superior acetabular defects can be dealt with by means of morsellized bone and medial perforations can be reconstructed by means of autogenous cortical and cancellous bone strips.

Clinical Examples

Case 1

The patient seen in Figure 5-41A was 73 when she presented with a loose acetabular component, 14 years after her initial cemented total hip replacement. There was a

significant superior intra-acetabular defect as well as an anteromedial perforation which measured 2cm. in diameter. Although there was proximal stress shielding, the femoral component was not loose by x-ray or by clinical examination at the time of surgery.

The medial perforation was filled with cortical and cancellous strips from the iliac crest, placed intrapelvically (through the defect). A large disc, fashioned from an allograft femoral head was contoured to occlude the defect and was placed within the acetabulum to push the center of rotation laterally. The rest of this allograft head was morsellized and mixed with autogenous morsellized bone, from the iliac crest to fill the irregular defects of the superior intra-acetabular area. A second very large femoral head was used against this morsellized bone. The superior intra-acetabular allograft was inherently stable because of its contact with the dome of the acetabulum and the morsellized bone but additional fixation was provided by two screws. An uncemented Harris-Galante acetabular component (Zimmer, Warsaw, IN) was fixed with four screws which provided additional stability to the allograft (Figure 5-41B). Approximately one fifth of the sintered surface of the acetabular component was in contact with living bone.

Ambulation with crutches was begun on the fourth postoperative day. X-rays taken just prior to discharge showed

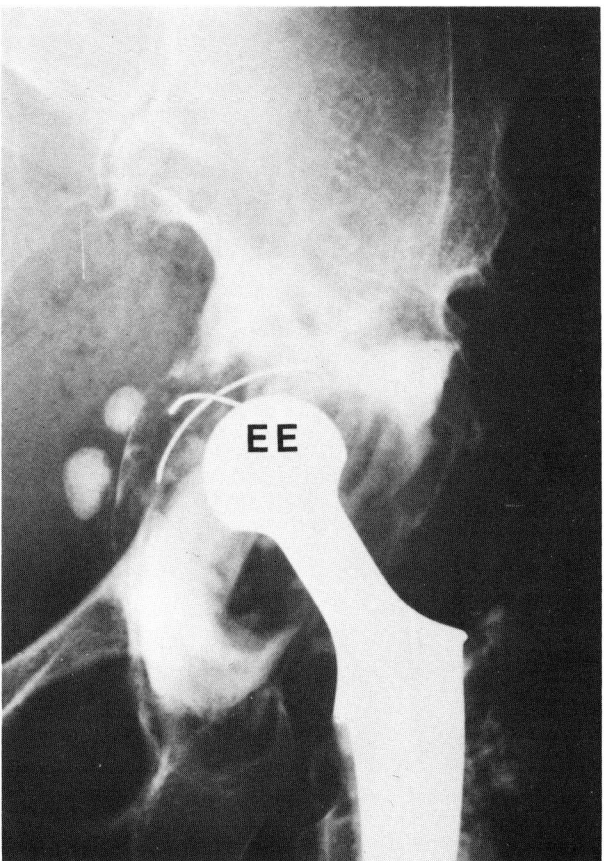

Figure 5-39A. This 53 year old woman presented with this loose acetabular component, twelve years after her primary total hip replacement for hip dysplasia. Note the striking osteolysis.

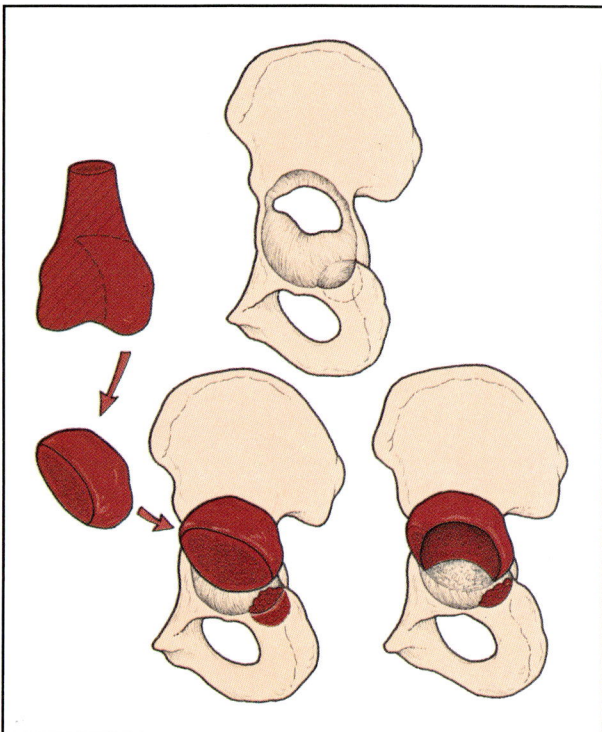

Figure 5-39B. The small posterior intra-acetabular defect in the ischium was packed with a mixture of autogenous and allograft morsellized bone. Cortical and cancellous strips were placed in the medial defect and then one large femoral condylar allograft was used to reconstruct the defects in the superior rim, the superior intra-acetabular area, and the perforation of the medial wall.

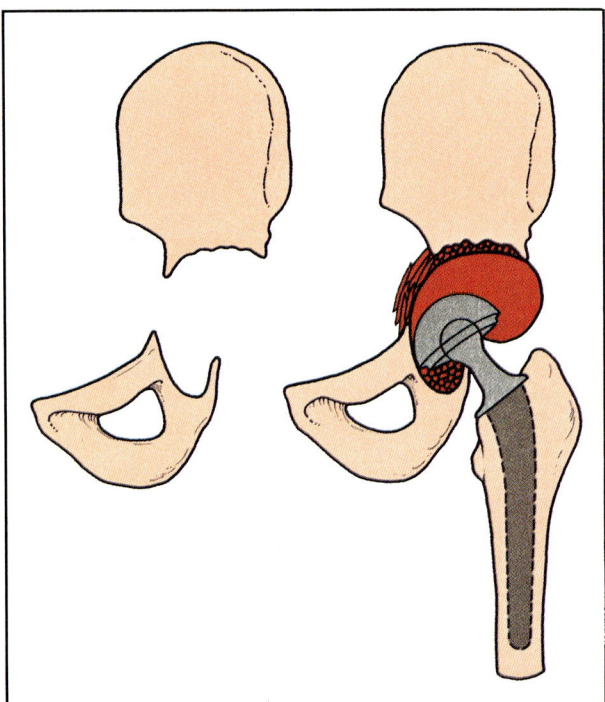

Figure 5-39C. Cancellous and cortical autograft strips from the ilium were used to graft the medial defect and a mixture of morsellized allograft and autograft bone was used in the superior and posterior intra-acetabular area before the femoral condylar allograft was inserted.

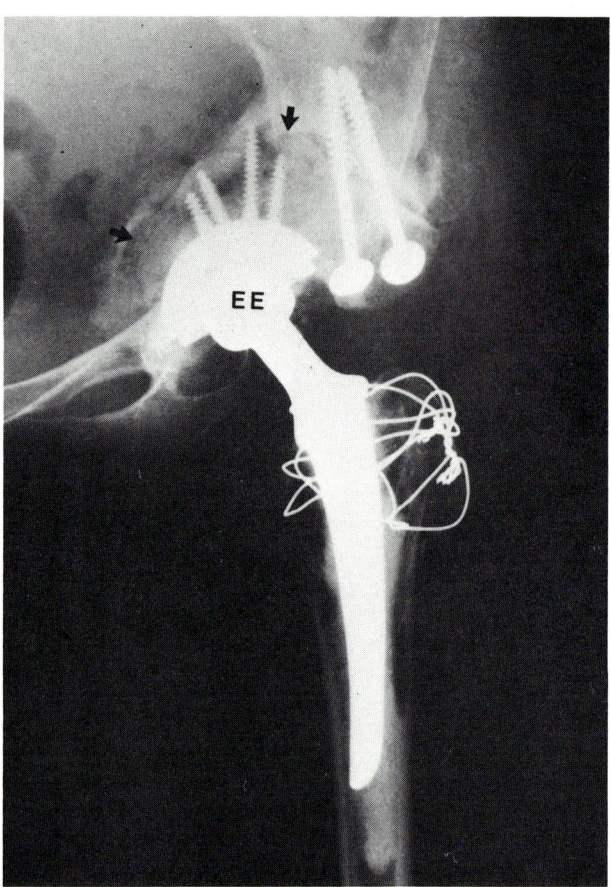

Figure 5-39D. Although there was lysis of the femur, the femoral component was not loose and was not changed. In this immediate post-operative x-ray, the area that was packed with morsellized bone (between the femoral allograft and the ilium) is evident. Some of the screws from the uncemented Harris Galante acetabular component (Zimmer, Warsaw, IN) aid in graft fixation.

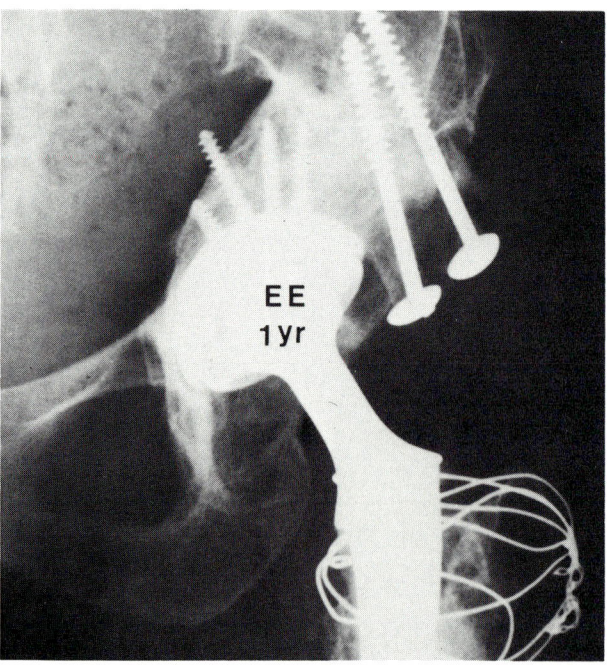

Figure 5-39E. At twelve months the graft appears to be incorporating well. The patient rates 98 on the Harris scale.

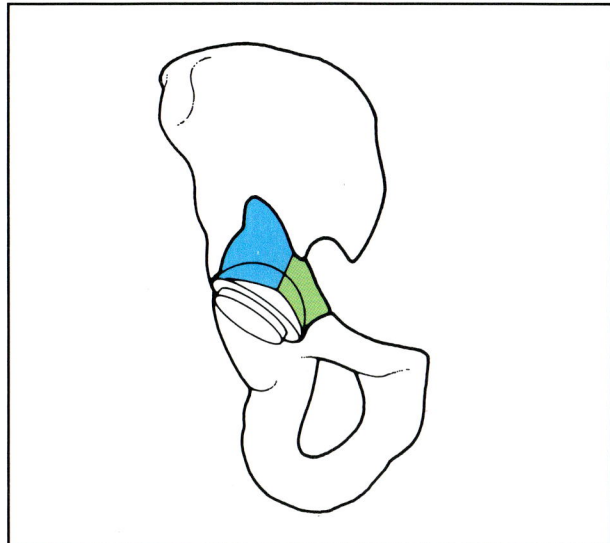

Figure 5-40. Superior intra-acetabular defects and perforations of the medial wall.

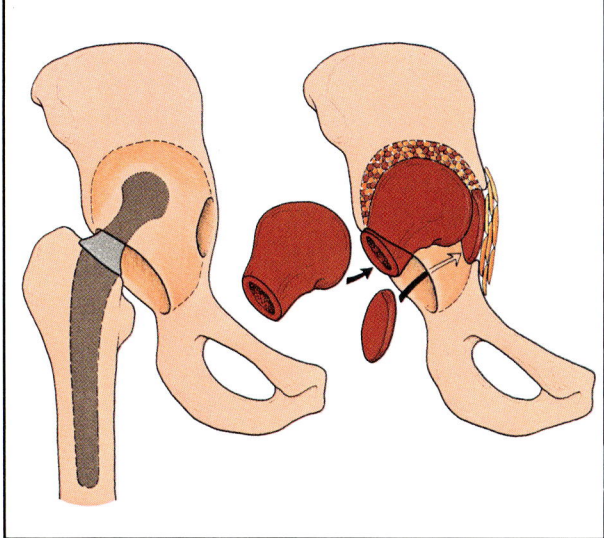

Figure 5-41B. The intact rim allowed containment of a large volume of mixed autologous and allograft morsellized cancellous bone which was impacted into the irregular surface of the roof of the major superior intra-acetabular defect. A large femoral head provided the structural strength to bring the center of rotation inferiorly. The medial perforation was filled with cortical and cancellous strips placed intrapelvically (through the defect) and a disc of allograft femoral head within the acetabulum was used to push the center of rotation laterally.

avulsion of the anterolateral crest of the ilium (Figures 5-41C and 5-41D), thus adding a lateral rim problem to the pre-existing superior intra-acetabular and medial wall defects. However, the patient was asymptomatic and the superior intra-acetabular graft and the acetabular component did not change position. Partial weight bearing (50 to 60 lbs) was continued. At eight weeks, x-rays showed no change and the patient used a cane for an additional month. X-rays at one year, seven months suggest that the acetabular component may have shifted more proximally and into more abduction along with the major superior intra-acetabular graft (Figure 5-41E). At followup of one year, eight months, the patient walks without support and without pain. She rates 94 but does have a mild abductor lurch, probably because of distal migration of the origin of the abductors when the crest avulsed.

Case 2

The patient seen in Figure 5-42A was 70 when she presented with loose acetabular and femoral components, four years after her first revision. Her complex femoral defect is discussed in the chapter on femoral problems (See Figure 6-17).

She had a modest superior intra-acetabular defect and a large medial perforation which was 2.5cm. in diameter. Cement and reinforcing mesh had protruded intrapelvically, and it was very difficult to remove this complex without damaging more acetabular stock. The Midas Rex (Midas Rex Institute, Fort Worth, TX) was extremely effective in cutting the composite of mesh and cement into small por-

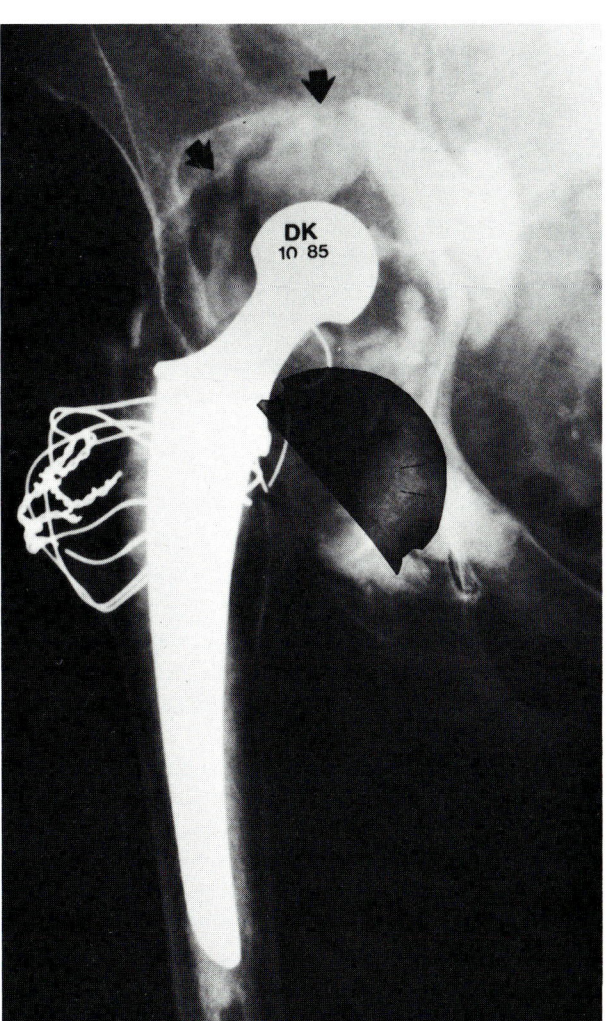

Figure 5-41A. This 73 year old woman presented with a loose acetabular component. The template points out the significance of the superior intra-acetabular defect. The perforation of the medial wall was 2cm. in diameter.

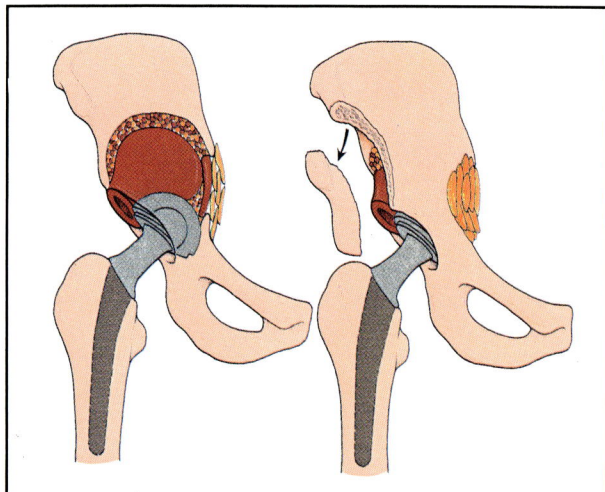

Figure 5-41C. Unfortunately, the anterior spine and anterior ilium avulsed, probably because the bone was weakened by harvesting of iliac crest strips. The defect was therefore converted to a superior rim defect as well as a superior intra-acetabular and a medial defect. Because the femoral head allograft was stable and provided both rim as well as superior intra-acetabular support, we elected to continue physical therapy and ambulation with crutches.

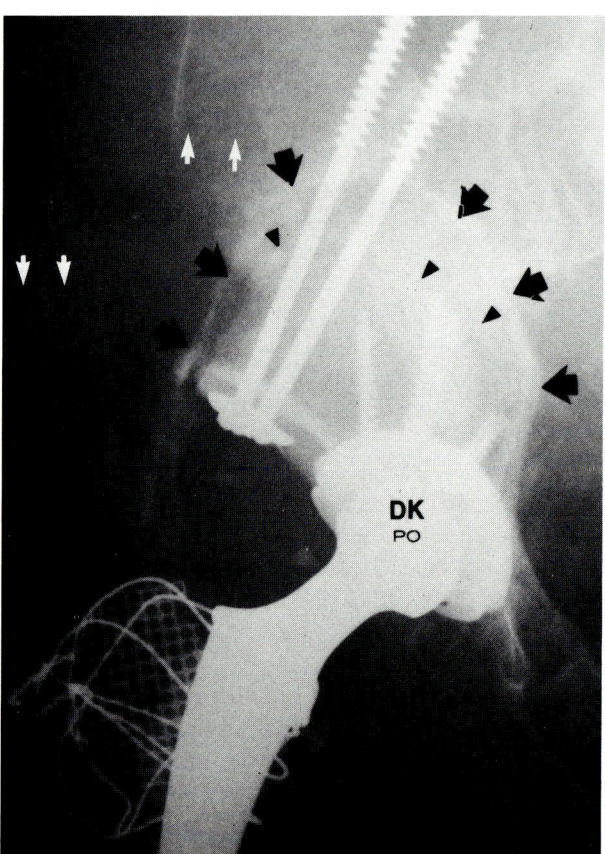

Figure 5-41D. X-rays at nine days show avulsion of the anterior spine and the anterior iliac crest (white arrows). The small black arrows outline the allograft femoral head. The large black arrows outline the superior intra-acetabular defect. Morsellized bone fills the space between. An uncemented acetabular component has 20% contact with living bone.

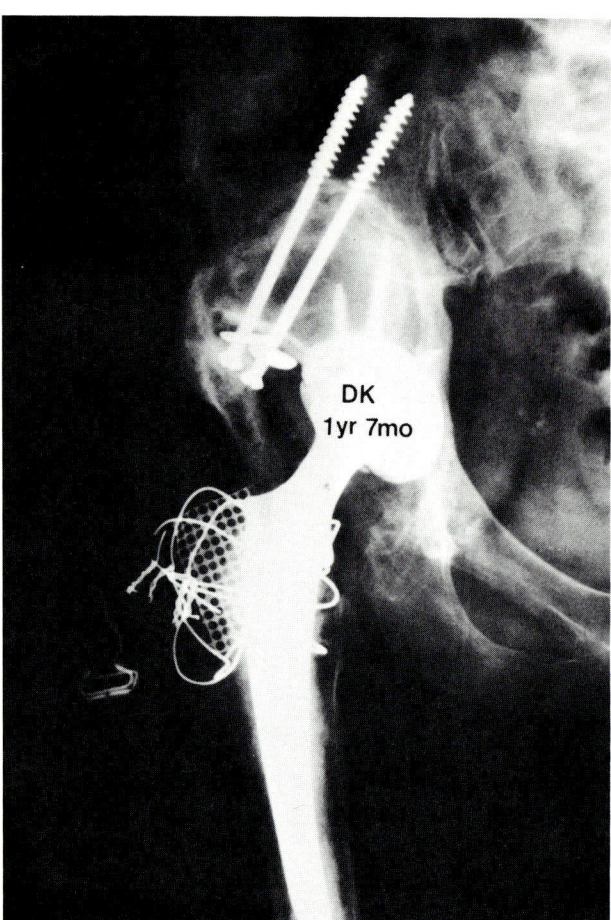

Figure 5-41E. At one year and seven months the grafts appear to be doing well. The medial defect appears to have healed. The avulsed anterior spine has united to the superior rim. The acetabular component probably has shifted into more abduction and, along with the major superior intra-acetabular graft, may have migrated superiorly (note the change in the relationship of the washers). However, the patient has no pain and walks without support. She does have a mild abductor lurch, probably because some of the abductor muscles are attached to the avulsed spine and crest. She rates 94.

tions that could eventually be retrieved. The medial perforation was occluded with cortical and cancellous strips from the iliac crest that were placed intrapelvically (through the defect). The superior acetabular defect was packed with a combination of autogenous and allograft morsellized bone (Figure 5-42B). An uncemented acetabular component was used. At seven weeks she was started on a cane (Figure 5-42C). At short followup of eight months, the medial wall of the acetabulum and the superior intra-acetabular area seem to be doing well (Figure 5-42D). She still uses a crutch for an unrelated ipsilateral foot problem but has no hip pain. She rates 88.

Case 3

The patient seen in Figure 5-43A was 74-years-old when she presented with loose acetabular and femoral components, two years following her first revision. Her complex

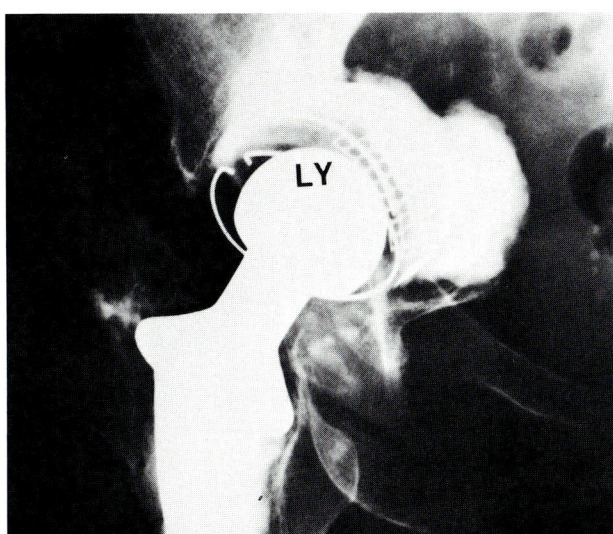

Figure 5-42A. This 70 year old woman presented with a loose acetabular component. The superior intra-acetabular defect was modest but the medial perforation was large (2.5cm.) and the cement and mesh were trapped within the pelvis. The Midas Rex (Midas Rex Institute, Fort Worth, TX) was extremely helpful in cutting the cement and mesh into small enough proportions to remove them without further damage to the medial wall.

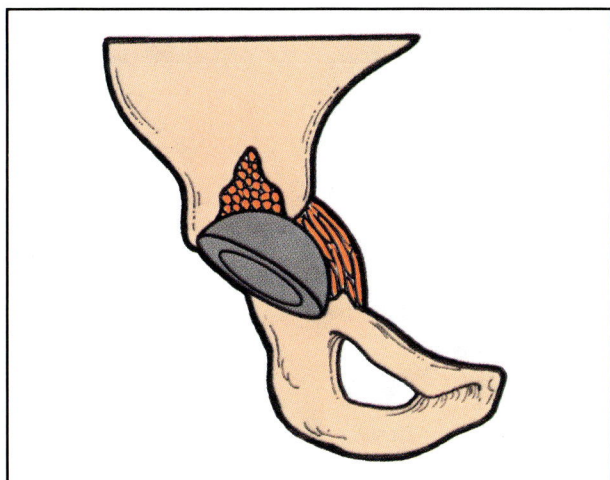

Figure 5-42B. The medial defect was filled with cortical and cancellous strips. The superior intra-acetabular defect was packed with a mixture of morsellized autograft and allograft cancellous bone.

femoral deficiency is discussed in the chapter on femoral reconstruction (See Figure 6-4).

The perforation of the medial wall defect was filled with cortical and cancellous strips from the iliac crest that were placed within the pelvis; the superior intra-acetabular defect was packed with a mixture of morsellized autogenous and allograft bone. The uncemented acetabular component had about 30% contact with living bone (Figure 5-43B).

At one year, the acetabular reconstruction appears to be doing well by x-ray (Figure 5-43C). This patient had a significant preoperative neurologic disorder characterized by choreiform and athetoid movements necessitating the

use of a walker for balance. Her rating is only 71 because of her neurologic status and limited walking tolerance. She has no pain, has been converted from a wheelchair existence to a household ambulator, and is pleased with her hip.

Global Deficiency (Figure 5-44)

Global defects (complex deficiencies of the anterior, superior and posterior rim, and the anterior superior and posterior intra-acetabular area) are surprisingly common. In our series there were ten patients (13%) with these complicated problems. The etiology in all cases was failure of a previously cemented total hip acetabular component.

Authors' Preferred Treatment. We prefer to use one of the transtrochanteric approaches for these extensive

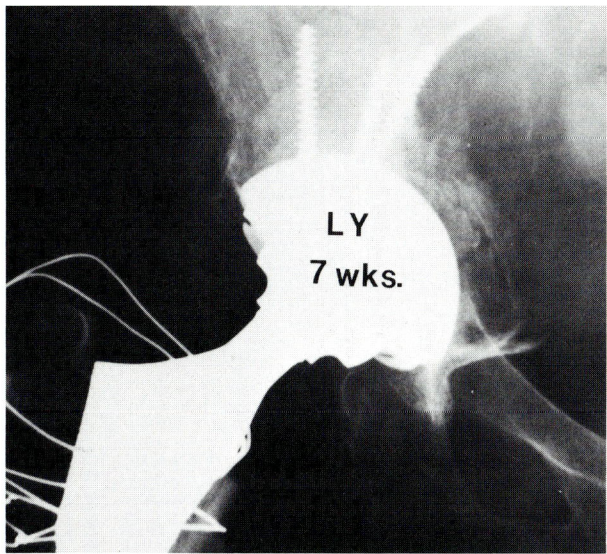

Figure 5-42C. At seven weeks, the acetabular grafts appear to be doing well and the patient was started on a cane.

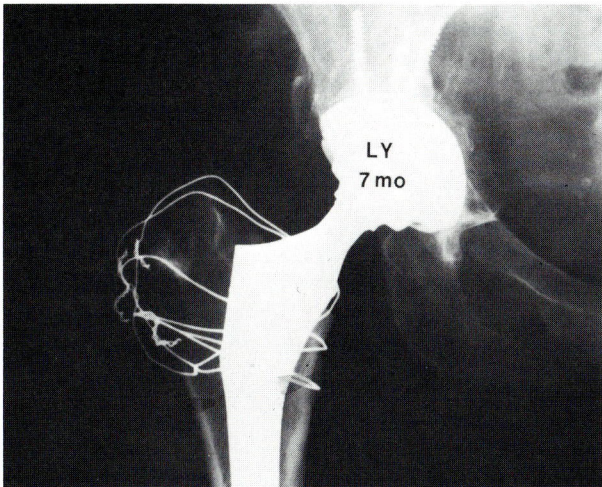

Figure 5-42D. At seven months, the acetabular reconstruction appears to be doing well. The patient still uses a crutch to protect an unrelated foot problem on the ipsilateral side, but can walk with a negative Trendelenburg gait without support. She rates 88.

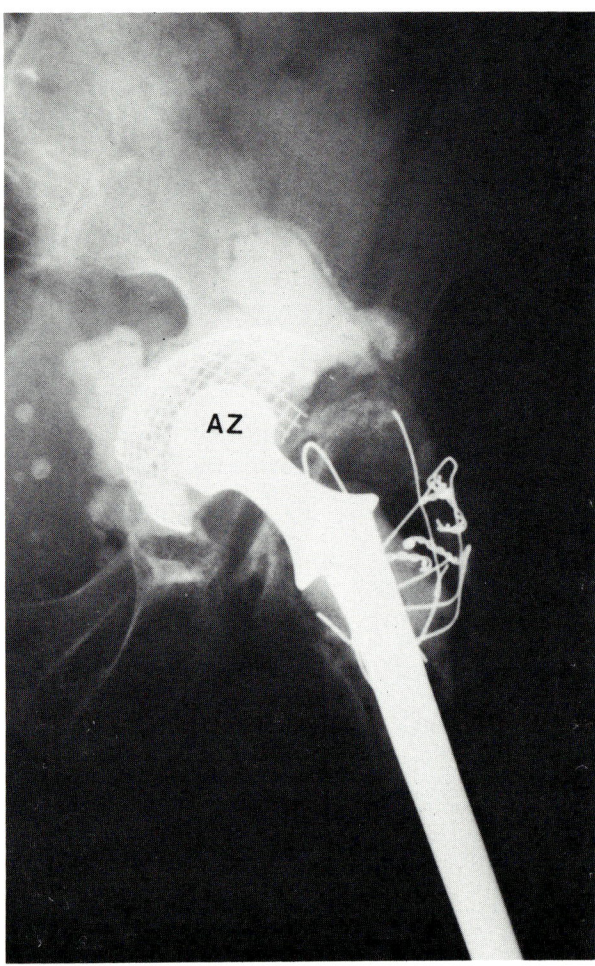

Figure 5-43A. This 74 year old woman had a 2.5cm. perforation of the medial wall. The superior intra-acetabular defect was also quite large, but there was bone available at the periphery that could support the new acetabular component.

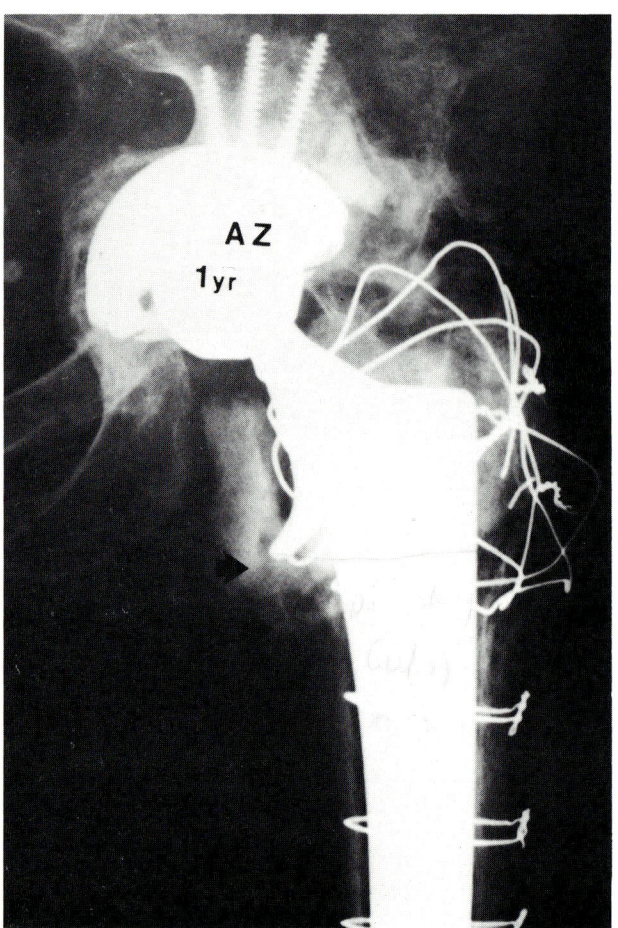

Figure 5-43C. The acetabular reconstruction appears to be doing well at one year. The patient had a severe neurological disorder pre-operatively and requires a walker for balance. She has limited motion because of heterotopic bone, but was converted from a wheelchair existence to a household ambulator. She rates only 71, but has no pain and is very pleased with her hip.

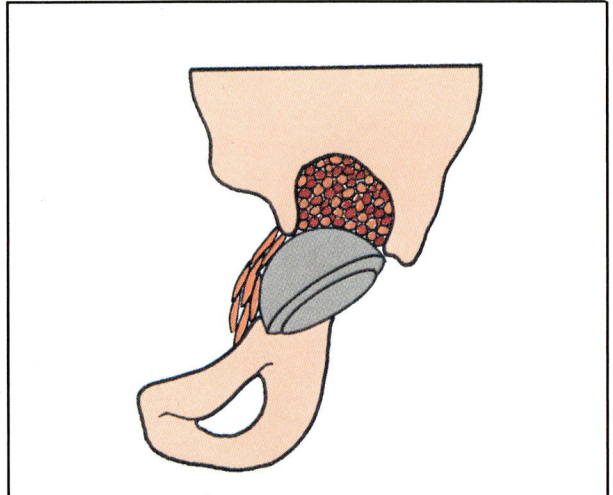

Figure 5-43B. The medial perforation was filled with cortical and cancellous strips from the ilium that were placed intra-pelvically. The superior intra-acetabular defect was packed with a mixture of autograft and allograft morsellized cancellous bone. An uncemented acetabular component was used.

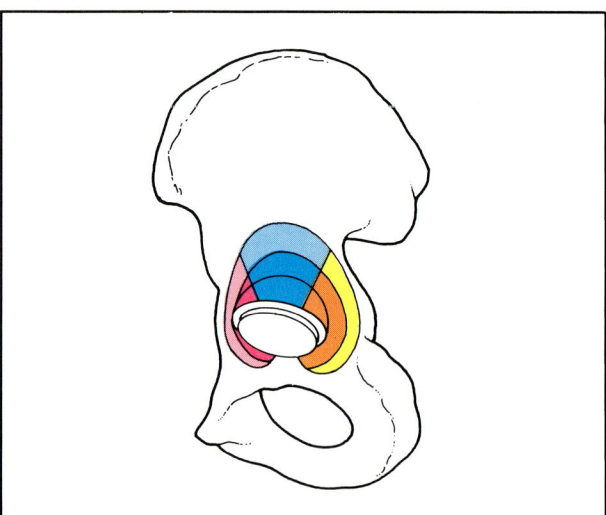

Figure 5-44. Global deficiency (complex deficiency of the anterior, superior, and posterior rim and the anterior, superior, and posterior intra-acetabular area).

defects. Since by definition, the superior rim and superior intra-acetabular area are lost, it is always necessary to reconstruct this defect with a solid graft. Because the patient's femoral head is almost always absent, an allograft is usually necessary. This graft must be large enough to reconstruct at least the superior rim and intra-acetabular bone stock but ideally provides material to reconstruct all the defects. It is possible with small defects to use a very large allograft femoral head to rebuild the acetabulum. Larger defects may need a distal femur or proximal tibia. As with all other allografts, we feel that it is important to use autologous bone from the iliac crest as well.

Although we initially felt that cement should be used if significant contact of a sintered surface with living bone could not be achieved, we now feel that uncemented acetabular components can be used almost routinely, even when less than one fifth of the surface is in contact with living bone.

Clinical Examples

Case 1

The patient whose x-rays are seen in Figure 5-45A was originally diagnosed as having pigmented villonodular synovitis. She was unsuccessfully treated by two prior mold arthroplasties. At the time of the last procedure, an extremely large cup was used. She presented with a stiff, painful hip at age 40. At the time of her operation, acetabular components large enough to fill the defect were not available. A very large allograft femoral head was reamed with a female cup reamer of the same outer diameter as her cup (Figure 5-45B). The graft was then placed into the deficient acetabulum and fixed with peripheral lag screws. It was then reamed in the usual fashion. X-rays immediately after her procedure (Figure 5-45C) clearly showed the line of demarcation between the graft and the acetabulum. Within a year, however, the graft seemed to be incorporating and the line was no longer obvious (Figure 5-45D). X-rays

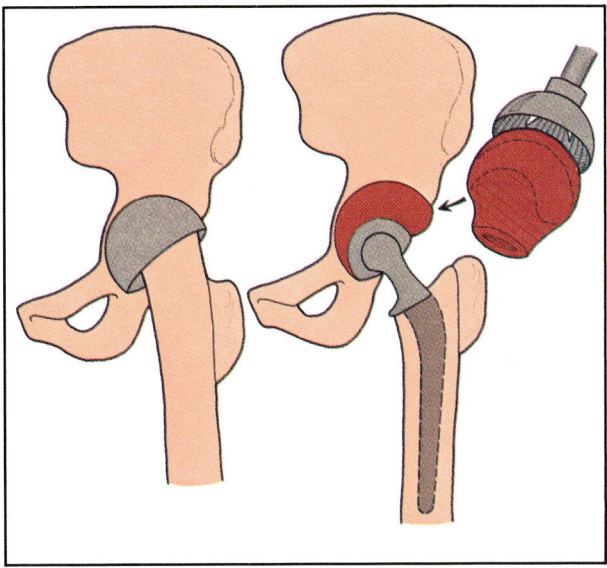

Figure 5-45B. A very large allograft femoral head was reamed with the female reamer that corresponded to the outer diameter of the cup.

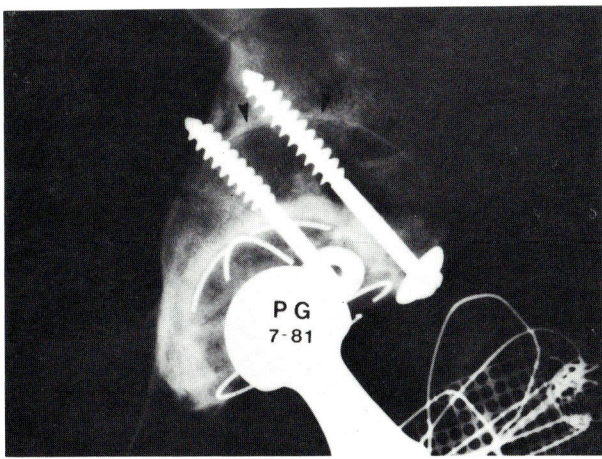

Figure 5-45C. Post-operative x-rays show the line of demarcation between the graft and the pelvis.

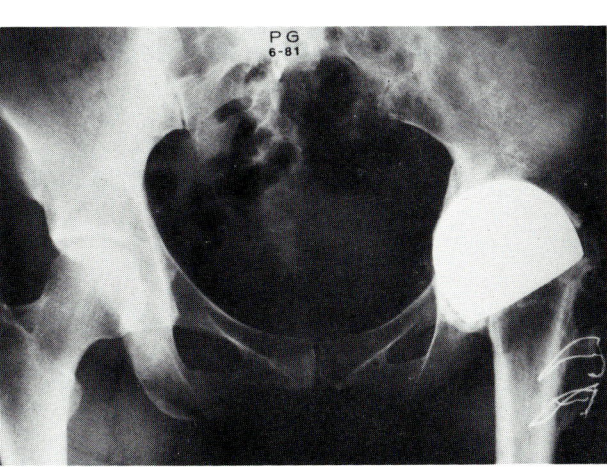

Figure 5-45A. This 40 year old woman had a painful left hip following two failed mold arthroplasties. At the time of her last procedure, a very large cup was used.

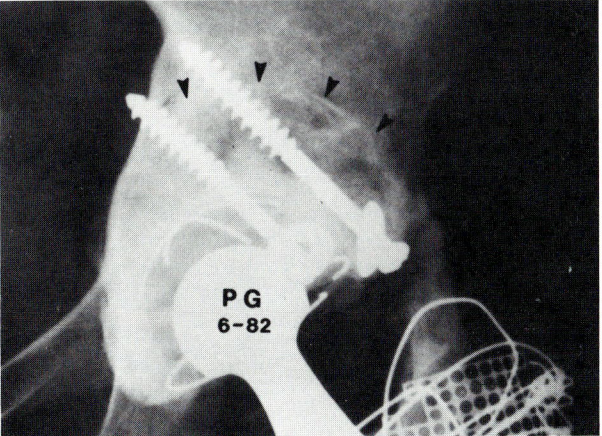

Figure 5-45D. Within one year, the interface is disappearing. Note the medial migration of the washers.

at five and one half years show that the graft appears to be doing very well (Figure 5-45E). At followup of six years, the patient has no pain in her hip but has limited motion because of the bar of heterotopic bone that is attached to the greater trochanter. Despite her poor motion, she is pleased with her function and rates 85. We plan to remove the heterotopic bone in the future. In this patient there was no contact of the acetabular component with living bone and cement was used. Faced with the same problem now, we would use a very large uncemented acetabular component without a bone graft. A longer neck on the femoral component would be necessary to re-establish the proper leg length.

Case 2

The patient seen in Figure 5-46A was 44 when he presented with pain and recurrent dislocation of his right hip. He had undergone a variety of operations following his original diagnosis of Legg-Calve-Perthes disease. These included a Moore prosthesis, an arthrodesis, four cup arthroplasties and three total hip replacements. At the time of his last revision, 75mm. outer diameter custon acetabular

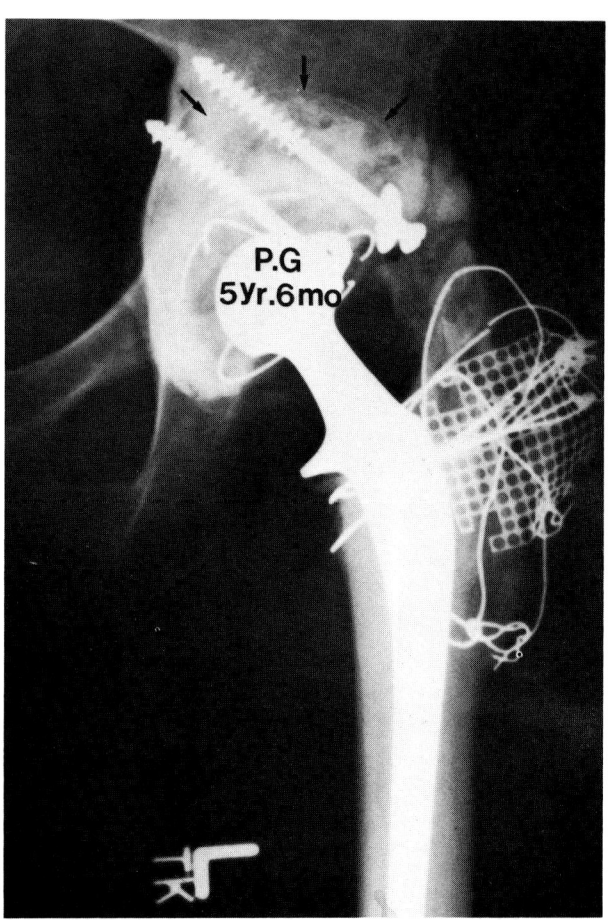

Figure 5-45E. At five years and six months, the graft appears to be doing well. Motion is limited because of the bar of heterotopic bone that extends upward from the greater trochanter, but the patient has no pain and has walked without support and with a normal gait since her two month office visit. She rates 85.

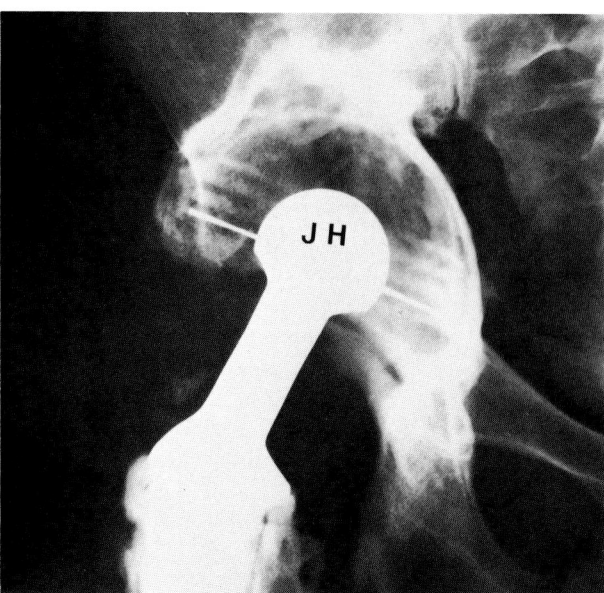

Figure 5-46A. This 44 year old man presented with a loose 75mm. custom acetabular ccmponent. Because the component was not flexed enough, he dislocated daily but could reduce the hip himself.

component and a 30cm. long stem cemented femoral component were used. Both components were loose. His complex femoral defect is discussed in the chapter on femoral problems (See Figure 6-8).

With acetabular defects of this magnitude, it is impossible to find a femoral head large enough to reconstruct the rim and we elected to use a distal femur including both condyles. Since a concave reamer of this magnitude was not available, the graft was shaped by means of an oscillating saw and the Midas Rex (Midas Rex Institute, Fort Worth, TX). The intercondylar notch was grafted with an additional block of allograft bone (Figure 5-46B). Fixation was achieved by the standard methods. Autograft from the iliac crest was added. Cement was used as there was no contact of the acetabular component with viable bone.

Bccausc of thc difficulty in removing a cemented long stem prosthesis that is well fixed distal to the isthmus and loose proximally, we did not change this component. Unfortunately the patient has thigh pain and rates only 72; however, the acetabular graft appears to be doing well by x-ray at short follow-up of one year, seven months (Figure 5-46C). We would now use a very large uncemented acetabular component without a graft but such components were not available at the time of the patient's surgery.

Case 3

The patient seen in Figure 5-47A was 62 when she presented with a Moore prosthesis that had migrated proximally to the level of the anterior spine. There was no bone available at the level of the original acetabulum except for the flat medial wall of the ilium. Her original diagnosis of slipped epiphysis was treated by fixation with a Smith-Petersen nail. She had two other childhood operations and

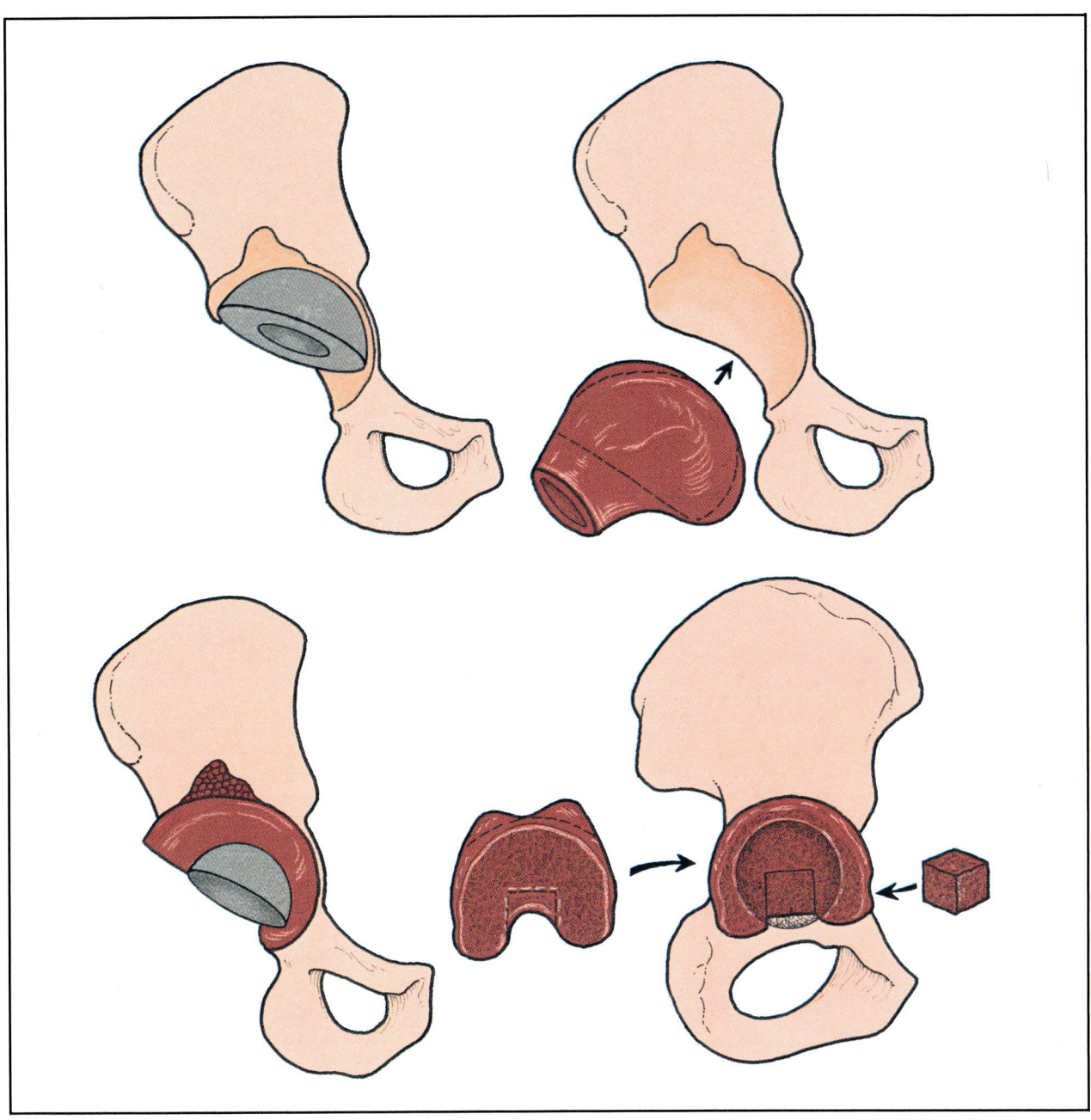

Figure 5-46B. A distal femur, includinb toh condyles, was used to reconstruct the rim and intra-acetabular defects. Morsellized bone was used to fill the small superior intra-acetabular defects. A block of allograft bone was used to fill the intercondylar notch. Since there was no contact of the acetabular component with living bone, cement was used.

then four cup arthroplasties with significant proximal femoral loss (Figure 5-47B). The final operation prior to her bone grafting procedure was the insertion of a custom long stem uncemented Moore prosthesis. She required two axillary crutches for the 22 years that this prosthesis was in place. Her complex femoral problem is discussed in the femoral reconstruction section (See Figure 6-19).

In this global acetabular defect, we used a distal femur with the inferior aspect of the condyles oriented laterally. The cortical bone of the distal shaft of the allograft femur was buttressed beneath the area of her false acetabulum and then the graft was fixed in the usual way. It was necessary to

use another allograft from the same femur to reconstruct the posterior acetabular rim (Figure 5-47C). Approximately one fifth of the uncemented acetabular component was in contact with living bone and the remainder with allograft. The acetabular component is abducted too much and the patient had three dislocations in the first six months but has been stable for the subsequent 16 months. At one year, ten months, the graft appears to be doing well (Figure 5-47D). The patient has normal motion and no pain but still has an abductor lurch because of abductor weakness. Her strength is improving but she still needs support for most walking. Because of carpal tunnel syndrome, the patient prefers to

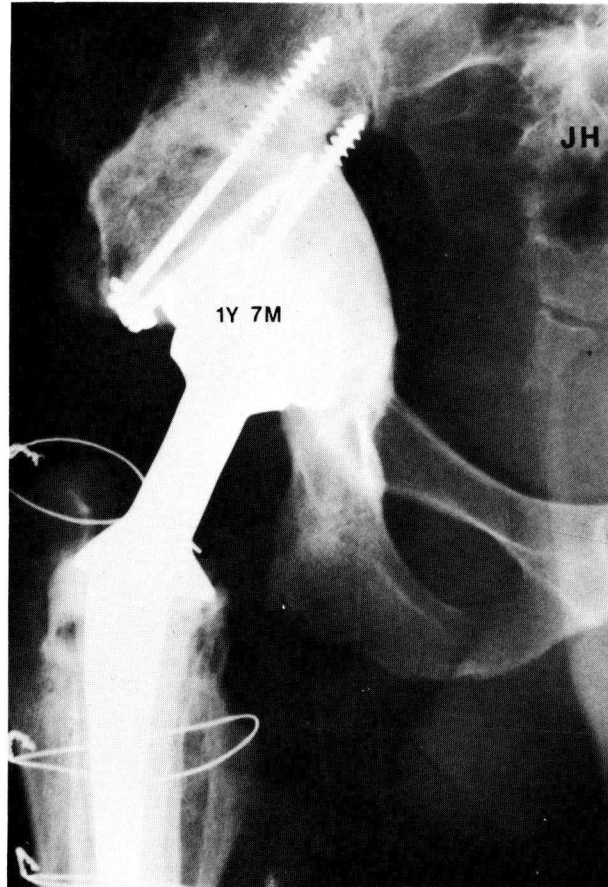

Figure 5-46C. At follow-up of one year and seven months, the acetabular graft appears to be incorporating. Unfortunately the patient still has pain in his thigh, probably due to a loose femoral component. He rates only 72 on the Harris scale.

use a crutch to a cane. However she ambulates as well with the cane as she does with the crutch. She is able to walk one half mile and rates 82.

Case 4

The patient seen in Figure 5-48A presented at age 37 with a loose acetabular component and a loose proximal femoral replacement component. Her care was further complicated by the fact that she had polio at age two with significant weakness of the ipsilateral lower extremity. At age 13, she had an arthrodesis of her hip which was successful until her early twenties when she fell and sustained a subtrochanteric fracture. Several attempts at attaining union were unsuccessful and a cemented long stem proximal femoral replacement prosthesis was inserted ten years prior to presentation for her current reconstruction. The acetabular component was revised twice and an attempt was made to rebuild the superior and posterior rims by means of cement, mesh, and wires. At least one of the wires impaled the sciatic nerve and destroyed what residual motor power she had left in that extremity. She was left with a flail extremity with intractable pain from her hip and from her sciatic nerve injury. She had a history of addiction to a

variety of narcotics but by the time of admission had been weaned to 12 60mg codeine tablets a day. Her sedimentation rate was 125 and aspiration proved that she had an alpha streptococcus infection. She refused hind quarter amputation. Her complex femoral problem will be discussed in the section on femoral grafts (See Figure 6-21).

Her infection was treated by removal of the components, extensive debridement, insertion of tobramycin-impregnated methylmethacrylate beads and six weeks of intravenous antibiotic therapy (Figure 5-48B). At six weeks, a distal femur was used to reconstruct the global rim, intra-acetabular, and medial wall deficiencies (Figure 5-48C). Due to her muscle weakness, a bipolar prosthesis was chosen because of its inherent stability. Her pelvis was so small that there was no room for screws at the periphery of the reamed acetabulum. The acetabular graft was therefore

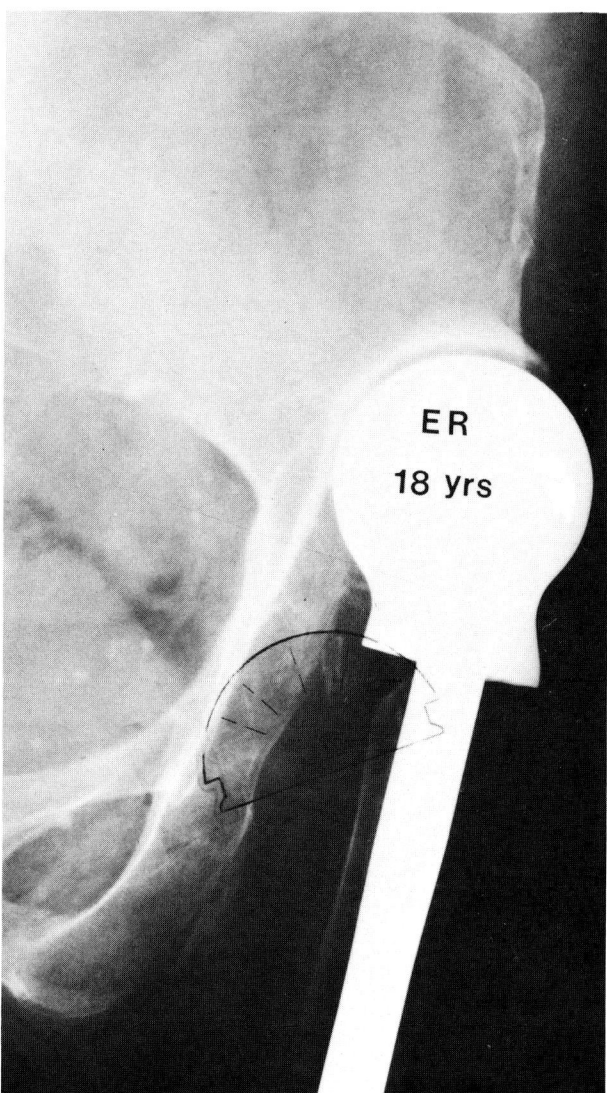

Figure 5-47A. After eighteen years, a custom long stem Moore prosthesis had migrated proximally to the level of the anterior superior spine. There is a global defect with complete loss of the entire rim and intra-acetabular area. Note the striking stress shielding of the femur.

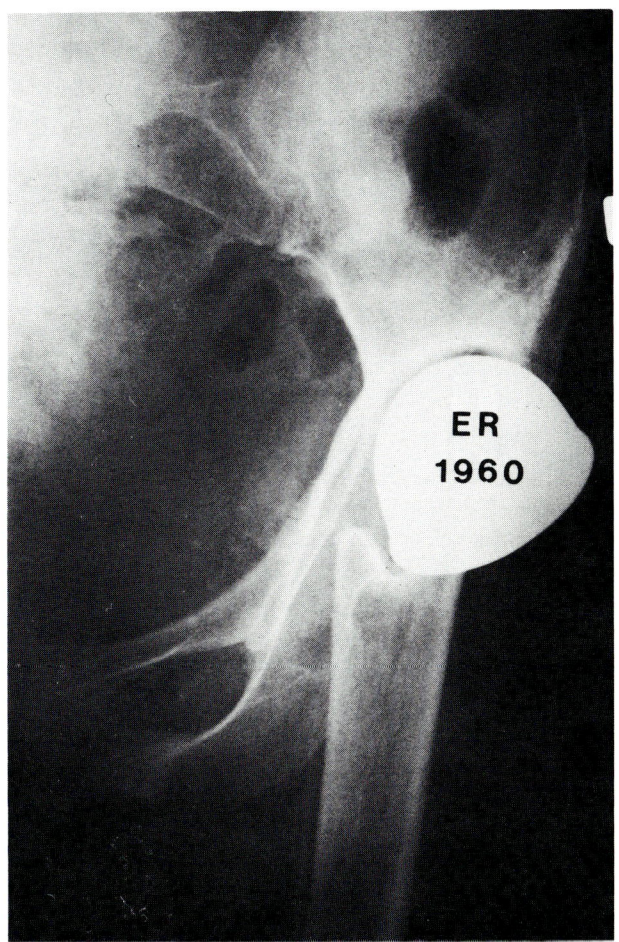

Figure 5-47B. There was significant acetabular erosion as well as proximal femoral bone loss after her last cup arthroplasty. The femoral cortices were somewhat thin even then.

reamed before it was placed in the patient. It was temporarily fixed with crossed K-wires and then held with three screws that were countersunk within the acetabulum.

At four months, the sedimentation rate was 11 and the patient was doing well (Figure 5-48D). At 12 months she fell and sustained an anterior dislocation (Figure 5-48E). A closed reduction was performed (Figure 5-48F). The patient was placed in an abduction brace for six weeks. At followup of 18 months there have been no further dislocations. The sedimentation rate remains normal. The patient has no hip pain. Her sciatic distribution pain improved when the K-wires were removed from the nerve but she still has residual pain in the sciatic distribution of her foot and takes an average of 20 codeine 30mg tablets each month. She will always require two axillary crutches because of total paralysis of the extremity and rates 74.

Case 5

The patient shown in Figure 5-49A was 24 when he presented with complex acetabular and femoral defects. At age 19 he sustained a posterior fracture-dislocation of his hip. An attempt at arthrodesis was unsuccessful. He then had a total hip replacement with two subsequent revisions, including a femoral head allograft to reconstruct the superior rim and intra-acetabular area. Unfortunately he developed a staphylococcal infection and required a resection arthroplasty. Reconstruction of his femur is discussed in the section on femoral defects (See Figure 6-18).

The acetabular defect extended to the anterior spine with total loss of the rim and intra-acetabular area and only the flat ilium remained. There was a small medial perforation as well. This global defect was dealt with by means of an

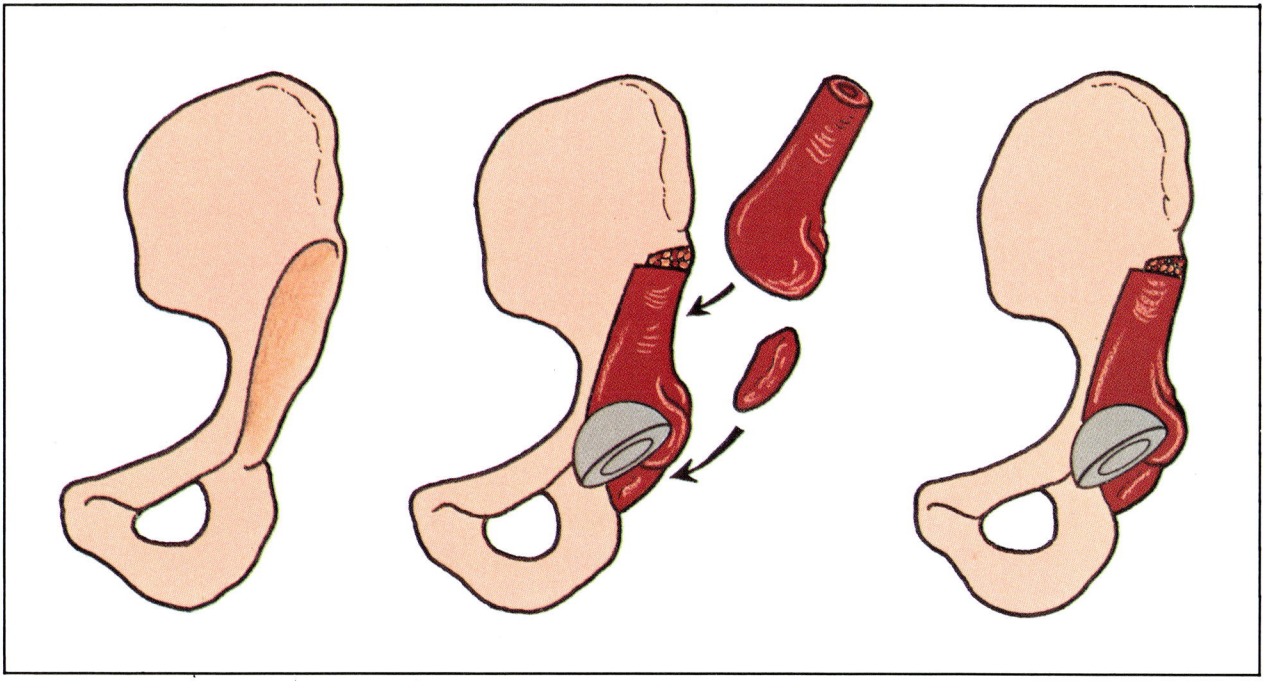

Figure 5-47C. A distal femur was butted against the superior aspect of her false acetabulum and provided superior intra-acetabular superior rim stock. A posterior rim and intra-acetabular deficiency required a separate allograft.

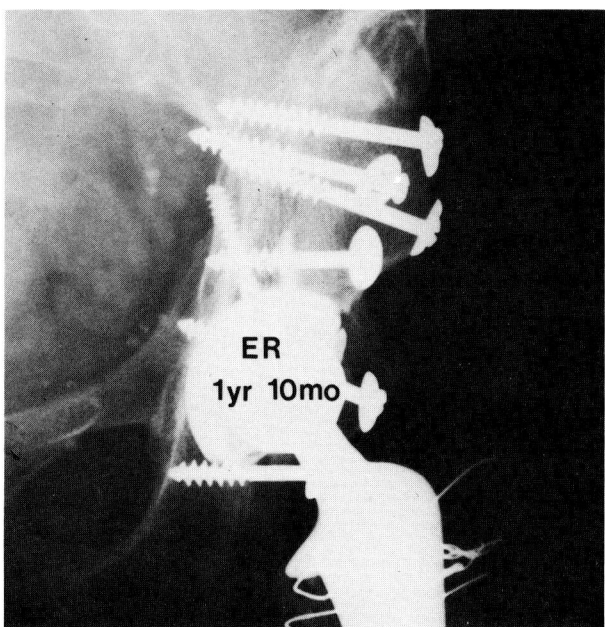

Figure 5-47D. The uncemented acetabular component is in contact with one-fifth living bone. Unfortunately, it was placed in too much abduction and the hip dislocated three times but has been stable for sixteen months. At one year and ten months, the graft appears to be doing well. The patient rates 82.

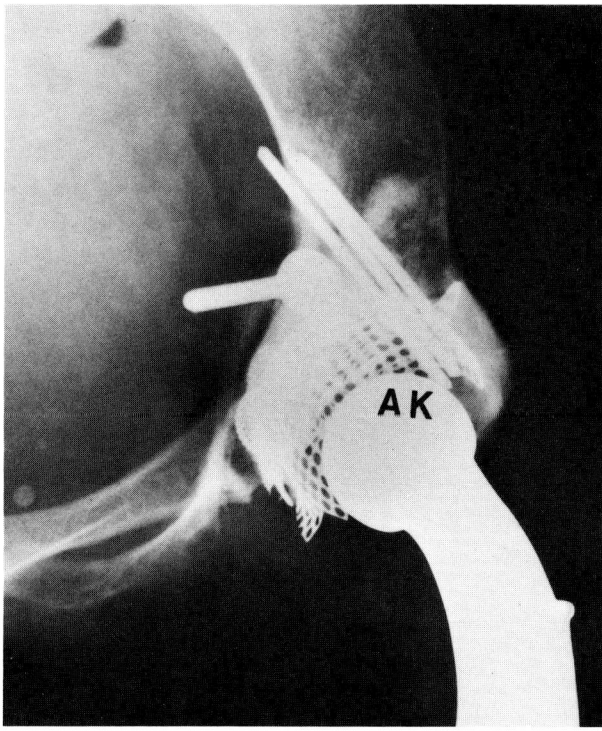

Figure 5-48A. This 37 year old woman with childhood polio had this acetabular component inserted ten years before presentation. The K-wires above the acetabulum had impaled the sciatic nerve and the combination of this injury and her polio caused this extremity to be completely flail. She had intractable hip pain as well as sciatic pain which radiated to her toes. She was addicted to twelve 60mg. codeine tablets a day. Aspiration proved she had an alpha streptococcus infection. There was global loss of the rim and intra-acetabular bone stock.

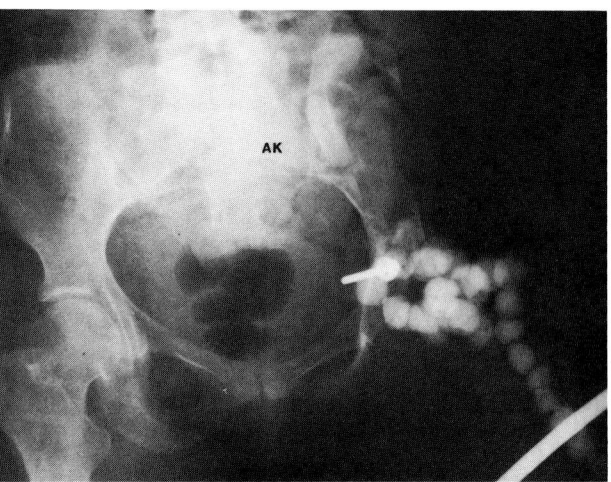

Figure 5-48B. The infection was treated by removal of the components, debridement, insertion of Tobramycin impregnated beads, and six weeks of intravenous antibiotics.

allograft proximal tibia positioned with the articular surface facing inferiorly (Figure 5-49B). It was wedged against the roof of his old acetabulum and was fixed with four screws. An uncemented Harris-Galante acetabulum (Zimmer, Warsaw, IN) was used and had less than one fifth of its surface in contact with living bone (Figure 5-49C).

Early in his postoperative course this patient dislocated on four separate occasions and subluxed repeatedly. At followup of one year, seven months, the acetabular graft is doing well but the acetabular component is loose and has shifted into abduction. There has been slight proximal migration of the component as well (Figure 5-49D). The patient has intermittent jolts of groin pain with certain position changes but does not take analgesics. He uses a cane for long walks because of abductor weakness. He rates 67 and is scheduled for revision.

Column Defects

Column defects consist of anterior or posterior rim and intra-acetabular defects in conjunction with major medial perforation, resulting in discontinuity between the iliac and the pubic and or ischial segments. Fortunately such extensive bone loss is not a very common problem and occurred in only one patient (1.3%) in our series. We have recently operated on two other patients with column defects but followup is too short to include them in this report.

Authors' Preferred Treatment. These extensive defects require extensive exposure and we prefer one of the transtrochanteric approaches. There is no alternative to solid bone grafting in these cases. Metallic devices, used alone or with cement, cannot be supported by the available bone. A single femoral head is rarely large enough; it is usually necessary to use two heads, a femoral condyle, or a whole acetabular allograft. Fixation can be provided by screws alone or screws in conjunction with an acetabular reconstruction plate.

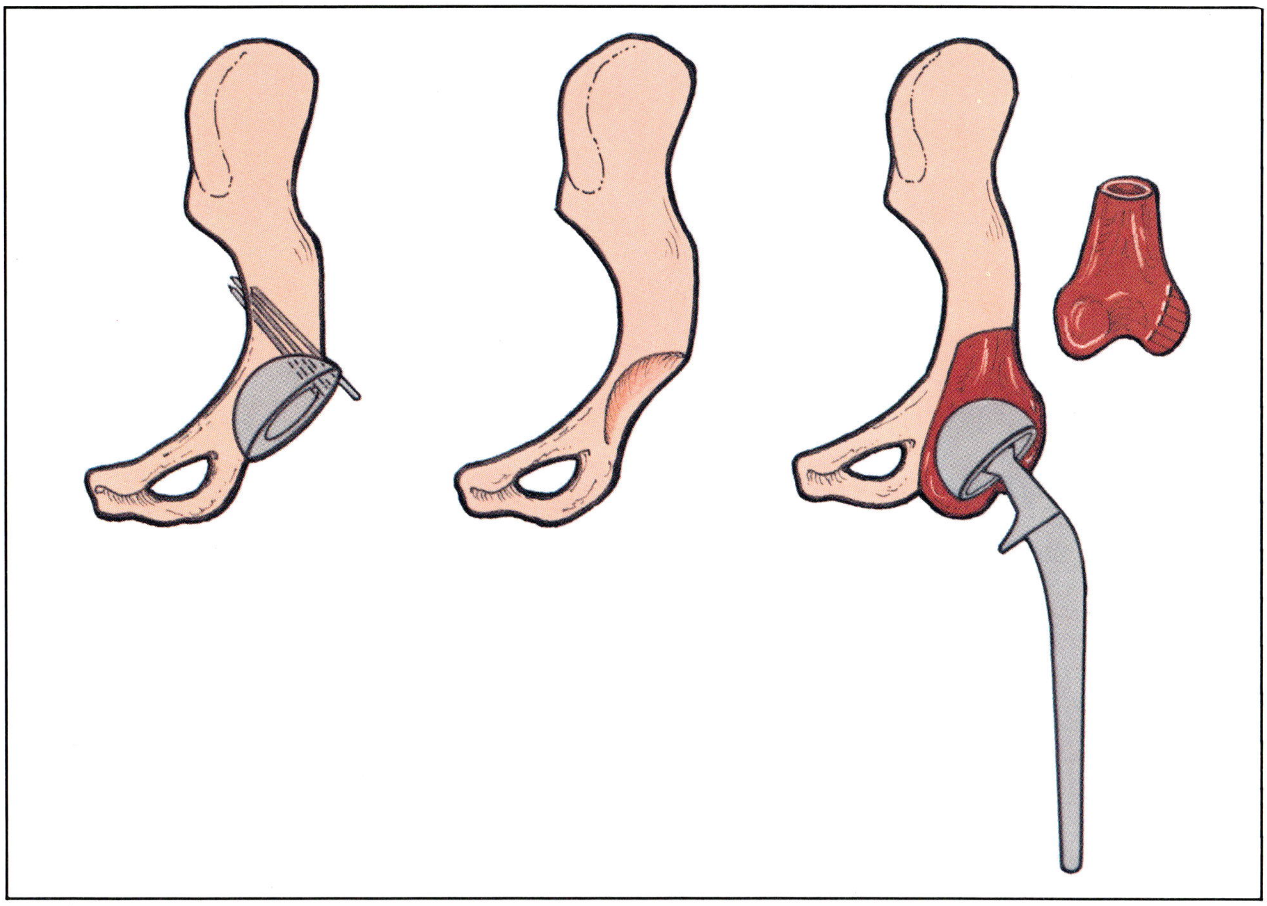

Figure 5-48C. A distal femur was used to reconstruct the intra-acetabular and superior rim bone. In view of her completely paralyzed extremity, a bipolar prothesis was used because of its inherent stability.

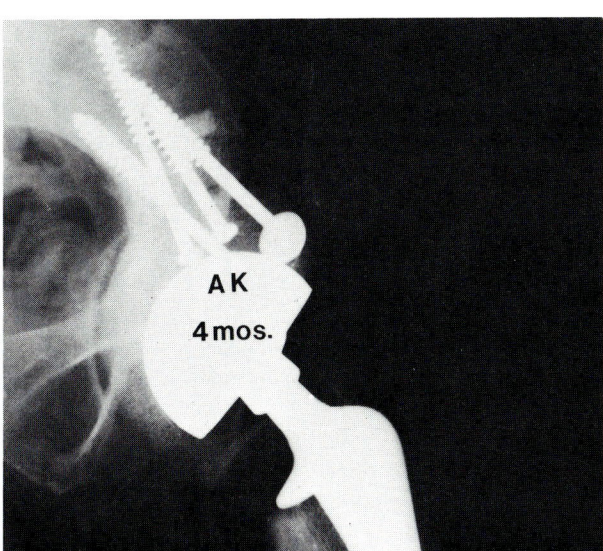

Figure 5-48D. At four months, the sedementation rate was 11. There is still a gap medially, but superiorly the graft appears to be uniting.

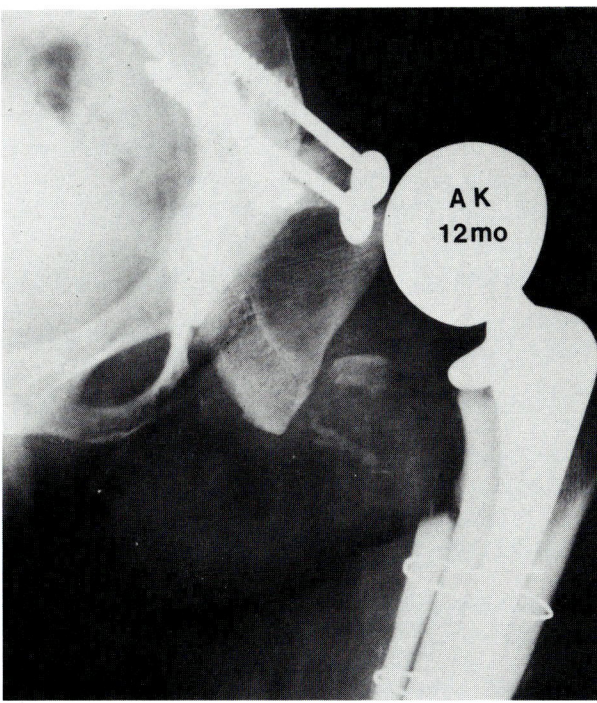

Figure 5-48E. Unfortunately she fell at one year and sustained an anterior dislocation of her hip. The dislocation allowed good x-ray evaluation of the acetabular graft.

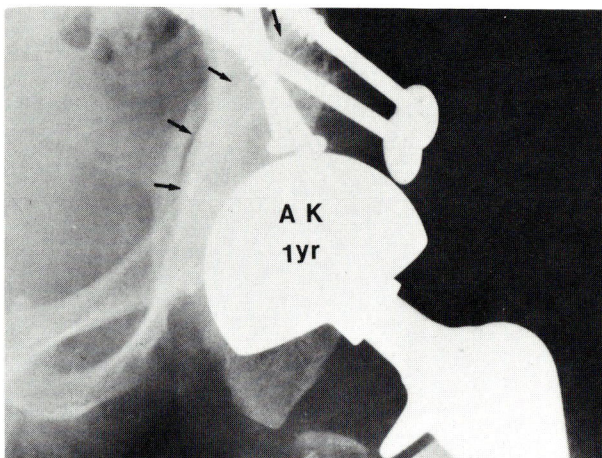

Figure 5-48F. Post-reduction films show that there is still a gap medially, but superiorly the graft appears to be uniting.

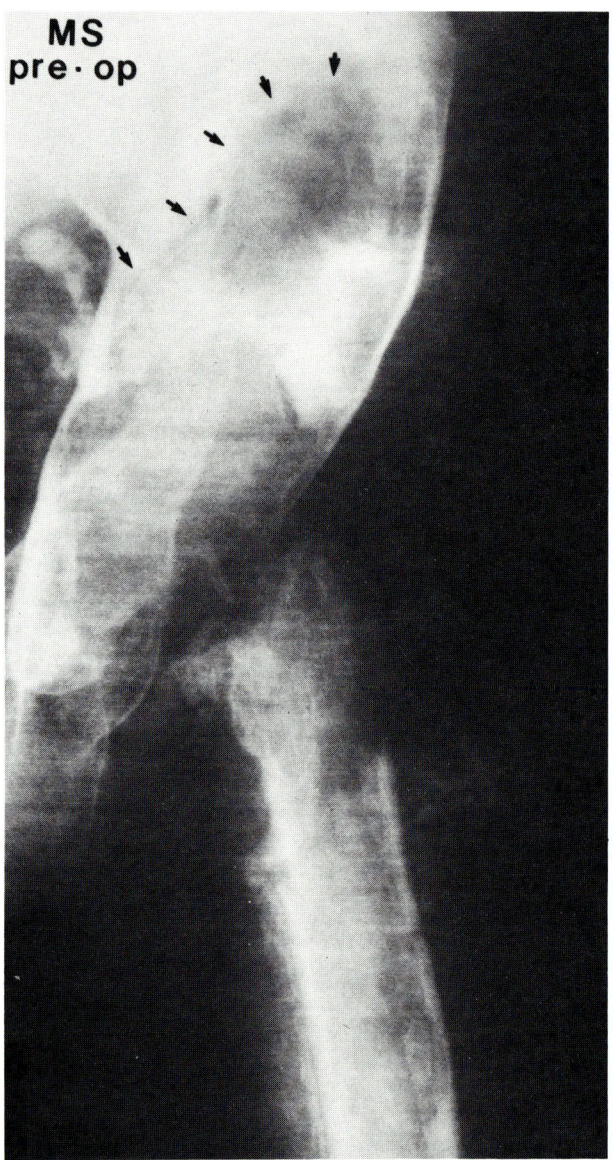

Figure 5-49A. This 23 year old man presented with complex acetabular and femoral defects following multiple hip operations culminating in a resection arthroplasty for staphlyococcus sepsis.

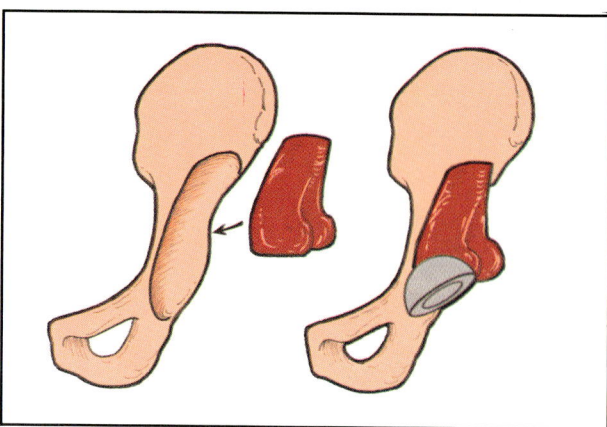

Figure 5-49B. An allograft proximal tibia was used to reconstruct the rim and the intra-acetabular area. The articular surface was oriented inferiorly, and proximally the diaphysis was wedged beneath the remnants of the false acetabulum.

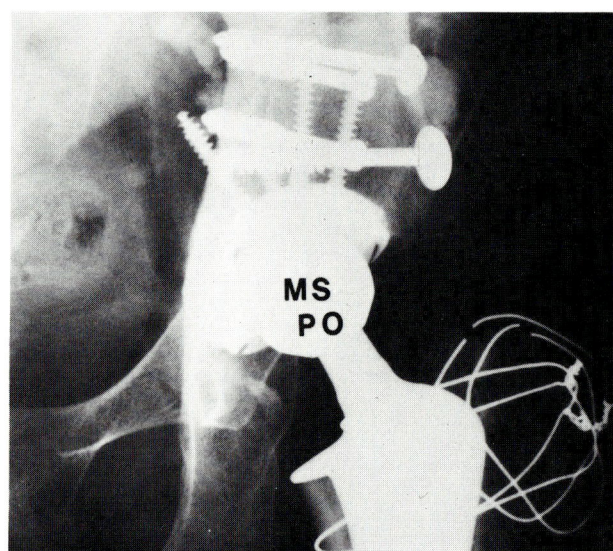

Figure 5-49C. The proximal tibial allograft provided enough stock to reconstruct the entire rim and intra-acetabular area. Less than one-fifth of the uncemented acetabular component was in contact with living bone.

Clinical Examples

Case 1

The patient seen in Figure 5-50A was 67 at the time of revision surgery for a loose acetabular and femoral component. A femoral perforation occurred when the cement was being removed. This defect was reconstructed by means of an onlay cortical strut and an uncemented femoral prosthesis was used.

There was a significant anterior rim and anterior intra-acetabular defect that in combination with a small medial perforation, comprised an anterior column defect (Figure 5-50B). This very large defect could not be filled with one femoral head and we elected to use two large allograft femoral heads. These were split so that two thirds of each of the two heads were preserved. When these grafts were

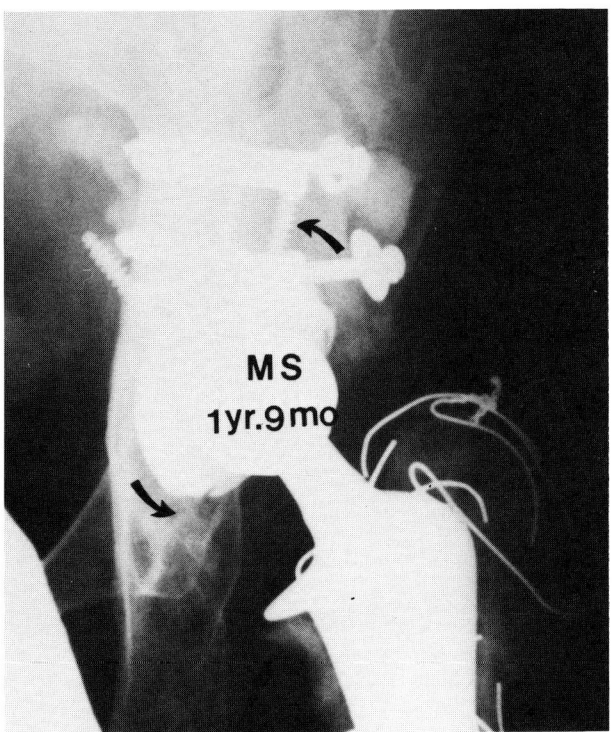

Figure 5-49D. At follow-up of one year and nine months, the acetabular graft appears to be doing well, but the acetabular component has shifted into abduction and has migrated proximally. The patient rates 67 and is scheduled for acetabular revision.

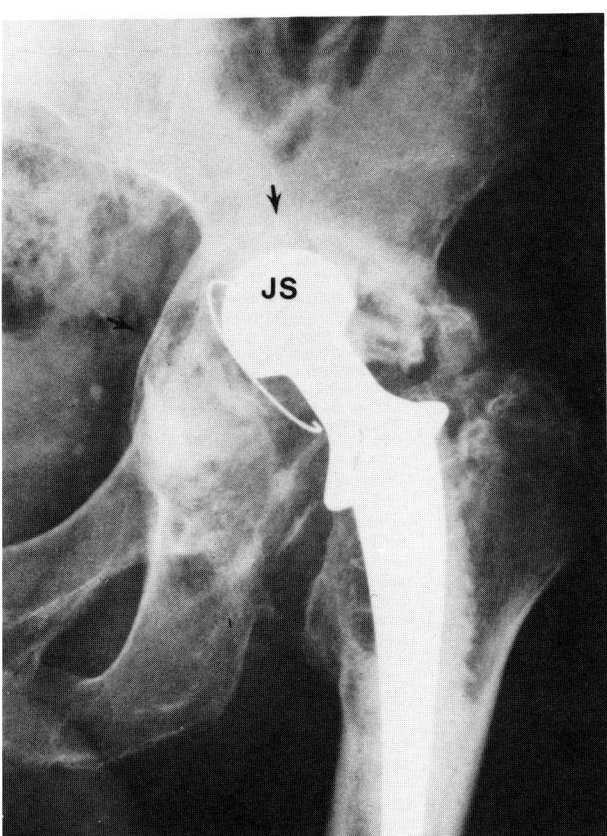

Figure 5-50A. This 67 year old man had a loose acetabular and femoral component.

combined, they provided a very large anterior posterior dimension (Figure 5-50C). Cancellous and cortical strips were used to repair the anterior and medial wall perforations and morsellized autogenous and allograft bone was used superiorly to fill the small irregularities (Figure 5-50D). After the posterior graft was placed in position, the second (anterior) graft was inserted and impacted. The two grafts were extremely stable, even before fixation with two extra cancellous screws in the periphery of the acetabulum.

This patient unfortunately had a significant cerebral vascular accident on the second postoperative day, leaving him with weakness of the ipsilateral upper and lower extremity and with major loss of speech and intellectual function. He slowly recovered and by eight weeks had no residual motor weakness but has some permanent intellectual and speech deficit. His hip recovered uneventfully despite this problem and by eight weeks he discarded crutches and has not used support for this hip since. He has psoriatic arthritis involving his opposite ankle and now uses a cane to protect this extremity. He has no pain in his operated hip and at short term followup of one year and three months his graft

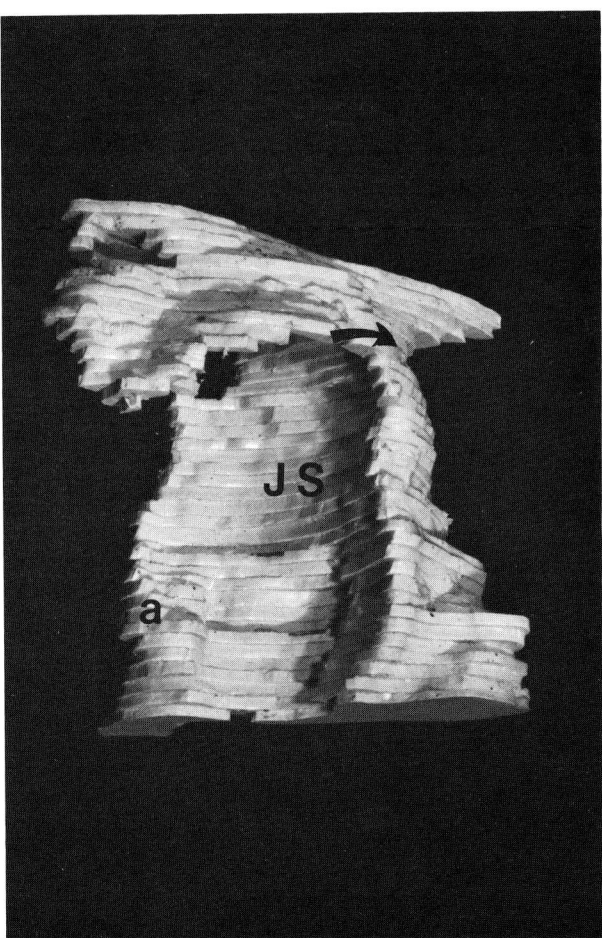

Figure 5-50B. A computer generated pre-operative model showed a large intra-acetabular defect as well as an anterior rim defect that, together with an anteromedial perforation, comprised an anterior column defect. The superior arrow points to the sciatic notch.

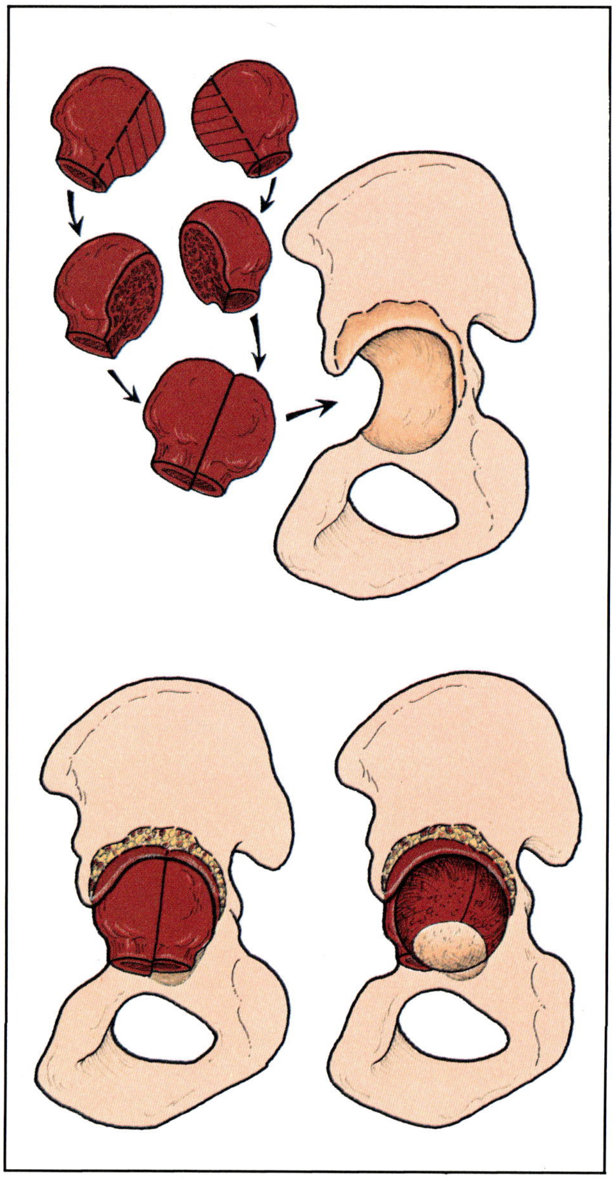

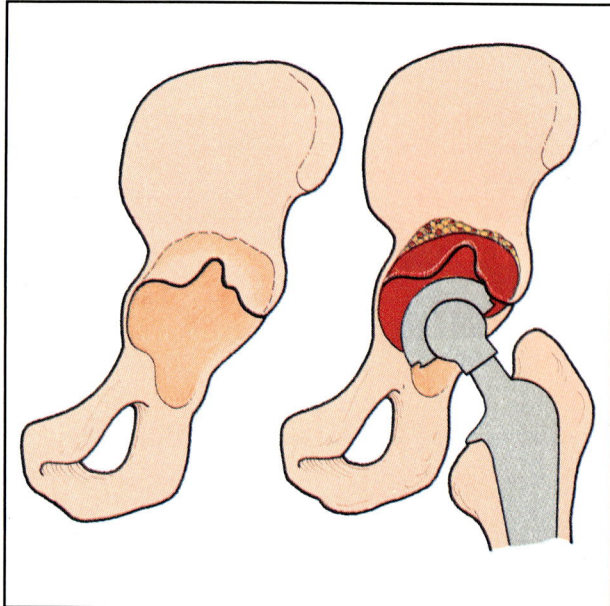

Figure 5-50C. Two femoral heads were used. Approximately one-third of each was discarded. Together they provided sufficient bone stock to reconstruct this very large defect. A mixture of morsellized cancellous autograft and allograft was first impacted into the roof of the intra-acetabular defect. Cortical and cancellous autograft strips were used to fill the medial perforation.

Figure 5-50D. A mixture of morsellized autograft and allograft bone was first placed in the intra-acetabular defects, and then two femoral heads were used to provide structural support for the uncemented acetabular component.

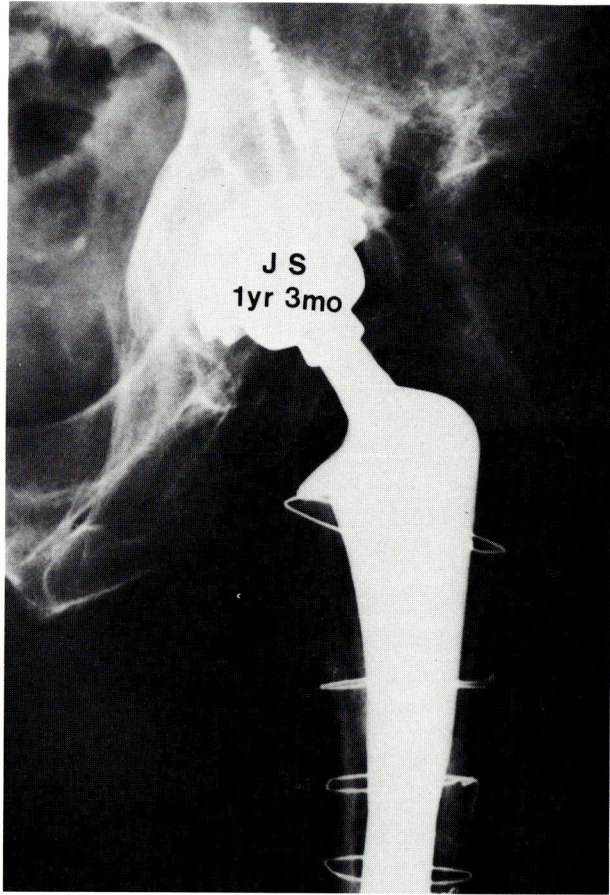

Figure 5-50E. The patient discarded all support at eight weeks. At follow-up of one year and three months, the acetabular grafts appear to be uniting and the patient rates 96. An onlay femoral cortical strut was used to reconstruct a femoral perforation.

appears to be doing well by x-ray (Figure 5-50E). He rates 96.

Summary of Authors' Preferred Treatment for Reconstruction of Acetabular Defects

In general, small contained defects can be managed by morsellized bone alone. Large defects in weight-bearing areas are best managed by solid grafts. If available, autografts are preferable to allografts. If allografts are necessary, we prefer to use autograft in addition. This can be in the form of morsellized bone, cortical and cancellous strips from the ilium or particulate bone obtained from acetabular reamers. Solid grafts must be buttressed against solid bone and if additional fixation is necessary, we prefer to use chrome cobalt or titanium screws to hold the graft against the buttress. These screws themselves do not bear weight and should be oriented in such a fashion that they will not interfere with impaction of the graft against the buttress.

Uncemented acetabular components can be used in virtually all instances. We prefer hemispherical acetabular components that are fixed with individual screws that often can help fix the grafts as well as the acetabular components. The large inventory of available modern components has allowed reconstruction of some very small or very large acetabuli that in years past would have required extensive grafting if older cemented components were used.

Rim Defects. In the past, standard cemented components were deeper, and mild superior rim defects often required grafting to provide coverage. More modern components have a lower profile and sometimes can be used without grafting in these circumstances, however, solid grafts, fixed with two or three cancellous screws, are necessary for all major rim defects. Major posterior rim defects may require an acetabular reconstruction plate, extending from the ischium to the ilium although we have not yet used this technique.[9]

Intra-acetabular Defects. Small cavitary defects that are surrounded by strong bone, can be filled with morsellized bone grafts. Large superior defects require solid grafts to return the center of rotation to the anatomic position. We do not hesitate to put a layer of morsellized bone graft between the solid graft and the dome of the patient's acetabulum. Large posterior intra-acetabular defects that are subjected to stresses with such functions as stair climbing or getting out of a chair, require solid grafts.

Protrusio Acetabulum. Deeper protrusio style cups can be used for minor defects. Very large protrusio problems may sometimes require a solid graft to move the center of rotation laterally but it is usually possible to fill the protrusio defect with morsellized bone and to slightly over ream the area where the anatomic acetabulum should be so that the new component has more peripheral support.

Medial Wall Perforations. If there is enough bone available so that the acetabulum can be reamed to accept a component which is large enough so that it cannot protrude through the defect, and is supported by the anterior and posterior columns and the acetabular dome, the defect itself can be grafted with cortical and cancellous strips from the iliac crest. These strips should be placed through the defect and against the iliacus. An uncemented acetabular component is preferred and acts as a mold for the grafts.

References

1. Capello, W.N., et al.: AAOS Classification System of Acetabular Deficiencies, exhibited at AAOS annual meeting, San Francisco, CA, Jan. 1987.

2. Harris, W.H., Crothers, O., Oh, I.: Total hip replacement and femoral head bone grafting for severe acetabular deficiency in adults. J Bone Joint Surg. 59A.752-759, Sept. 1977.

3. Harris, W.H.: Allografting in total hip arthroplasty: In adults with severe acetabular deficiency including a surgical technique for bolting the graft to the ilium. Clin Orthop 162:150, 1982.

4. Engh, C., Bobyn, J.: Biological Fixation in Total Hip Arthroplasty. Slack, Inc., Thorofare, NJ, 1985.

5. Bierbaum, B: Acetabular revision arthroplasty, p. 107. In Turner, R.H., Scheller, A.O. (eds): Revision Total Hip Arthroplasty. Grune and Stratton, Inc. NY, 1982.

6. Chandler, H.P., Penenberg, B.L.: Autografts and Allografts in Total Hip Replaceeent, AAOS Sci. exhibit, Atlanta, 1984.

7. Hodge, W.A., et al.: Human In Vitro Acetabular Pressure Measurement: A One-Year Update, Transactions of the 32nd Annual Orthopaedic Research Society Meeting, New Orleans, LA, Feb. 1986.

8. Gerber, S., Harris, W.H.: Femoral head autografting to augment acetabular deficiency in patients requiring total hip replacement. A minimum five year and average seven year follow-up study. J Bone Joint Surg 68-8: 1241-1248, Oct. 1986.

9. Borden, L.: Personal Communication

10. Borja, F.J., Mnaymneh, W.: Bone allografts in salvage of difficult hip arthroplasties. Clin Orthop 197:123, 1985.

11. Trancik, T.M., et al.: Allograft reconstruction of the acetabulum during revision total hip arthroplasty. Clinical radiographic and scintigraphic assessment of the results. J Bone Joint Surg 68A:527, April 1986.

12. Jasty, M., Harris, W.H.: Total hip reconstruction using frozen femoral head allografts in patients with acetabular bone loss. Orth Clin No Am 18:291, April 1987

13. Scott, R.D.: Use of bipolar prosthesis with bone grafting for acetabular reconstruction. Contemp Orthop 9:35, 1984.

14. Murray, W.: Use of bipolar prosthesis and bone graft in acetabular reconstruction. Presented in Palm Springs, 1986.

15. Hastings, D.E., Parker, S.M.: Protrusio acetabuli in rheumatoid arthritis. Clin Orthop 108:76, 1975.

16. Salvati, E.A., Bullough, P., Wilson, P.D.: Intrapelvic protrusio of the acetabular component following total hip replacement. Clin Orthop 111:212, 1975.

17. Ranawat, C.S., Dorr, L.D., Inglis, A.E.: Total hip arthroplasty in protrusio acetabuli of rheumatoid arthritis. J Bone Joint Surg 62A:1059-1065, Oct. 1980.

18. Sotelo-Garza, A., Charnley J.: The results of Charnley arthroplasty of the hip performed for protrusio acetabuli. Clin Orthop 132:12, 1978.

19. McCollum, D.E., Nunley, J.A., Harrelson, J.M.: Bone grafting in total hip replacement for acetabular

protrusio. J Bone Joint Surg 62A:1065-1073, Oct. 1980.

20. Heywood, A.W.B.: Arthroplsty with a solid bone graft for protrusio acetabuli. J Bone Joint Surg 62B:332-336, Aug. 1980.

21. Morley, D.C., Jr., Schmidt, R.H.: Protrusio acetabuli prosthetica. Orthop Review, 15(3):41-47, 1986.

22. Hirst, P., et al.: Bone grafting for protrusio acetabuli during total hip replacement. A review of the Writhington Method in 61 hips. J Bone Joint Surg 69B:229-233, Mar. 1987.

23. Mendes, D.G., Roffman, M., Silbermann, M.: Reconstruction of the acetabular wall with bone graft in arthroplasty of the hip. Clin Orthop 186:29, 1984.

24. Cameron, W.U.: Four methods for reconstruction of acetabular floor deficiencies. Orthop Review 14(9):71, 1985.

Six

Hugh P. Chandler, M.D.
Brad L. Penenberg, M.D.

Femoral Reconstruction

Although our initial experience with bone grafting techniques was with acetabular reconstruction, in recent years we have begun to see an increasing number of complex femoral deficiencies. These are most commonly associated with failed implants. The solution in the past has been to use more cement in conjunction with larger and longer stems.[1] As with acetabular defects, failure of such reconstructions occurs relatively early and the second or third revision will be much more difficult than the first. A new iatrogenic problem has been created by these techniques. We have named this "Cemented Long Stem Disease." It is caused by a cemented stem that extends distal to the isthmus and is characterized by severe osteopenia of the proximal femur with proximal loosening of both the cement-prosthesis and the cement-bone interfaces. However, in many cases the distal cement remains adherent to the stem, making extraction very difficult as the cement mass is too large to pass proximally through the isthmus.

There are now many long stem prostheses available that can be used without cement. If sintering extends distal to the metaphysis, stress shielding will occur and extraction becomes very difficult (Figures 6-1A and 6-1B). We have seen significant stress shielding of the femoral cortex even in the presence of smooth surfaced long stem devices (Figures 6-19A and 6-19B). Unlike intramedullary rods which are flexible, the stems of all femoral components are extremely rigid and do not allow the cortices to see normal bending stresses. For this reason we prefer to reconstruct

the bone with grafts and to use conventional length, proximally sintered components whenever possible.

Material

In our series, there were 16 isolated femoral grafts and another 27 combined femoral and acetabular grafts making a total of 43 hips in 37 patients that had femoral grafts. There were 23 females and 14 males with an average age of 60 (range 25 to 77 years). The average followup was 19 months (range six months to five years, seven months).

Forty of the 43 femoral grafts were required in revision operations. There were 34 revisions for failed total hip replacements, three for resection arthroplasties, two for failed Moore prostheses and one for a failed cup.

Methods

Although we prefer to use autogenous bone if available, the majority of these patients required their grafts for revision surgery and their femoral heads were not available. The bone source was therefore autogenous in two (iliac crest in one and the proximal fragment of a fractured femur in the other) and allograft in 41 (femoral heads in seven and formal harvests in 34). Allografts were frozen at $-80°C$. In the past three years, all allografts have been supplemented with autografts from the iliac crest or from the patient's femoral head. Finely morsellized autograft bone obtained from acetabular reamings or from reaming cancellous portions of an allograft were frequently mixed with autologous blood and used to fill interstices between the allograft and the host femur.

Femoral Defects

As with the acetabulum, we have outlined a classification of femoral defects based on femoral anatomy. The types of femoral defects that we have encountered in our series are outlined below:

Table 6-1

1. Calcar deficiency
    A. Intramedullary
    B. Total deficiency
2. Trochanteric deficiency
3. Cortical thinning
4. Cortical perforation
5. Femoral fractures about or below the stem of a femoral component
    A. Fractures of the patient's femur
    B. Fatigue fracture of an allograft
6. Circumferential deficiency of the metaphysis and proximal diaphysis
    A. Loss of the trochanter and metaphysis with a thin shell of the diaphysis remaining
    B. Total loss of the proximal femur

Calcar Deficiency

Calcar defects are commonly seen in revision surgery. In our series there were four isolated calcar defects (10%) and an additional seven hips with a combination of calcar and other femoral defects, making a total of eleven hips (26%) with calcar problems.

Calcar bone loss was associated with failed cemented total hip replacement in ten hips and failed Moore prosthesis in one. Calcar resorption may be caused by proximal stress shielding in the presence of cemented femoral components that are well fixed distally, by mechanical pressure from a loose varus femoral component, or by the foreign body reaction generated by particulate debris of either cement or polyethylene.[2] We have reinforced the stress shielded-calcar in two patients who had well-fixed femoral components. The other nine patients with major calcar problems had a loose cemented femoral component.

Review of Literature. At the time of revision, the femoral component ideally should be placed in neutral or slight valgus; however, with significant calcar resorption, there is usually a large gap medially if the revision prosthesis is correctly positioned into valgus. In the past, many

surgeons have filled this medial space with cement but the longevity of this construct is questionable and further bone loss is very likely. Harris has developed a Calcar Replacement Prosthesis (Howmedica, Rutherford, NJ) which must be used with cement.[3] Metal intramedullary cylinders have been developed to fill this defect (Joint Medical Products Corp., Stanford, CT) and are designed to be used without cement. Calandruccio and McConnell have advocated the use of a femoral head shaped like a napkin ring and placed over the proximal femur to reconstruct the calcar.[4] Bargar et al. have described their experiences with an iliac crest graft used to reconstruct the intramedullary calcar loss in dogs and humans.[5] In 1984, we first presented our experiences with the use of an allograft femoral head to reconstruct the

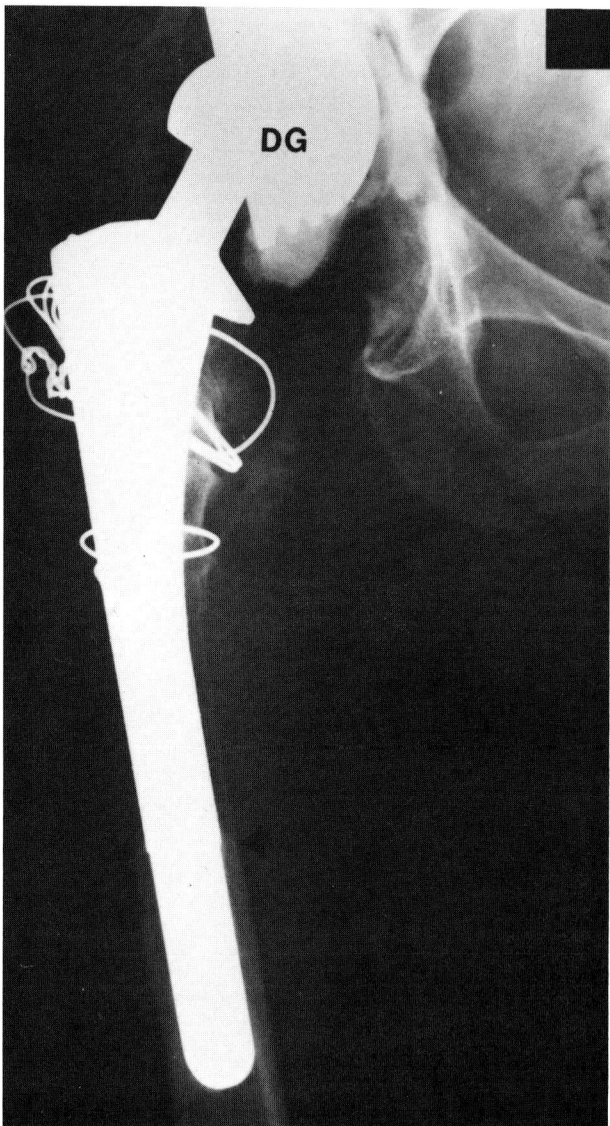

Figure 6-1A. If sintering extends distal to the metaphysis, proximal stress shielding will occur. Note the dramatic loss of the proximal femoral bone. Distal to the sintered surface, the forces are again transferred to the cortex. This patient was sent to us because of a loose acetabular component. In the long term, the femur will be a much more challenging problem.

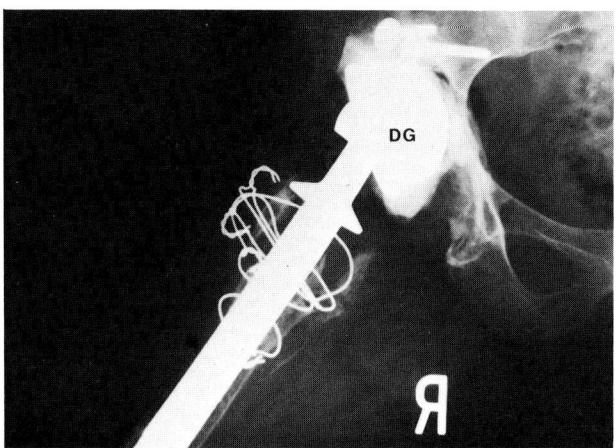

Figure 6-1B. The anterior cortex has disappeared.

intramedullary calcar defect.[6] There are two clinical patterns of calcar deficiency. The first is *calcar intramedullary deficiency* with a thin peripheral medial cortical rim remaining, and the second is *total loss of the calcar* with no remaining bone above or at the lesser trochanter.

Treatment

Calcar Intramedullary Deficiency. In our series, there were seven hips (17%) with calcar intramedullary deficiencies. Six were isolated and one had an associated loss of the greater trochanter. The etiology in every case was a loose cemented femoral prosthesis that had subsided and fallen into varus.

Any surgical approach can be used as the exposure need not be extensive. We prefer to use the direct lateral approach unless associated problems require a more extensive exposure.

Since this defect always occurs in conjunction with a failed femoral stem, the patient's femoral head is not available. If the problem is caused by a failed Moore prosthesis (without cement) the defect is narrow enough so that a full thickness iliac crest graft is sufficient.[5] In the presence of lysis about a loose cemented total hip component, however, the defect is almost always too wide for the iliac crest and a larger graft is usually necessary. An allograft femoral head and neck can be shaped like a cylinder with the neck oriented distally (Figure 6-3). This cylinder is impacted into the medullary canal and then the new canal is formed laterally by means of a high-speed burr. Although we used two transverse screws through the cortex of the proximal femur in our first case, we now feel that screws are unnecessary and disadvantageous because they may prevent the graft from impacting.

Clinical Examples

Case 1

The patient seen in Figure 6-2A was 64 and weighed 270 lbs when he presented with a loose femoral component that had subsided into varus. A thin medial shell of calcar still remained. An allograft femoral head was shaped to fit within the proximal femur and then a lateral channel for the prosthesis was made with a high speed burr (Figure 6-2B). Cement was used because cementless prostheses were not commonly available at the time of his surgery (1982). However, cement intrusion into the nonbleeding cancellous bone of the allograft was excellent. In this circumstance, cement fixation was much better than it would have been had cement been used against the smooth eburnated bone of the calcar rim itself. X-rays remain unchanged at five years, one month (Figure 6-2C) and at followup of five years, three months the patient rates 98. He still weighs 270 lbs.

Case 2

The patient whose x-rays are seen in Figure 6-3A was 79 when she presented with a painful loose Moore prosthesis that had been inserted one year, ten months prior to revision. Immediate postoperative x-rays following the Moore prosthesis were not available and it is not clear whether the calcar was inadvertently removed at the initial operation or

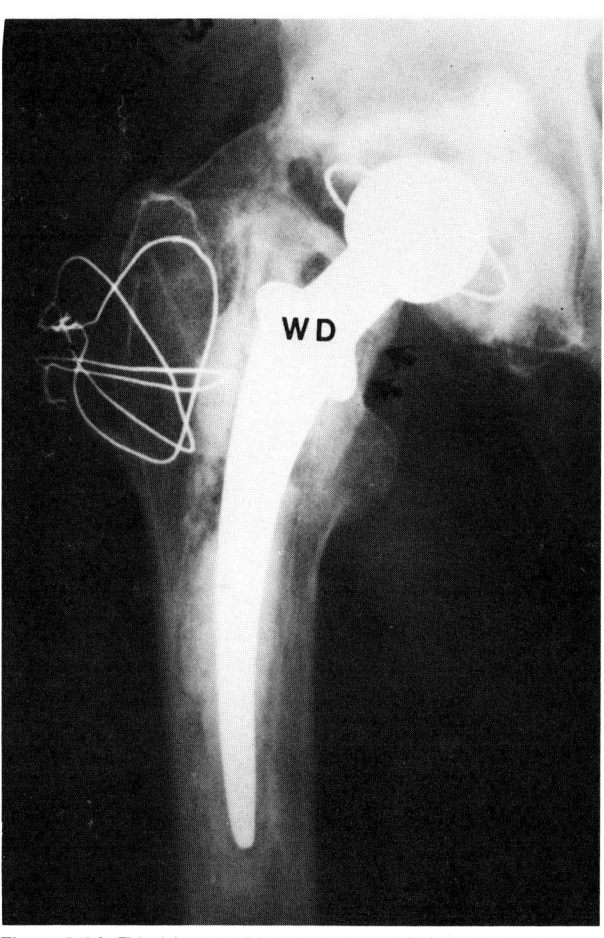

Figure 6-2A. This 64-year-old man weighed 270 lbs. when he presented with this loose femoral component 11 years after his original total hip replacement for osteoarthritis. Note the medial position of the proximal portion of the femoral component with loss of the intramedullary calcar bone. A thin medial shell of calcar remained.

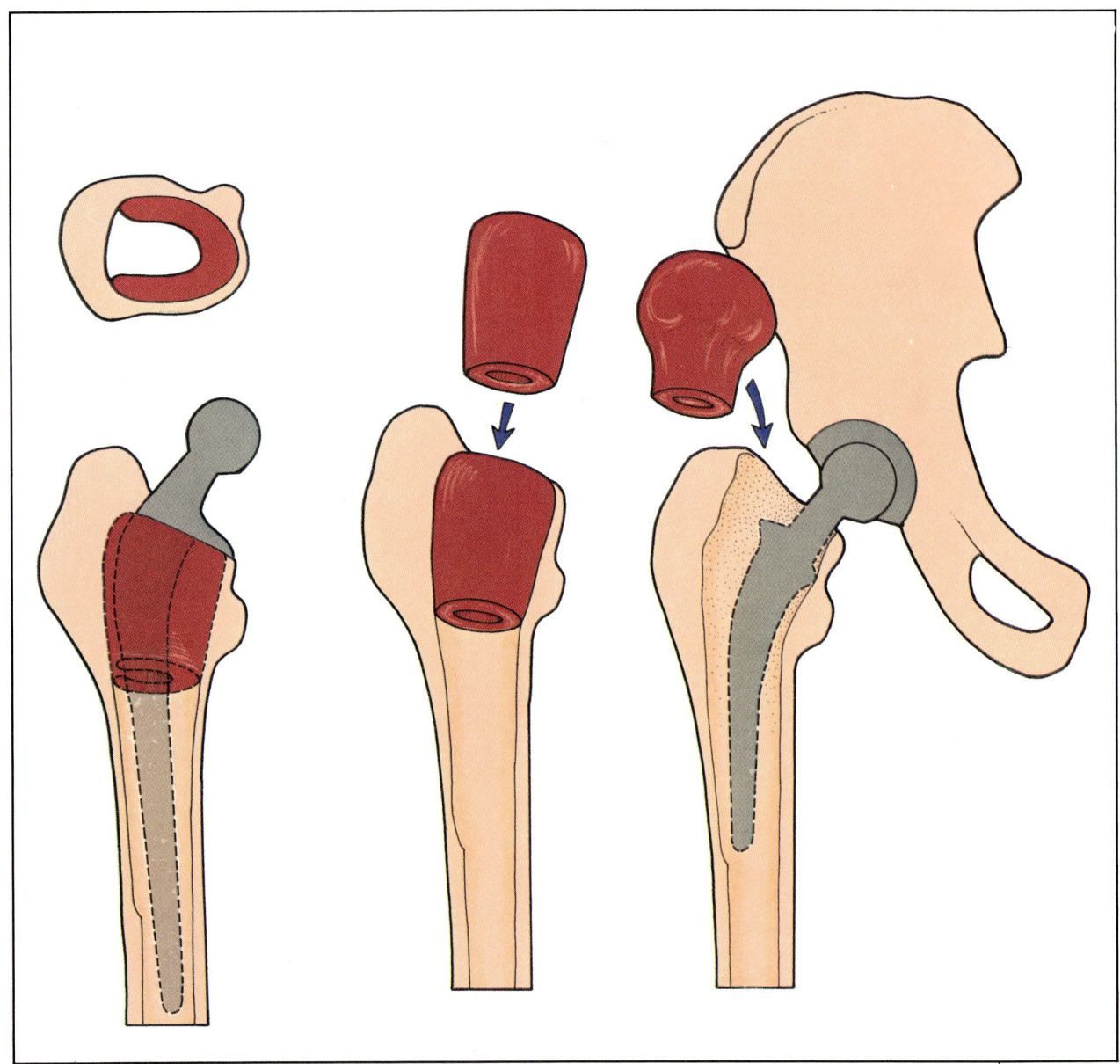

Figure 6-2B. An allograft femoral head was shaped like a cylinder and impacted into the old medullary canal and then the new canal was created laterally by means of a high-speed burr after the graft was in place. Femoral rasps were used to finish the femoral preparation.

had eroded secondary to subsidence and varus positioning of the component. In addition to the femoral loosening problem, the acetabular cartilage had also eroded. The intramedullary calcar defect created by the uncemented Moore prosthesis was narrow and could be reconstructed by a full thickness autogenous iliac crest graft (Figure 6-3B). Cement was used because of the patient's age. At one month the graft is in good position (Figure 6-3C) and there is little change at three and one half years except for some radioluciency of the graft, probably secondary to revascularization and stress shielding (Figure 6-3D). At followup of three years, eight months, the patient considers her hip to be normal and she rates 96.

Total Calcar Deficiency. In our series there were four patients (10%) with total calcar deficiency. All were sec-ondary to a varus, loose, cemented total hip replacement and all were associated with thinning or perforation of the lateral cortex at or distal to the tip of the stem of the femoral component.

Since exposure of the femoral shaft is necessary to reconstruct these associated defects, either the trochanteric slide or the vastus slide is the preferred approach. If maximum exposure of the acetabulum is also necessary, the trochanteric slide is our choice. If less exposure is necessary on the acetabular side, we prefer the vastus slide.

The calcar from an ipsilateral allograft femur is the ideal source of bone to reconstruct the deficient calcar. Although we have used an isolated calcar graft, we now feel that it is best to use the allograft calcar in conjunction with a distal cortical strut. We prefer a collared femoral component so

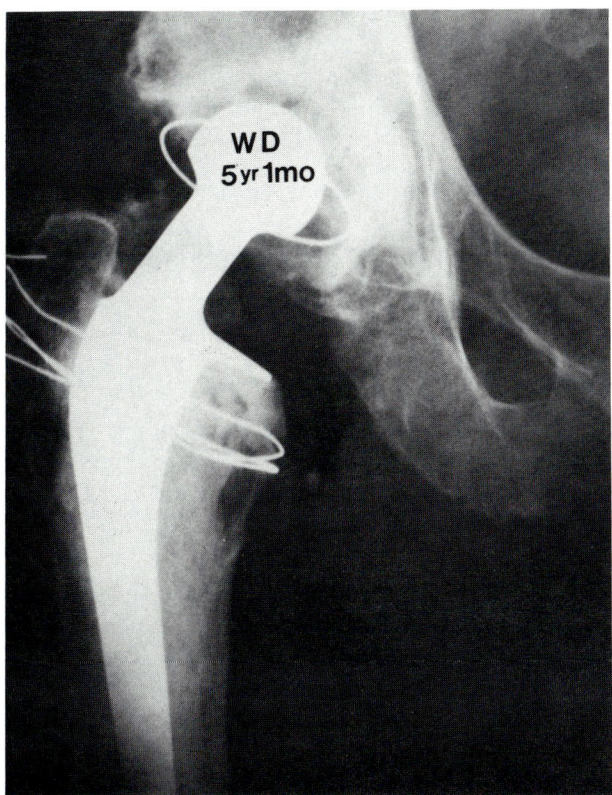

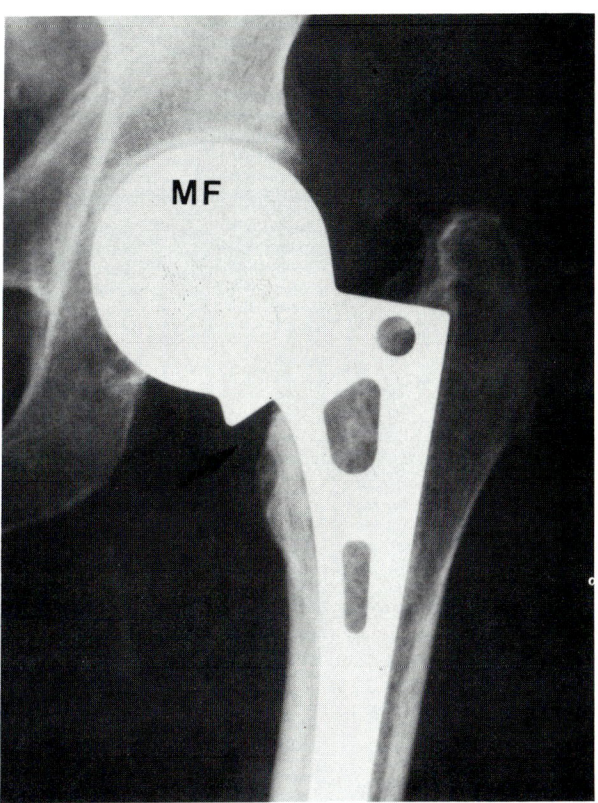

Figure 6-2C. At five years, one month the graft appears to have incorporated. There is a faint radiolucent line between the graft and the lesser trochanter. The patient rates 98.

Figure 6-3A. This 79-year-old woman had left hip pain one year, ten months after insertion of a Moore prosthesis in treatment for a femoral neck fracture. There is erosion of the acetabular cartilage, loosening of the stem and loss of the intramedullary aspect of the calcar.

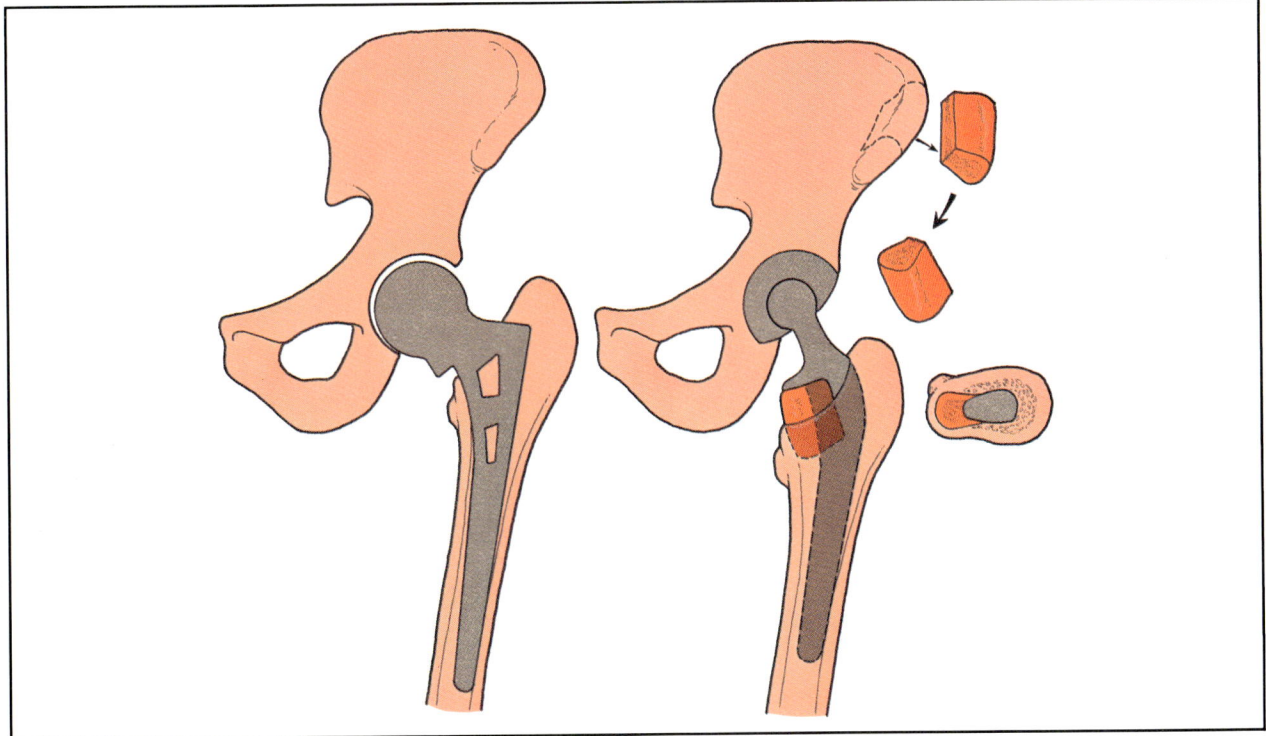

Figure 6-3B. A full thickness iliac crest graft was wide enough to reconstruct the intramedullary calcar loss and allowed the new femoral component to be placed in a valgus position.

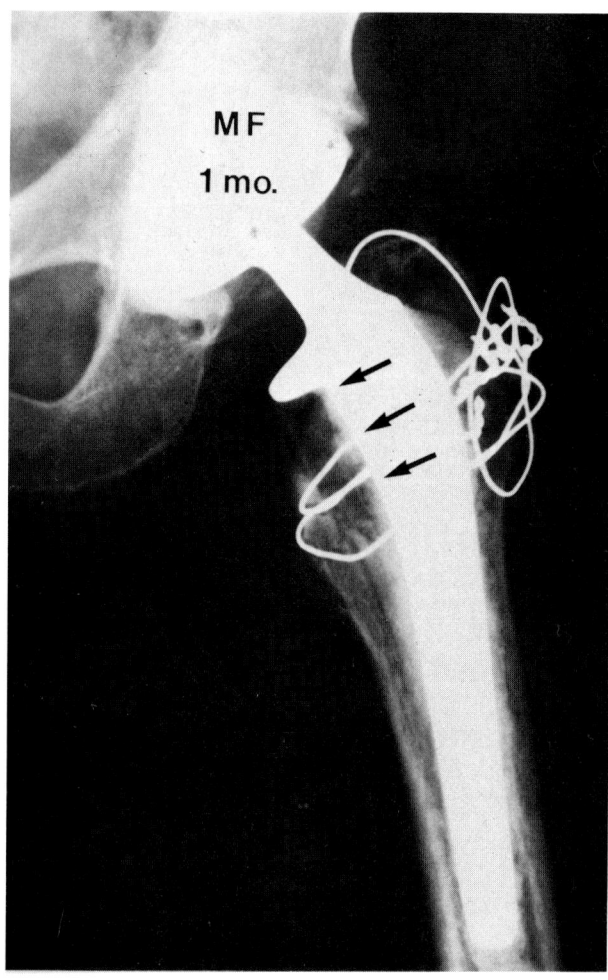

Figure 6-3C. X-rays at one month show the graft is in good position and the component is well-supported in valgus.

that the calcar graft is impacted into its bed. Cement is not necessary or desirable unless there are other specific reasons to use it. A long stem is not necessary.

Clinical Examples

Case 1

The patient whose x-rays are seen in Figure 6-4A was a 74-year-old woman who had her original total hip replacement performed because of degenerative arthritis. Failure of this device was associated with severe calcar resorption. On the first revision, the surgeon elected to rebuild the calcar with cement and used a cemented long stem component. As would be predicted, this failed quickly and she presented to us two years after her revision suffering from cemented long stem disease. The component had subsided and was loose proximally but distal to the isthmus the cement was firmly adherent to the stem (Figure 6-4B). Her acetabular problem has been previously described (Figure 5-43).

Because the distal cement mass was too large to pass through the isthmus (Figure 6-4B), a window in the lateral distal femur was made so that the cement could be separated

from the prosthesis (Figure 6-4C). The window was replaced after the cement and prosthesis were removed, and the window and the thin stress-shielded lateral cortex were reinforced by a large onlay cortical graft. Autograft strips were placed over the window and at the junction of the allograft and the patient's femur. The calcar was reconstructed by an allograft from the calcar of an ipsilateral allograft femur (Figure 6-4D). In retrospect, it would have been better to include a medial cortical strut as well. An uncemented Bias component (Zimmer, Warsaw, IN) was used. We would now use a standard length uncemented prosthesis.

The graft appears to be doing well by x-ray at one year (Figure 6-4E) but there is significant heterotopic bone formation. The onlay graft used to reinforce the distal window appears to have united (Figure 6-4F). The patient had a pre-existing neurologic problem characterized by uncontrolled athetoid and choreiform motions. She has limited motion with flexion to only 70° and requires a walker for balance because of her neurologic problems. Despite her rating of

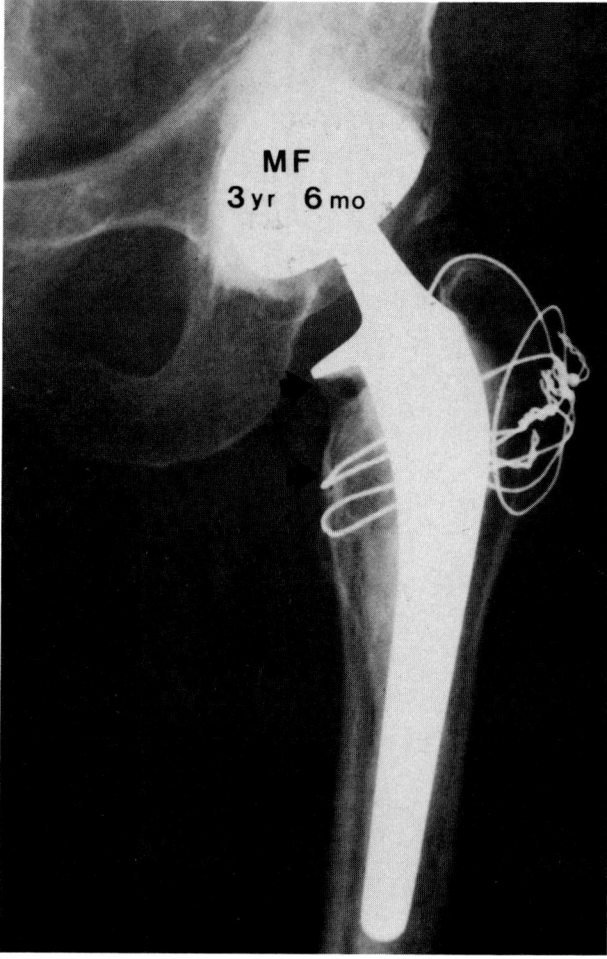

Figure 6-3D. At three and one half years, the graft appears to have incorporated. Although there may be some radiolucency of the graft beneath the collar from revascularization and/or stress shielding, the cemented component has not shifted and there is no sign of loosening. The patient rates 96.

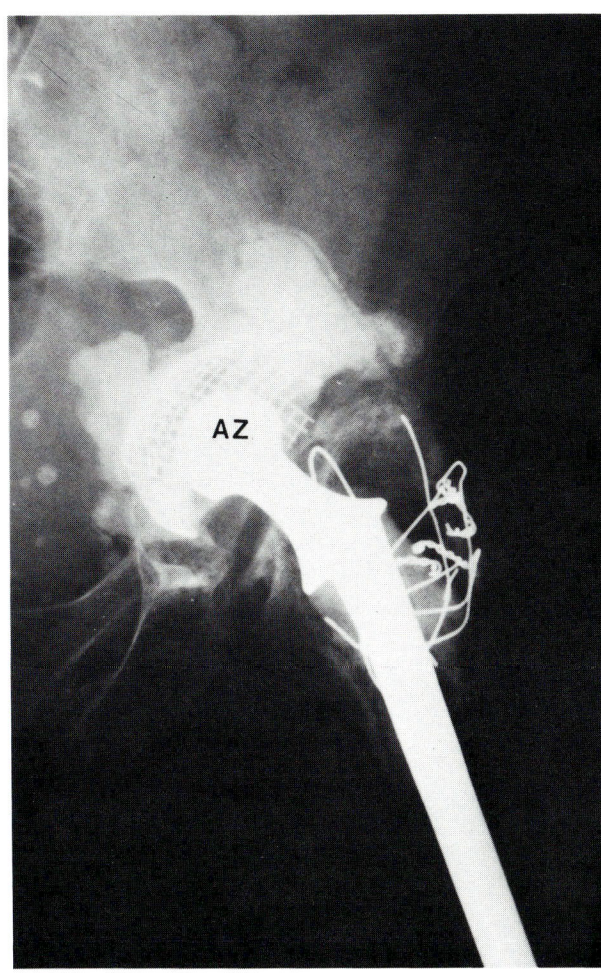

Figure 6-4A. This 74-year-old woman had a loose acetabular component as well as a loose long stem femoral component that had subsided. At the time of her first revision, the surgeon had elected to rebuild the calcar with cement. Failure occurred in two years. Note the proximal stress shielding of the femur secondary to the cemented long stemmed femoral component.

only 71, she has no pain and is pleased with her hip and has been converted from a wheelchair existence to a household ambulator.

Case 2

The patient whose x-rays are seen in Figure 6-5A was 69 when she presented with a failed total hip replacement, 12 years after her original surgery. She had a loose acetabular component with a combined medial and superior intra-acetabular defect. Autogenous strips from the iliac crest were used for the medial defect and a mixture of morsellized autogenous and allograft bone were used for the superior intra-acetabular defects. The acetabular component is uncemented.

The distal tip of the prosthesis has caused striking thinning of the overlying lateral cortex of the femur that was reconstructed with a cortical onlay graft. However, her major problem was in the calcar region where the collar of the loose prosthesis had caused significant erosion. The

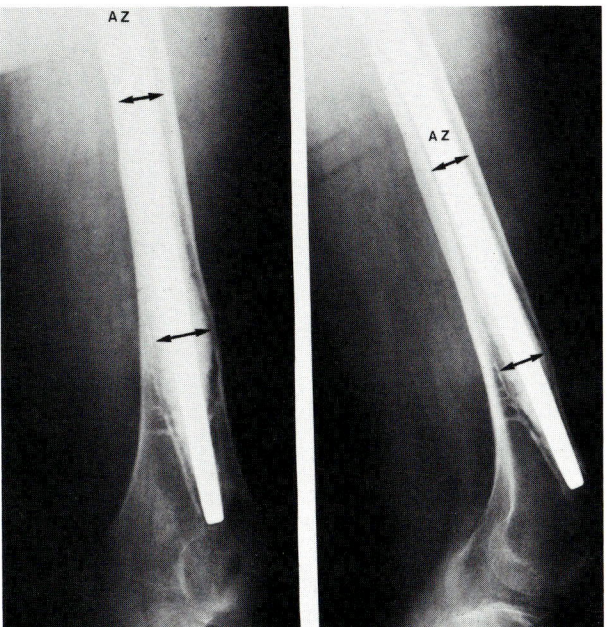

Figure 6-4B. This 74-year-old woman had a long stem cemented component inserted for revision of a failed total hip replacement 12 years ago. The prosthesis was loose and had subsided but the cement distal to the isthmus was firmly attached to the stem and could not pass through the isthmus. Note the stress shielding of the femur.

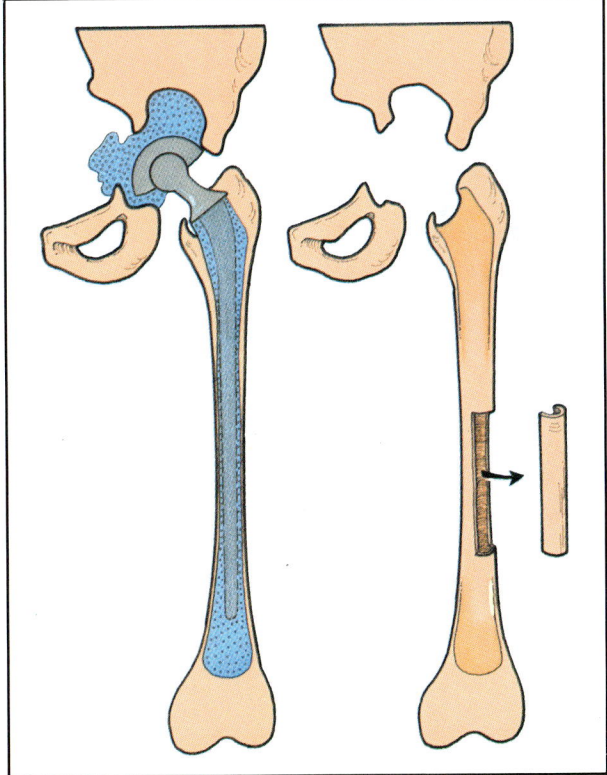

Figure 6-4C. The calcar had resorbed. The long stem cemented component was loose proximally and had subsided. Distal to the isthmus the cement was firmly adherent to the stem. Since the mass of the cement was too large to pass through the isthmus, it was necessary to make a window so the cement could be separated from the prosthesis.

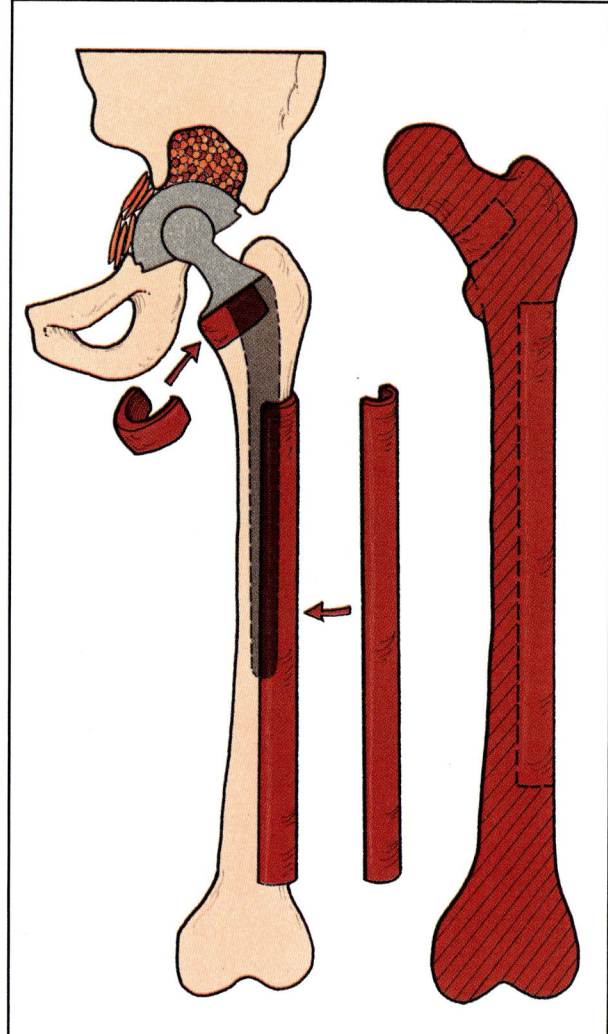

Figure 6-4D. The calcar was reconstructed with a calcar from an ipsilateral femoral allograft. The window was replaced and a large lateral onlay graft was used to protect the window and to reinforce the thin lateral cortex of the femur. Autograft strips from the iliac crest were added to both allografts.

calcar was absent and the lesser trochanter was eroded (Figure 6-5B). Reconstruction of the calcar was performed by means of a large medial allograft which combined the ipsilateral calcar, lesser trochanter and 4″ of the proximal medial cortex. An uncemented prosthesis was used. The collar helped stabilize the calcar graft by direct impaction (Figure 6-5C). Autogenous strips were placed about the junction of the allografts and the patient's femur. This patient discarded crutches at six weeks and began to use a cane. The grafts appear to be doing well by x-ray at five months (Figure 6-5D). At followup of one year, the patient has no pain but still requires a cane for long walks outside. She rates 86.

This particular graft appears to have a significant place in calcar and proximal medial femoral reconstruction and we have used it on four other cases in recent months but followup is too short to include in this series.

Trochanteric Deficiencies

Deficiency of the greater trochanter did not occur as an isolated problem in any patient in our series; however, combined with other defects, it was present in 11 patients (26%).

It was associated with a failed hip arthroplasty in all patients. One patient had a cup arthroplasty, one had a failed Moore prosthesis; two had resection arthroplasties; and three had failed total hips.

Review of Literature. The importance of the greater trochanteric lever arm is well recognized. Without this lever, there is not only significant functional abductor weakness but also greatly increases forces through the hip joint if the patient walks without support.[7] Lateral transfer of the greater trochanter, if possible, will improve the mechanics of this system. We have found two reports in the literature specifically describing augmentation of the greater trochanteric lever system in total hip replacement using bone grafts.[8,9]

Authors' Preferred Treatment. The trochanteric

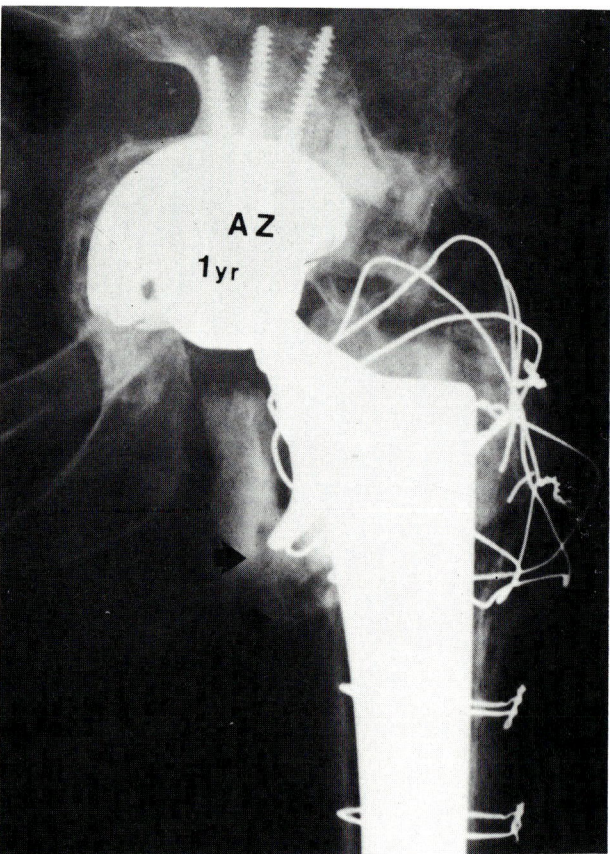

Figure 6-4E. The calcar graft is outlined by the arrows. In retrospect we should have used a medial strut as well (Figure 6-4C). Because of heterotopic bone, flexion is limited to only 70°. The patient has a significant pre-existing neurologic disorder characterized by uncontrolled athetoid motions. She requires a walker because of her neurologic problems but has no pain and was converted from a wheelchair existence to a household ambulator. She rates only 71 but is very pleased with her hip.

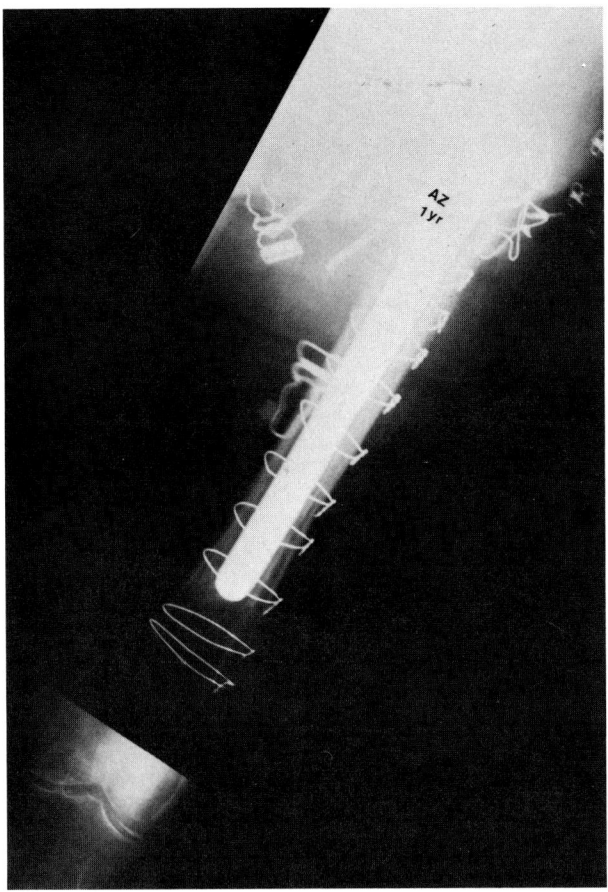

Figure 6-4F. At one year the onlay graft used to reinforce the distal window appears to have united to the shaft.

slide is the approach of choice whenever the trochanter is deficient and reconstruction with a graft is anticipated. The double pedicle blood supply from the abductors and from the quadriceps aids in union between the trochanteric fragment and the avascular graft. The quadriceps tends to inhibit proximal migration of the trochanter until union occurs. Often trochanteric augmentation is incidentally provided by proximal femoral replacement with an allograft that includes the greater trochanter, but we have used a bone graft specifically for the purpose of increasing the abductor moment arm in three patients.

If an isolated trochanteric defect is present, a femoral head can be used. If there is an associated deficiency of the proximal cortex, an allograft trochanter with the lateral cortex is preferred.

Clinical Examples

Case 1

The patient whose x-rays are seen in Figure 6-6A was 60 when he presented with a failed total hip replacement, 12 years after his original total hip replacement. He had undergone several surgical procedures following a slipped epiphysis at age 15. These included a surgical arthrodesis which was successful for over 20 years and then a Moore

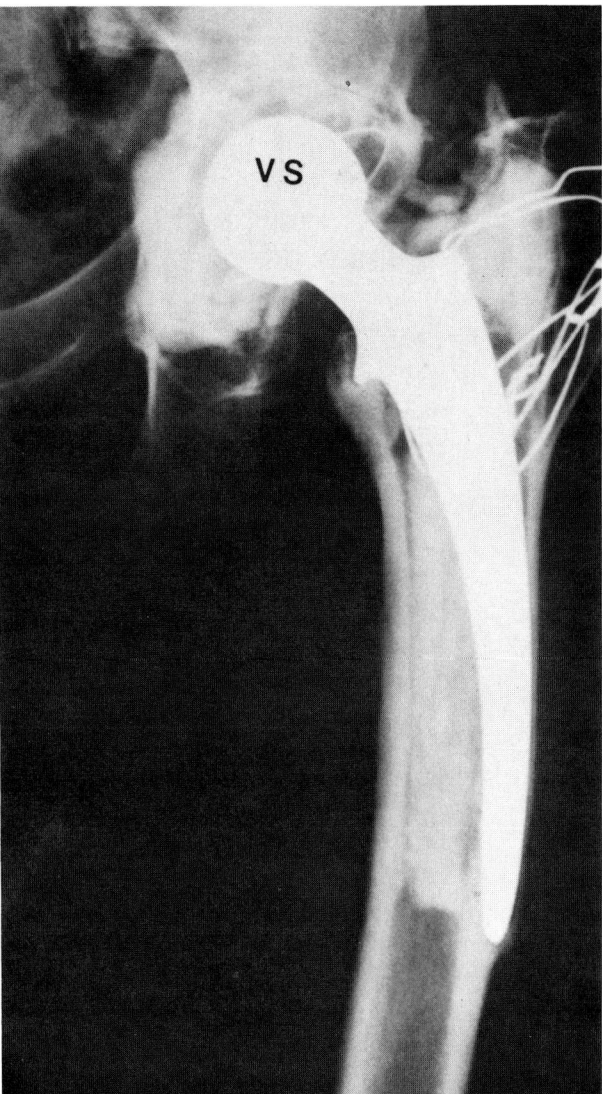

Figure 6-5A. This 69-year-old woman presented with a loose varus component, twelve years after her original total hip replacement for degenerative arthritis. The calcar is absent and even the lesser trochanter has been eroded. There is significant lateral cortical thinning at the distal stem of the femoral component.

prosthesis was inserted a year prior to his initial total hip replacement. There was just a wafer of bone in the trochanteric region and a severely compromised abductor lever system. Preoperatively he had a striking abductor lurch which was secondary to abductor weakness, a deficient both abductor moment arm, and pain. It is rare that femoral defects are isolated, and this man presented with both an intramedullary calcar deficiency and a greater trochanter deficiency.

The hip was exposed by means of the trochanteric slide. One allograft femoral head was utilized to provide intramedullary calcar bone stock (see section on intramedullary calcar reconstruction). This was our first reconstruction of intramedullary calcar defect and we used two transverse screws through the cortex of the patient's femur to fix the intramedullary graft. We now feel that such screws are

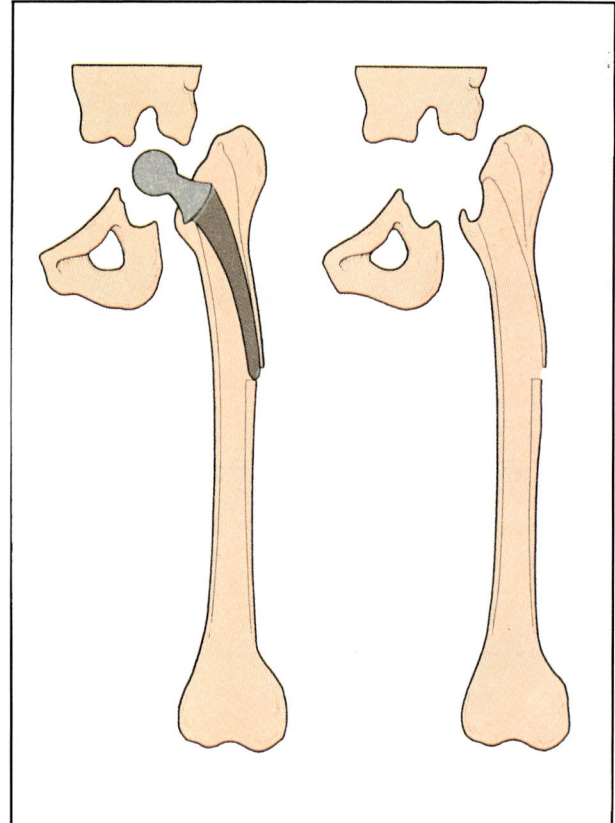

Figure 6-5B. There was complete loss of the calcar and the lesser trochanter was eroded. The distal tip of the prosthesis had caused significant thinning as well as a perforation of the lateral cortex of the femur. There was a perforation of the medial wall of the acetabulum as well as a superior intra-acetabular defect.

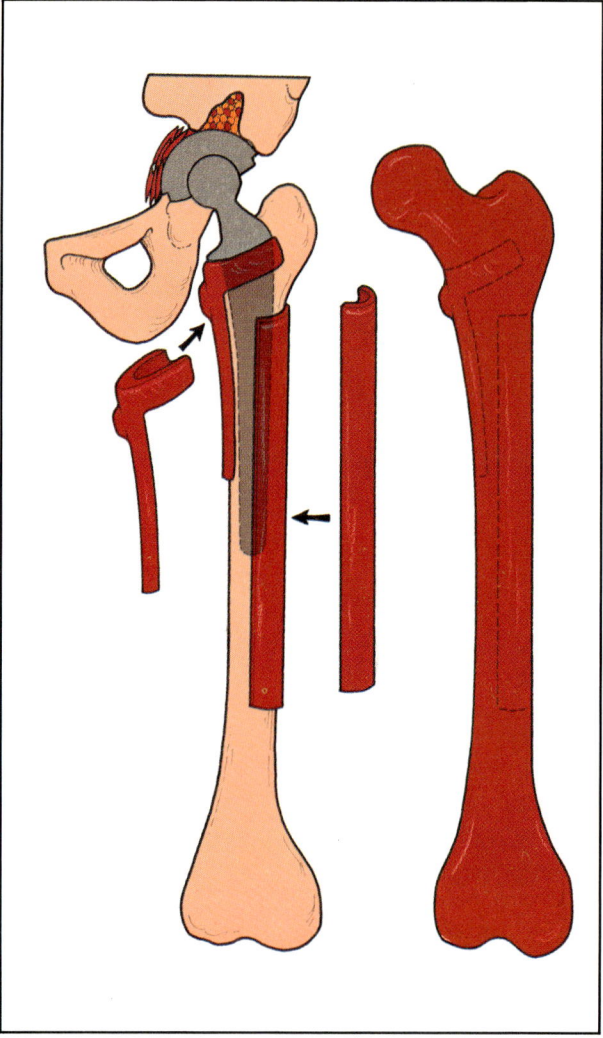

Figure 6-5C. An allograft which included the calcar, lesser trochanter, and a medial cortical strut was used to reconstruct the calcar region. An onlay graft was used to reconstruct the perforation of the lateral femur. Cortical and cancellous strips were placed in the medial acetabular defect and morsellized autograft and allograft were packed into the superior intra-acetabular defect.

undesirable, despite the fact that the graft appeared to have united in this patient. A second allograft femoral head was split in half and wired to the femur to provide a greater trochanter (Figure 6-6B). The patient shifted from crutches to a cane at eight weeks and by one year discarded support and walked without a limp. X-rays at four years appeared satisfactory (Figure 6-6C). The patient rated 92 and walked without support and without a limp. Unfortunately, at four years, three months he developed a hematogenous hip sepsis (*Staphylococcus aureus*) which required a resection arthroplasty (Figure 6-6D). Both grafts appeared structually viable and well vascularized when biopsied at the time of the resection arthroplasty and union of the grafts had clearly taken place. There was some resorption of the proximal portion of the trochanteric graft. The patient is currently without evidence of infection and awaits another revision.

Case 2

The patient whose x-rays are seen in Figure 6-7A was 61 when she presented with a painful shaft arthroplasty. She had undergone two previous cup arthroplasties for congenital dislocation of the hip. She had a dramatic abductor lurch, in part because of both poor abductor muscle biomechanics and in part because of pain. There was a superior

intra-acetabular and a superior rim defect. The calcar and both trochanters were absent (Figure 6-7B). An allograft femoral head was used to reconstruct her acetabulum and a second allograft femoral head was shaped like a napkin-ring to provide calcar support and a trochanteric lever system (Figure 6-7C). The trochanteric slide approach was used. There was no trochanteric fragment but the quadriceps and the abductor were left in continuity and a chair staple was used to attach them to the trochanteric graft.

Unfortunately the femoral component was cemented in too much varus and the inferior screw of the acetabular graft is too transverse. The femoral graft initially looked quite satisfactory (Figure 6-7D) but at four years, seven months it had disappeared, possibly because it has not stressed (Figure 6-7E). She fell and sustained an anterior dislocation and was revised because of a loose acetabular component at five years, two months. The architecture of the acetabulum was intact and an uncemented acetabular component was used without further grafting. The femoral component was loose and the entire femoral allograft had disappeared. Because the remaining proximal femur was damaged when the cement was removed, a portion was resected and a proximal femur was used with a butt joint and a side strut (Figure 6-7F).

We still feel that a greater trochanter augmentation graft is worthwhile but the napkin-ring configuration used in this case for calcar reconstruction is not helpful (at least in conjunction with cemented prostheses) because the graft appears to resorb if it is not stressed. Faced with this patient's original problem, we would now use a large uncemented acetabular component without an acetabular graft and would use a proximal femoral replacement allograft with a distal lateral strut, placing her deficient proximal femur within the metaphysis of the allograft femur (Figures 6-18C and 6-19C).

Case 3

The patient whose x-rays are seen in Figure 6-8A was a 43-year-old man whose acetabular reconstruction was described previously (Figure 5-46). He had pain and recur-

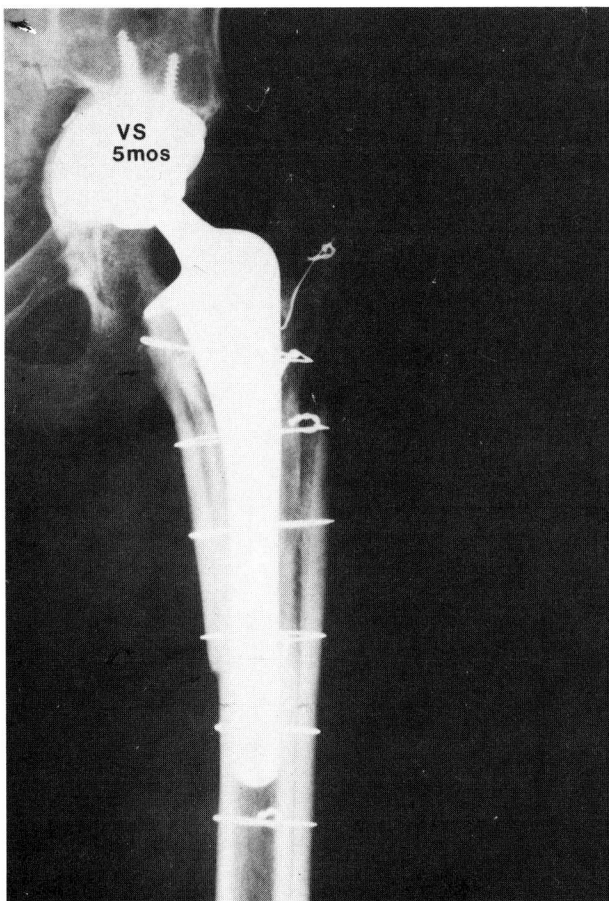

Figure 6-5D. Both the acetabular and femoral grafts appear to be doing well by x-ray at five months. Neither component is cemented. The patient has no pain at followup of one year but still uses a cane for long outside walks. She rates 86.

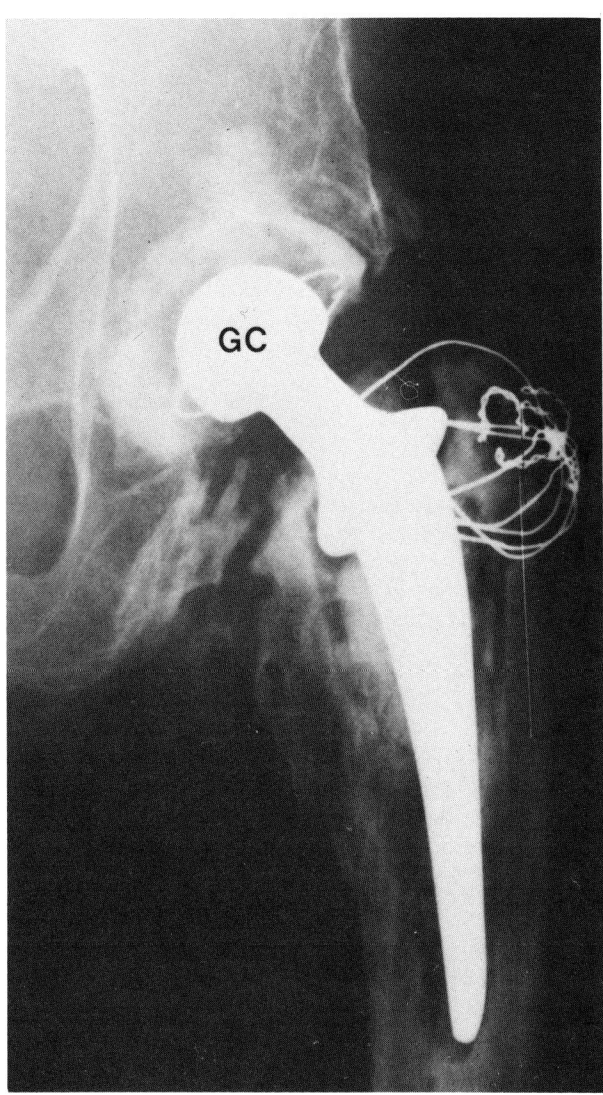

Figure 6-6A. This 60-year-old man had a loose femoral component 12 years after total hip replacement. The femoral component has subsided into varus and he has a calcar intramedullary defect. The greater trochanter is a thin wafer and there is no trochanteric lever system. He had a profound abductor lurch in because of the absent trochanter, weak abductor muscles, and in part due to pain.

rent dislocation of his right hip. Both the acetabular and femoral components were loose. The greater trochanter is absent. The patient had a marked abductor lurch, in part because he had no abductor lever system and in part because of pain. Bilateral cemented long stem disease was present with proximal loosening and cortical resorption. The distal cement remained firmly fixed to the stem and could not pass proximally through the isthmus (Figure 6-8B). Because his left femur was shattered in the process of removing the long stem prosthesis (Figure 6-20B), we were reluctant to remove the right prosthesis and elected to reinforce the proximal femur with onlay cortical grafts which included the greater and lesser trochanters. A trochanteric slide was used. The abductors and quadriceps were kept in continuity and were later wired to the allograft greater trochanter. A

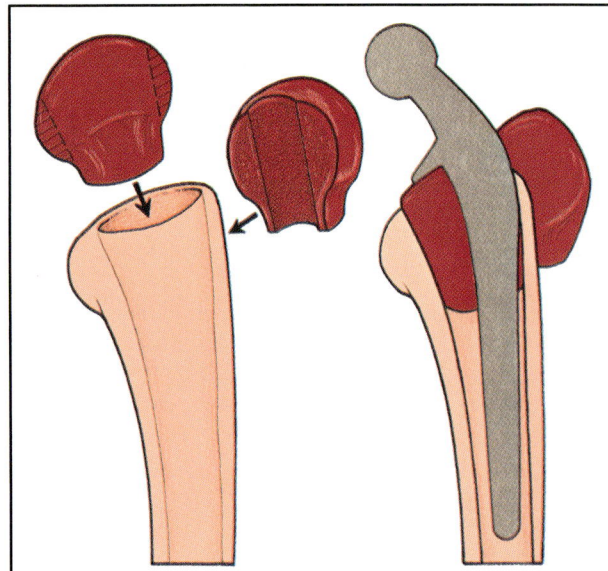

Figure 6-6B. One allograft femoral head was used to reconstruct the intramedullary calcar defect; a second allograft femoral head was split and wired to the proximal lateral femur to provide a greater trochanter. A trochanteric slide was used for exposure and the wafer of the patient's greater trochanter was placed over the greater trochanter of the allograft.

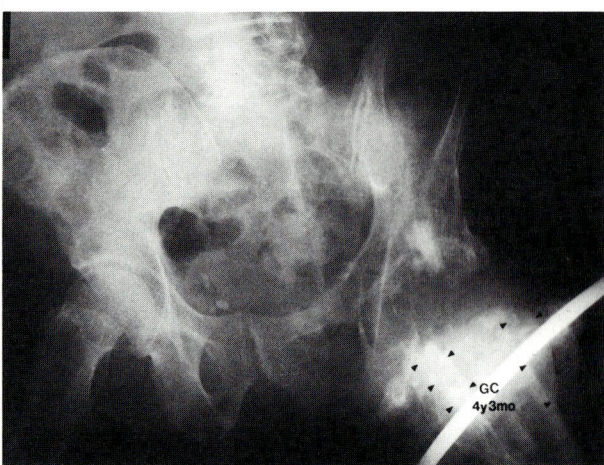

Figure 6-6D. Unfortunately the patient developed hematogenous *Staphylococcus aureus* hip sepsis at four years, three months and required a resection arthroplasty. Both the calcar intramedullary and the trochanteric augmentation grafts (outlined by arrows) had united and bled freely when biopsied.

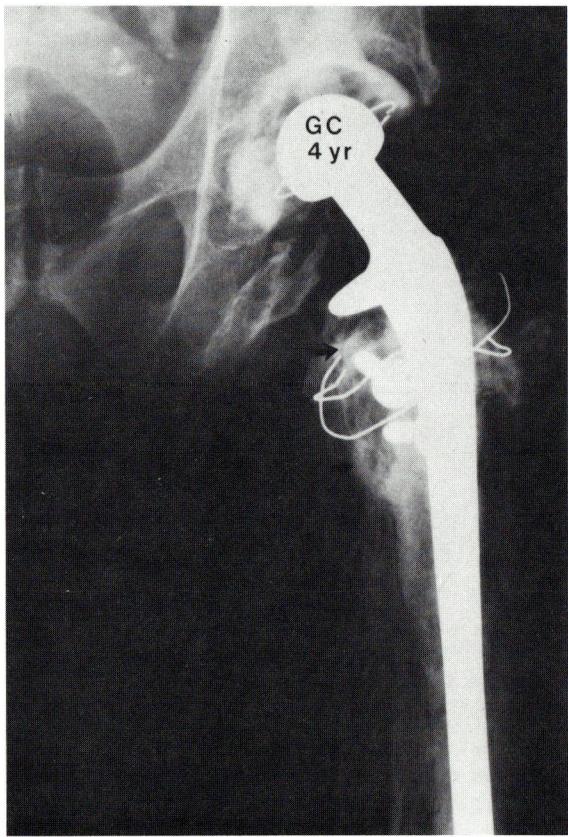

Figure 6-6C. Although there was a radiolucent line about the acetabular component, x-rays of the femur appeared satisfactory at four years. The patient walked without support and with a negative Trendelenburg gait. He rated 92.

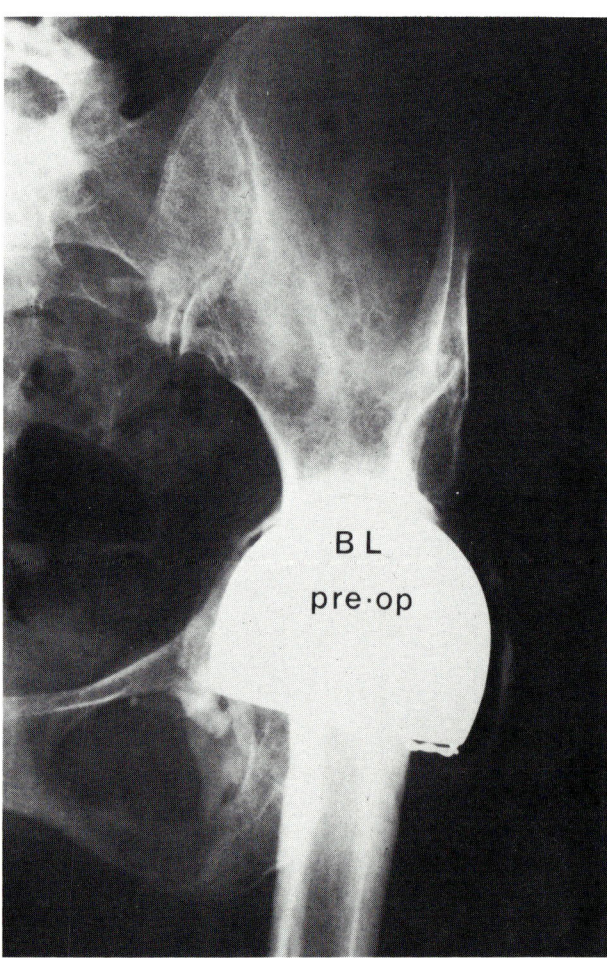

Figure 6-7A. After two cup arthroplasties, this 61-year-old woman presented with a shaft arthroplasty. There was no trochanteric lever system and she had a dramatic abductor lurch, because of poor abductor muscle biomechanics and pain.

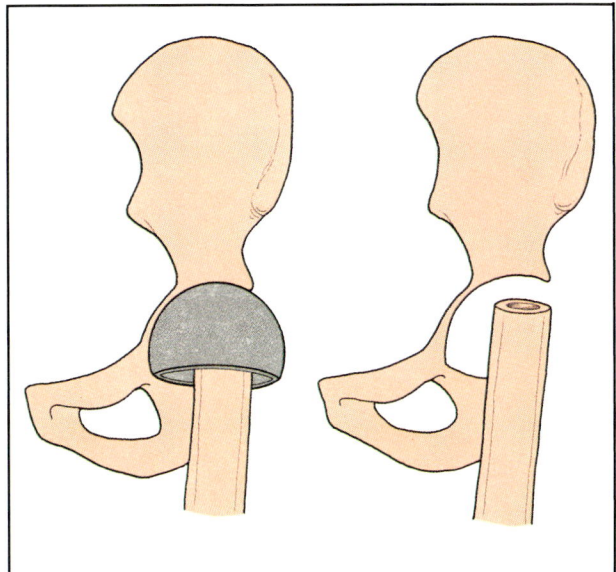

Figure 6-7B. There was a superior intra-acetabular and a superior rim defect as well as absence of the calcar and trochanters.

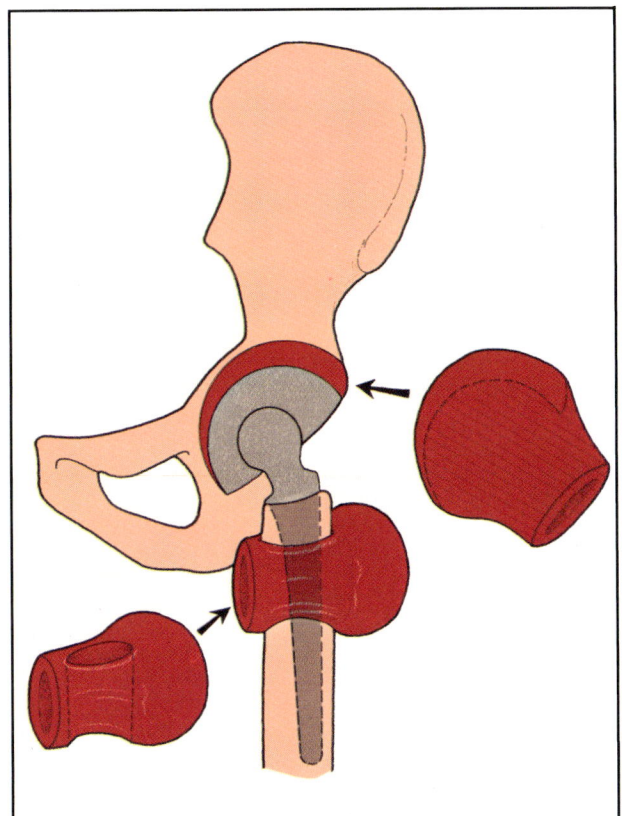

Figure 6-7C. One femoral head was used to reconstruct the ace-tabulum and another was shaped like a napkin ring to provide calcar reinforcement and a greater trochanter. A trochanteric slide was used, leaving the abductors in continuity with the vastus lateralis. This musculotendinous sleeve was fastened to the trochanteric graft by means of a chair staple.

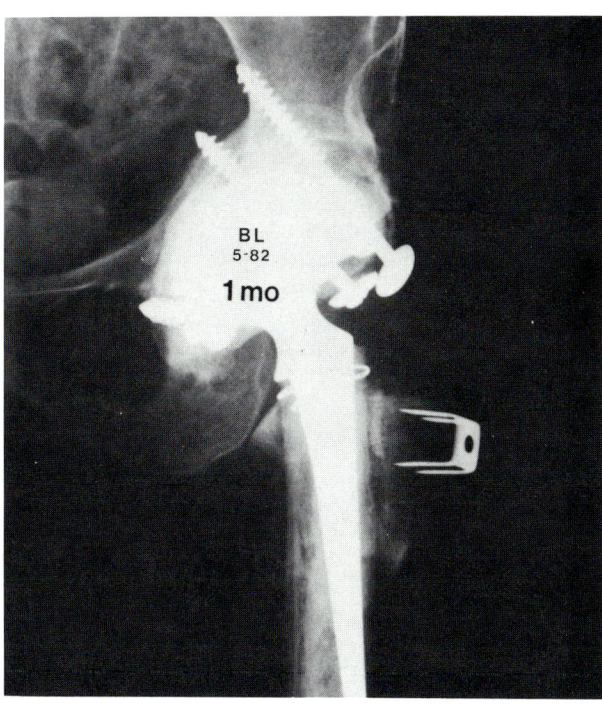

Figure 6-7D. X-rays one month postoperatively appear satisfactory.

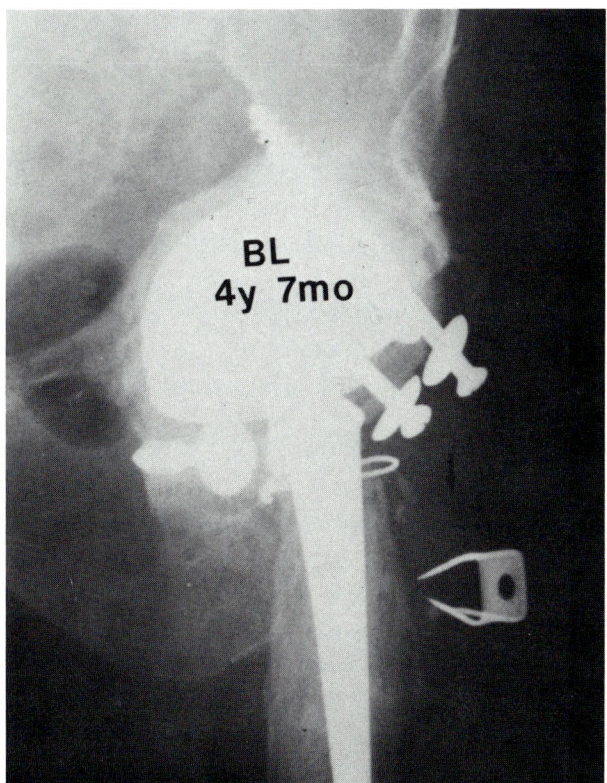

Figure 6-7E. X-rays at four years, seven months show that the femoral graft had disappeared. When the patient was revised at five years and two months for acetabular loosening, the entire femoral graft had resorbed. We no longer feel that this reconstruction is of value (at least with cemented femoral components) because the graft is not stressed. The transverse inferior acetabular screw may have contributed to failure of the acetabulum by preventing impaction and remodeling of the acetabular graft.

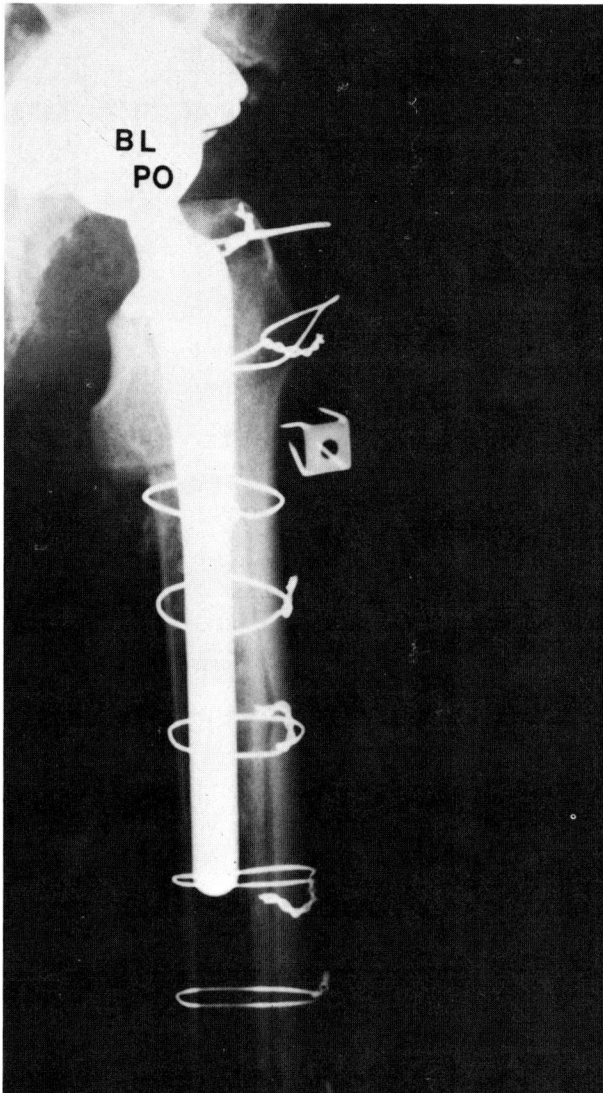

Figure 6-7F. An uncemented acetabular component was used at revision. No further acetabular grafting was necessary. A major femoral allograft was necessary to reconstruct the deficient proximal metaphysis and trochanter. The technique was similar to that seen in Figure 6-22F.

right proximal femoral allograft was split in half and the insides of the grafts were contoured to the outside of the patient's proximal femur (Figure 6-8C). The grafts were fixed with cerclage wires. Cortical and cancellous strips from the iliac crest were added. Both allografts reinforced the stress shielded proximal femur and the lateral graft provided a greater trochanter.

At one year, seven months, the grafts appear to be incorporating (Figures 6-8D and 6-8E). The patient walks without support and has strong abductor power but is disappointed because he still has pain in his thigh, surely from the proximably loose long stem component. He rates 70. We are contemplating revision of the femoral component. It will probably be necessary to window the distal femur (as in Figure 6-4C), in order to remove the cement and then hopefully a conventional length uncemented femoral device

can be used with its sintered surface against the shell of living bone of the proximal femur which has been reinforced by the cortical onlay grafts.

Cortical Thinning

Cortical thinning occurred as an isolated problem in only two patients (5%). It was present in combination with other femoral defects in ten other cases. We therefore had a total of 12 hips (28%) with problems related to thinning of the femoral cortex. In all instances, this defect was associated with a failed cemented femoral component. The lateral femoral cortex was most commonly involved.

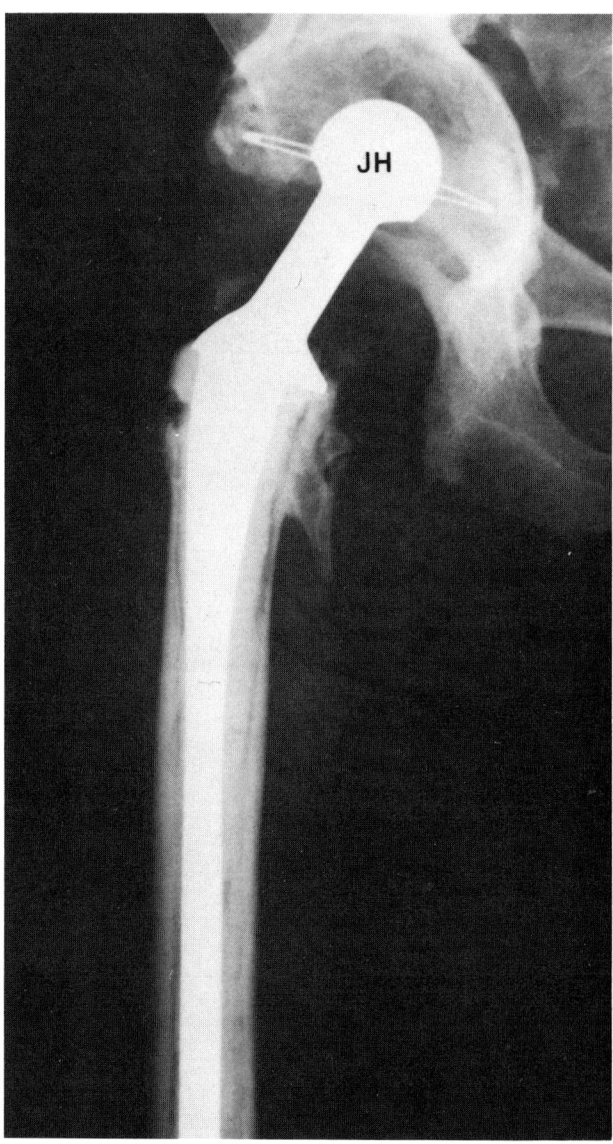

Figure 6-8A. This 43-year-old man had recurrent dislocation of his hip because of a malpositioned acetabular component and had pain from both a loose acetabular and loose femoral component. There is no greater trochanter. The proximal femur has undergone significant resorption and at surgery the component toggled proximally but the cement was well fixed distally. This is a classic example of cemented long stem disease.

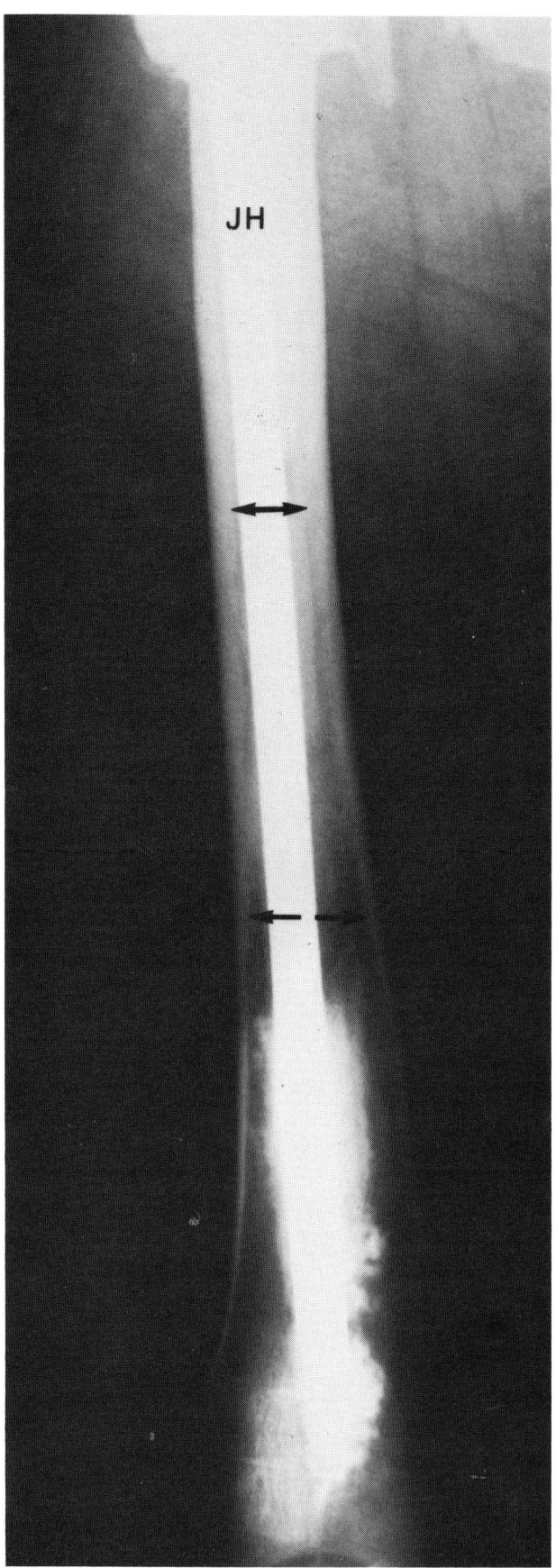

Figure 6-8B. The distal cement is well fixed to the stem and can not pass proximally through the narrow isthmus.

Review of Literature. Turner and others have advocated cemented long stem components in all femoral revision total hip replacement surgery and particularly in association with significant cortical compromise.[10,11] We have found no reports in the literature concerning the use of onlay cortical allografts to reinforce areas of cortical thinning.

Treatment. For reasons previously mentioned, we feel that a cemented long stem component has many disadvantages, including the danger that cortices that are already thin will undergo even further stress shielding because of the thick construct of metal and cement.

Our preference is to use onlay cortical allografts that extend at least 8cm. proximal and distal to the weak area. As with all allografts, we feel that autografts should be added to aid in union of the allograft. The medullary surfaces of the allografts are contoured to match the outer circumference of the patient's femur and the grafts are fixed to the recipient femur by multiple cerclage wires. In the past we have used #18 Vitallium wires (Howmedica, Rutherford, NJ), but more recently found that #16 Luque wires (Zimmer, Warsaw, IN) break less frequently when being tightened. It is preferable to twist the cerclage wires rather than to tie knots because it is difficult to tie knots tightly. We prefer to use the Harris wire tightener (Codman and Shurtleff, Inc., Randolph, MA). Wires are tightened sequentially and frequently a previously tightened wire will become loose when adjacent wires have been tightened. All loose wires must be replaced so all wires are equally tight at the termination of the procedure. Great care must be taken to avoid trapping soft tissue, especially the sciatic nerve, when passing the wires. We have found a bone hook with a small hole in its tip to be the easiest and safest device for passing wires around the femur (Figure 3-25).

The revision component should normally be uncemented and of standard length. The decision whether a longer stem is necessary should not be influenced by the area of cortical thinning because cortical onlay grafts provide enough strength so that early weightbearing can be allowed as long as there are no other contraindications.

Clinical Examples

Case 1

The patient whose x-rays are seen in Figure 6-9A was 46 when he presented with a loose acetabular component and significant thinning of the proximal lateral cortex of the femur related to a loose femoral component that had fallen into varus. He had undergone multiple previous operations following his initial fracture dislocation 18 years previously. These included three cup arthroplasties, a Moore prosthesis and a total hip. The acetabular reconstruction has been previously discussed (Figure 5-20).

Reconstruction of the femur was accomplished by means of a full thickness femoral allograft strut which was used to reinforce the lateral cortex and was held in place with cerclage wires (Figure 6-9B). Although there was also an

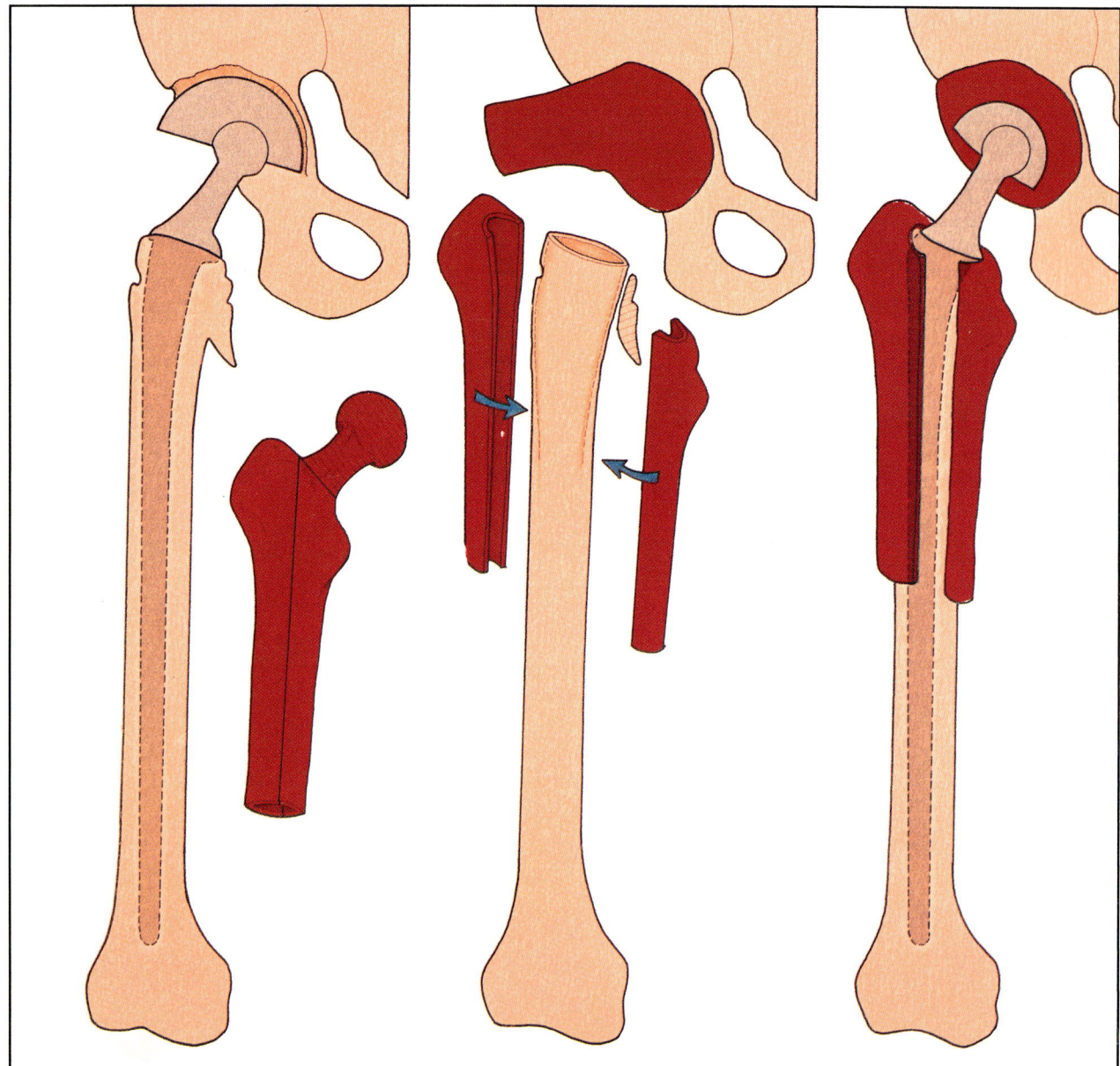

Figure 6-8C. A distal femur was used to reconstruct the acetabulum. A proximal allograft femur was split in half and the inner surfaces of the grafts were contoured to match the outer surface of the patient's femur. These grafts provide cortical reinforcement and the lateral one improves the abductor moment arm.

associated calcar intramedullary defect, this proved to be minor. There was adequate bone left in the calcar region to support the calcar of the cementless femoral prosthesis. This intramedullary calcar defect was packed with auto-genous iliac crest bone. Autogenous cortical and cancellous bone strips from the iliac crest were also placed about the onlay cortical allograft. During one of the previous operations, transection of the abductors had occurred. These were repaired at the time of his bone grafting procedure. In order to allow reattachment of the greater trochanter to the trochanteric bed, the gluteus medius and minimus attachment to the iliac wing had to be entirely released and the abductor mechanism slid 2cm. distally on its neurovascular pedicle.

The patient was protected with two axillary crutches for eight weeks and then used a cane, which he discarded three months after his revision. He is now one and one half years since surgery. X-rays suggest early incorporation of the onlay graft (Figure 6-9C). The patient walks without support but has a mild abductor lurch. He works full-time as an automobile mechanic. He has no pain and rates 92.

Case 2

The patient whose x-rays are seen in Figure 6-10A was a 64-year-old man who had had a total hip replacement eight years previously for degenerative arthritis. There was significant resorption of the proximal lateral femur associated with subsidence of the femoral component. Exposure was

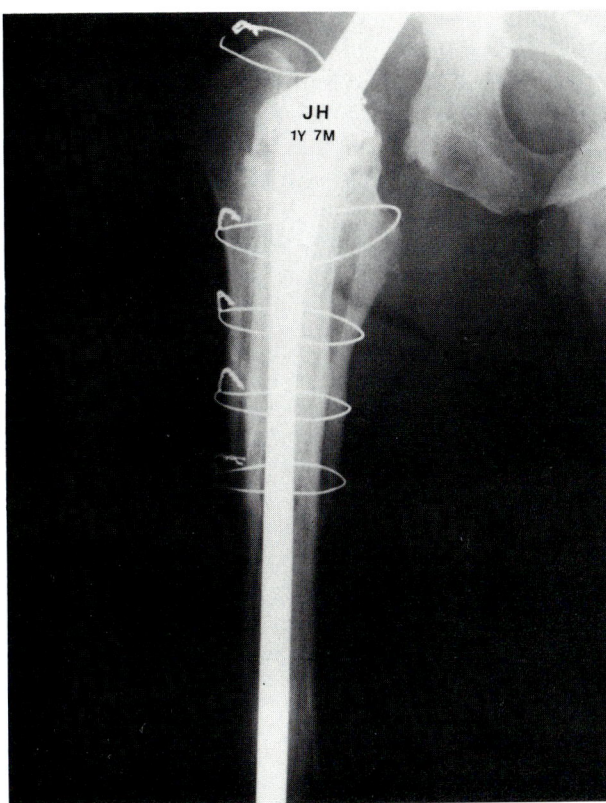

Figure 6-8D. At one year, seven months, the grafts appear to be incorporating. The patient has strong abductor power and walks without support, but is disappointed because he still has thigh pain because the femoral component is still loose. He rates 70 and we are contemplating revision of the femoral component.

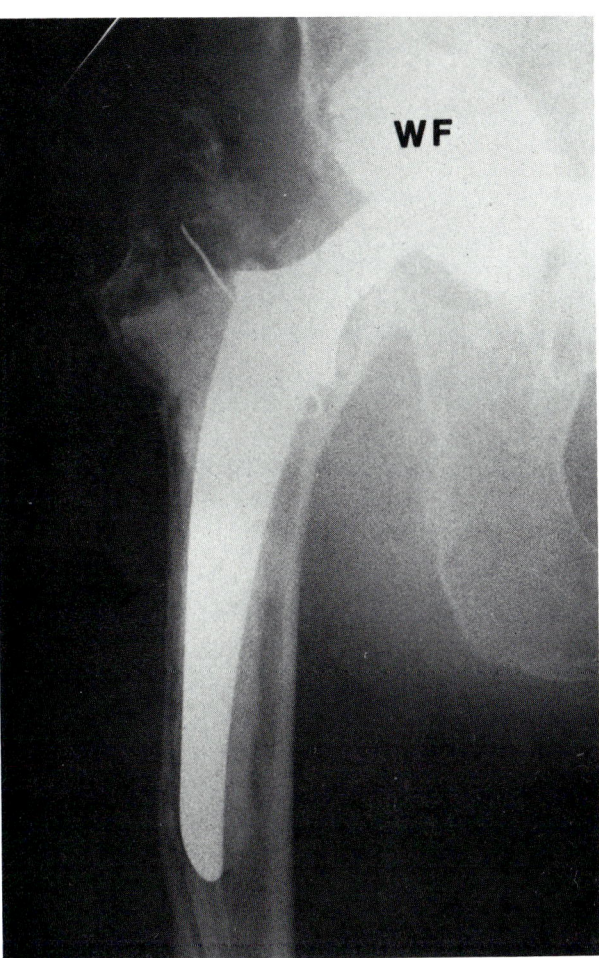

Figure 6-9A. This 46-year-old man had a loose cemented femoral component that had subsided into varus. There was major thinning of the lateral cortex. The calcar intramedullary defect was less significant than might appear from this x-ray.

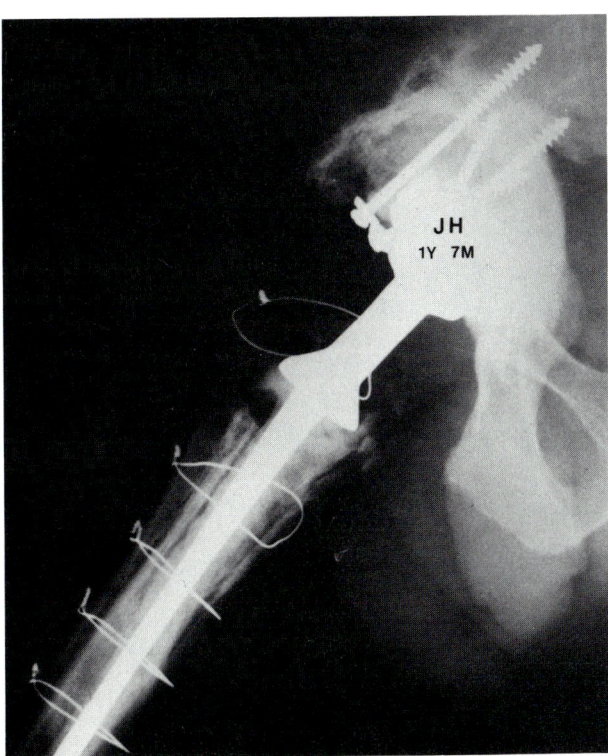

Figure 6-8E. The grafts appear to be doing well at one year, seven months.

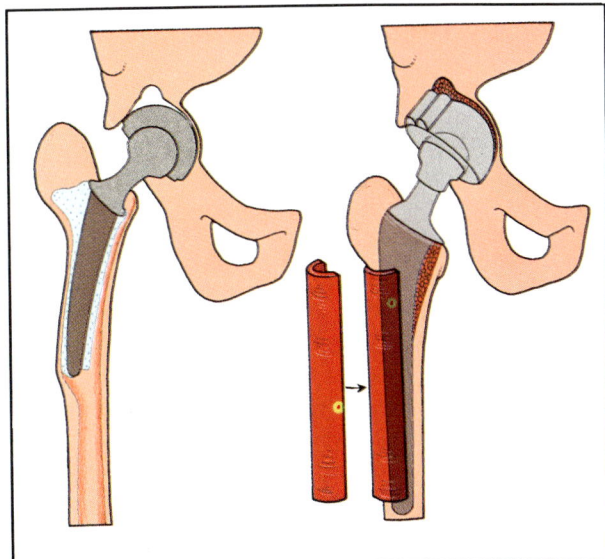

Figure 6-9B. The calcar of the uncemented femoral component rested on an area of intact calcar. Cancellous iliac crest bone was used within the calcar, beneath the collar. A cortical onlay graft was used to reinforce the thin lateral cortex.

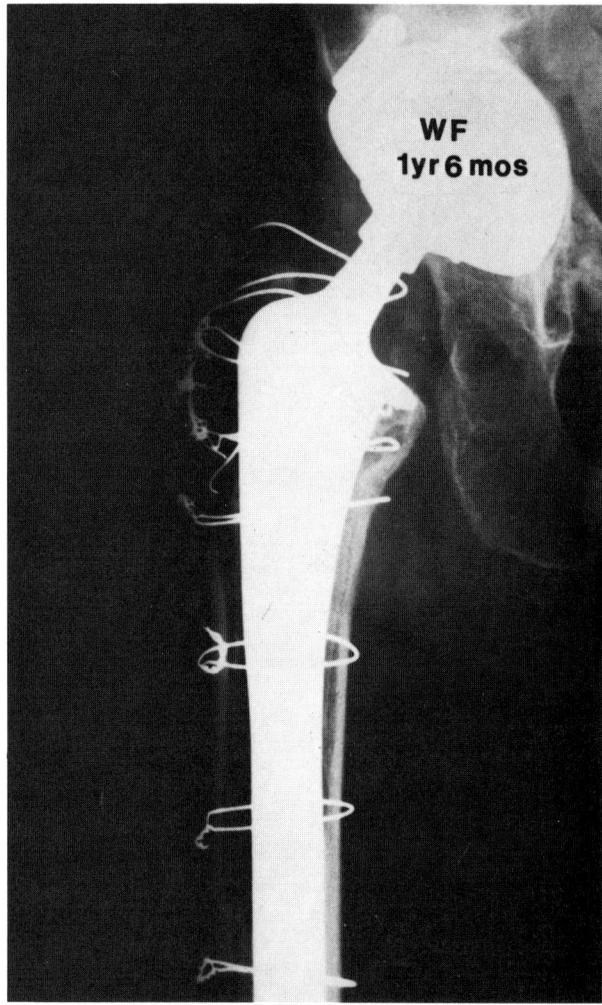

Figure 6-9C. X-rays at one and one half years appear satisfactory. Note that the uncemented femoral stem extends slightly distal to the defect and is engaged in the normal distal medullary canal. At followup of one and one half years, the patient works successfully as an automobile mechanic. He has no pain and walks without support but has a mild abductor lurch. He rates 92.

obtained by means of the trochanteric slide. The lateral cortex was very thin and at the time of revision, an allograft onlay cortical graft was used to reinforce the weakened lateral cortex of the femur. Cement was not used on the acetabular or femoral side. X-rays at two months show that the onlay graft is in good position and the standard length component engages the normal canal distally (Figure 6-10B). At this time the patient was shifted from crutches to a cane, which he used for another month. X-rays at two years show that the distal end of the graft has rounded off and the greater trochanter has united proximally to the allograft (Figure 6-10C). At follow-up of two years and five months the patient rates 100.

Cortical Perforation

In our series, five patients (12%) had isolated femoral perforations and four others had a perforation in conjunc-

tion with another femoral defect, making nine patients (21%) with cortical perforations.

In all cases, a failed cemented total hip replacement femoral component was present. Cortical defects may occur from lysis secondary to a loose component or may be created at the time of revision, either inadvertantly or by the use of an elective window to remove cement.

Review of Literature. Studies have demonstrated that stresses will normalize approximately two cortical diameters below the level of compromised bone.[13,14] As with cortical thinning, it therefore has been recommended that a cemented stem bypass the perforation by a distance of 110mm.[12] Most authors have advocated autogenous grafting as well and crutch protection for at least six months.[15,16]

Authors' Preferred Treatment. We prefer to replace a window if it is available and to graft the area with autogenous cancellous and cortical strips from the ilium. A large cortical onlay graft, contoured to fit the outside of the

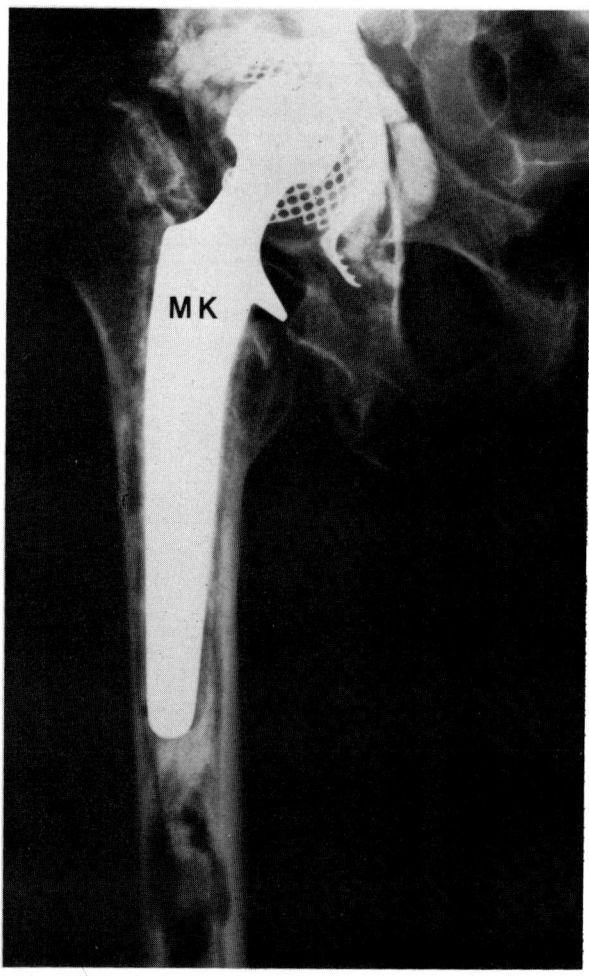

Figure 6-10A. This 64-year-old man had his original total hip replacement eight years previously. There is subsidence and varus positioning of the component. Although there was some loss of the calcar, this was not significant enough to require reconstruction. The major problem was thinning of the lateral femoral cortex.

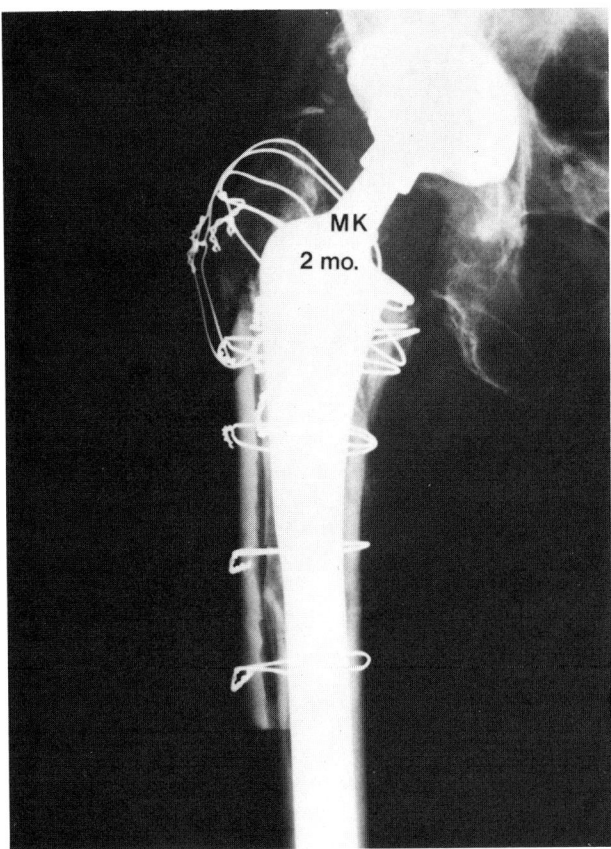

Figure 6-10B. X-rays at two months show the lateral onlay graft is in good position. Note that the standard length uncemented stem engages the normal distal medullary canal. Neither component is cemented.

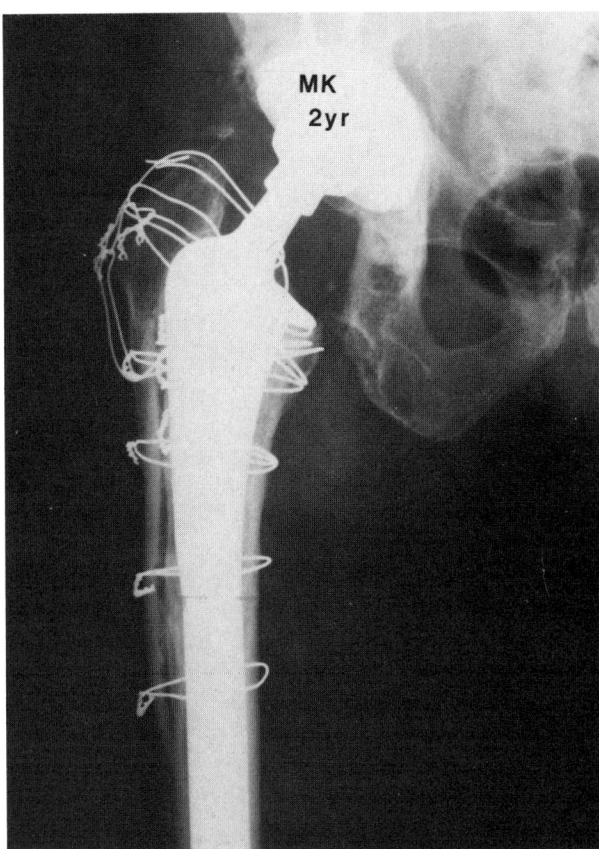

Figure 6-10C. X-rays at two years show that the distal end of the graft has rounded off and the greater trochanter appears to have united to the allograft. At followup of two years, five months, the patient rates 100.

patient's femur, should cover at least one half of the circumference of the recipient femur and should extend at least 8cm. distal, and if possible, the same distance proximal to the defect. The graft is held in place by multiple cerclage wires. In addition to grafting the defect beneath the allograft, we routinely add cortical and cancellous strips to the junction of the allograft and the host bone. Standard length uncemented components are adequate, even if they do not bypass the perforation. We do not protect these femurs any longer than primary hips and allow full weight-bearing as tolerated by six weeks. We have not had a fracture in 21 cases of thinning or perforation that have been followed at least six months.

Because of these encouraging early results with allograft cortical struts, we now do not hesitate to make an elective window anteriorly if distal cement is difficult to remove because it does not take long to fashion a protective graft and postoperative management is then not affected by the window.

Clinical Examples

Case 1

The patient whose x-rays are seen in Figure 6-11A was 62 when she presented to us in 1981 with a resection arthro-

plasty which had been performed four years previously. She had a femoral neck fracture ten years before that was fixed with pins. These were later removed. She developed avascular necrosis and a total hip replacement was performed. Five months later, a resection arthroplasty was performed because of a *Staphylococcus epidermidis* infection. The previous surgeon removed a large window, leaving a proximal femoral perforation which was approximately 20cm. in length and comprised more than one third of the circumference of her femur. She also had superior rim and superior intra-acetabular defects, which required an acetabular allograft.

A trochanteric slide was used for exposure. A large cortical onlay allograft was fashioned from a donor femur and fixation was provided by cerclage wires (Figure 6-11B). Six years ago we were not as confident about the strength of onlay grafts as we are now and used a cemented long stem prosthesis. X-rays at one month (Figure 6-11C), compared with x-rays at three years, seven months show that the graft is remodeling and the sharp distal end has blended with the patient's femur (Figure 6-11D). X-rays at five years, nine months show that the graft has not only united to the patient's femur, but is participating in the dramatic stress shielding of the femur secondary to the cemented long stem prosthesis (Figure 6-11E). Despite the worrisome cortical

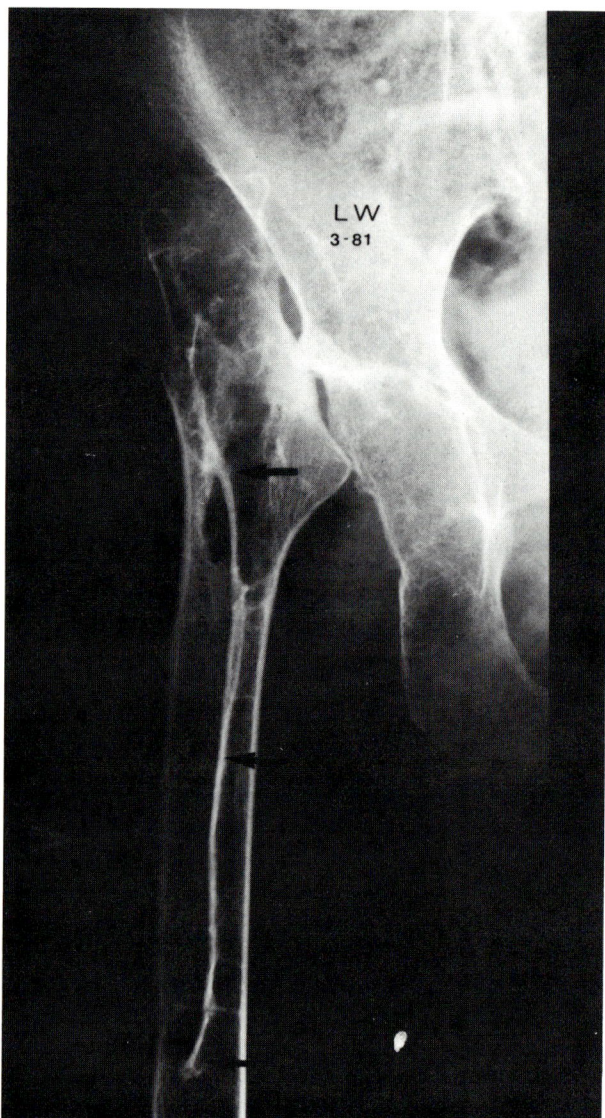

Figure 6-11A. This 62-year-old woman had a resection arthroplasty performed four years previously because of a septic *Staphylococcus epidermidis* hip. She had superior rim and superior intra-acetabular defects as well as a large femoral window.

femoral bone loss, the patient rates 100 and is delighted with her function. However, if the femoral component ever needs to be revised she will probably need a major allograft replacement of the proximal two thirds of her femur. We now feel that there is no indication for a cemented long stem prosthesis except, perhaps, in the terminal cancer patient who needs a short term palliative reconstruction.

Case 2

The patient whose x-rays are seen in Figure 6-12A was 53 when she presented with a resection arthroplasty that was performed because of a *Staphylococcus epidermidis* infection of a total hip replacement. In the process of removing the femoral cement, the referring surgeon was aware that the lateral shaft had been perforated (Figures 6-12B and 6-12C). Three months after the resection arthroplasty, the sedimen-

tation rate returned to normal, there was no sign of infection and a revision was performed.

As anticipated, a lateral perforation measuring 2cm.×3cm. was found when the hip was approached by means of the trochanteric slide approach. A large onlay femoral cortical allograft was used to reinforce the femur after the defect was grafted with autogenous strips from the iliac crest. Because the acetabular component was unstable, it was cemented. However, we would now use an uncemented component with screws. A standard length uncemented femoral component was used. The distal tip extended to the upper margins of the graft and was well proximal to the defect (Figure 6-12D). Partial weightbearing with a walker was started on the fourth postoperative day.

This patient has severe Parkinson's disease and had eight posterior dislocations over the following four months. The hip was reduced by closed methods on each occasion. After an adductor tenotomy and an anterior obturator neurectomy, the hip has remained stable without further dislocation the past two years. The graft appears to have united by x-ray at two years, four months (Figure 6-12E). Because of Parkinson's disease, the patient is still quite incapacitated and requires a walker for balance. She has full motion and no pain but at two years, ten months rates only 74 because of the functional limitations imposed by her Parkinson's disease.

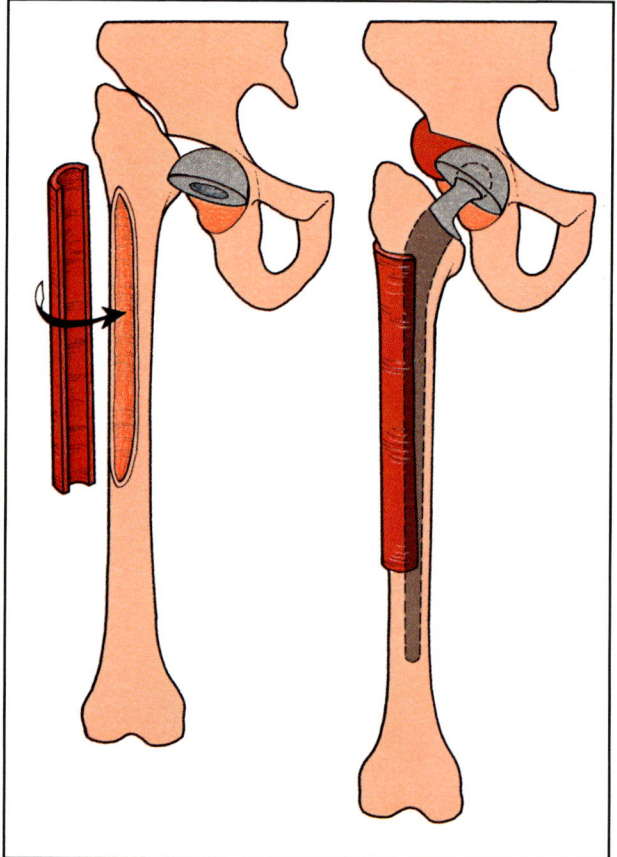

Figure 6-11B. A large femoral cortical onlay allograft was used to cover the defect.

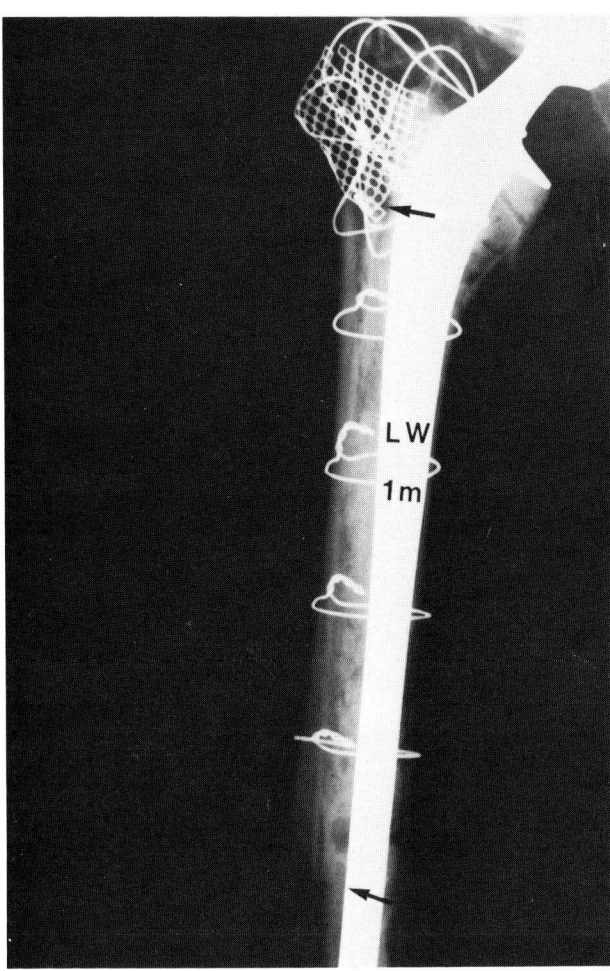

Figure 6-11C. At one month the graft can be seen on the lateral surface of the patient's femur. The arrows point to the proximal and distal end of the graft. Note that the distal end of the graft is square.

Case 3

The patient whose x-rays are seen in Figure 6-13A was 76 when she presented with a resection arthroplasty. A total hip replacement had been performed two years previously as treatment for degenerative arthritis. She had persistant pain and developed a draining sinus. Despite a sedimentation rate of over 100, cultures remained negative. A resection arthroplasty was performed with extensive debridement of obviously infected material. There was a 2cm.×2cm. perforation in the lateral femur 2cm. below the greater trochanter and the sinus tract extended to this defect. In the process of removing the distal femoral cement, a second 5cm.×1cm. long perforation of the femur occurred posterolaterally. Tobramycin-impregnated methylmethacrylate beads were inserted and the patient was treated with antibiotics for two months prior to her definitive revision procedure (Figure 6-13B).

At the time of reconstruction, autogenous grafts were first harvested from the iliac crest and then the iliac crest incision was closed before the hip was explored in order to avoid potential contamination of the donor site. An allograft femoral head was used to reconstruct the extensive superior

rim and superior intra-acetabular defect. A large onlay femoral cortical allograft was used to protect the femur after the perforations were grafted with strips from the iliac crest. Uncemented components were used for both the acetabulum and femur. The standard length femoral component extended just beyond the distal perforation. Antibiotics were continued for one month. Crutches were discarded at eight weeks. At one year, the grafts appear to be doing well by x-ray (Figure 6-13C). At followup of 14 months the sedimentation rate is 15. The patient uses a cane for balance purposes only on long outside walks and rates 96.

Femoral Fractures About or Below the Stem of a Femoral Component

In our series, there were four patients (11%) who had a femoral fracture about or below the stem of a femoral

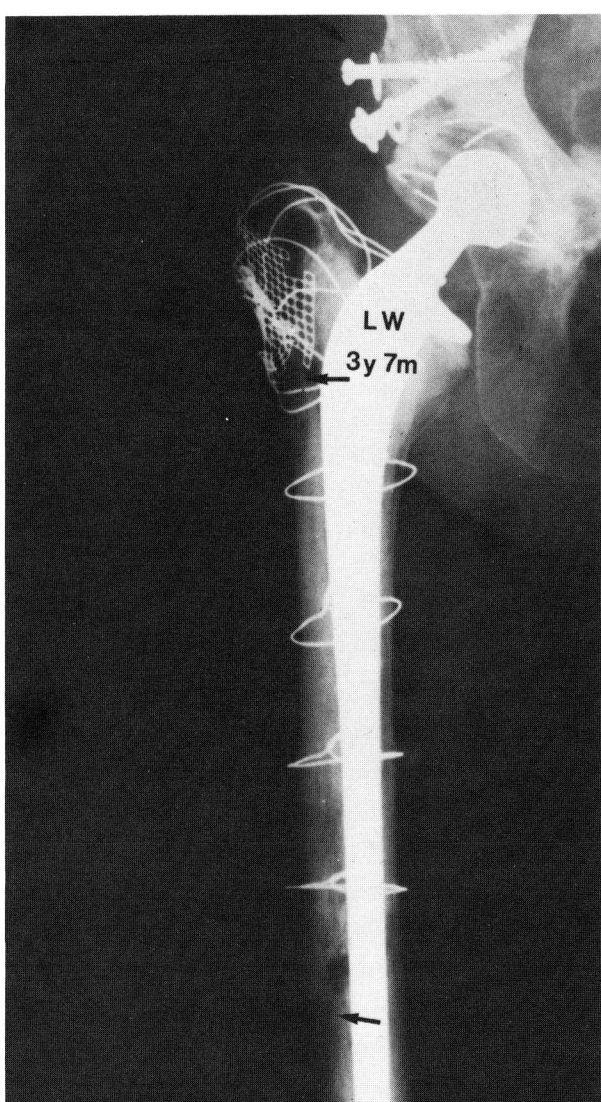

Figure 6-11D. X-rays at three years, seven months show that the distal end of the graft has now become rounded and the graft probably has united.

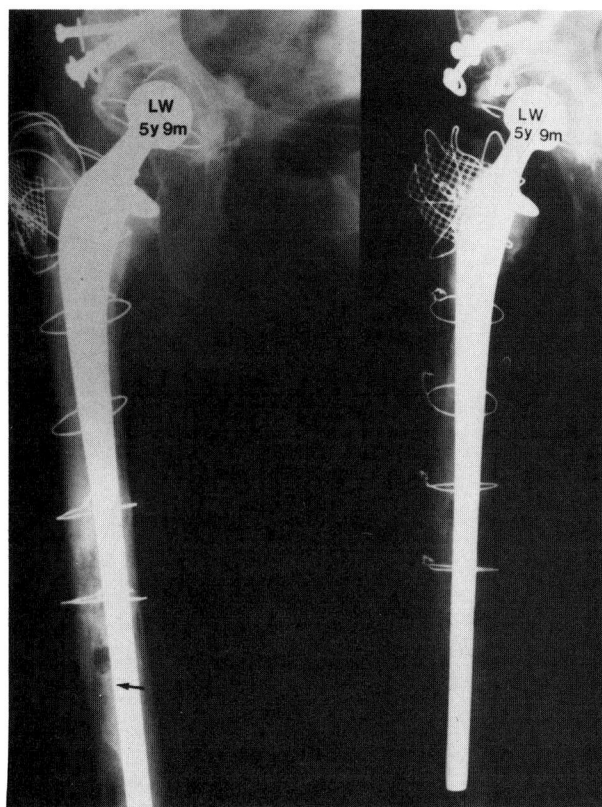

Figure 6-11E. At five years, nine months, the graft appears to be showing stress shielding along with the rest of the femur. The patient rates 100 but would need an allograft of the entire femur if the component ever had to be changed.

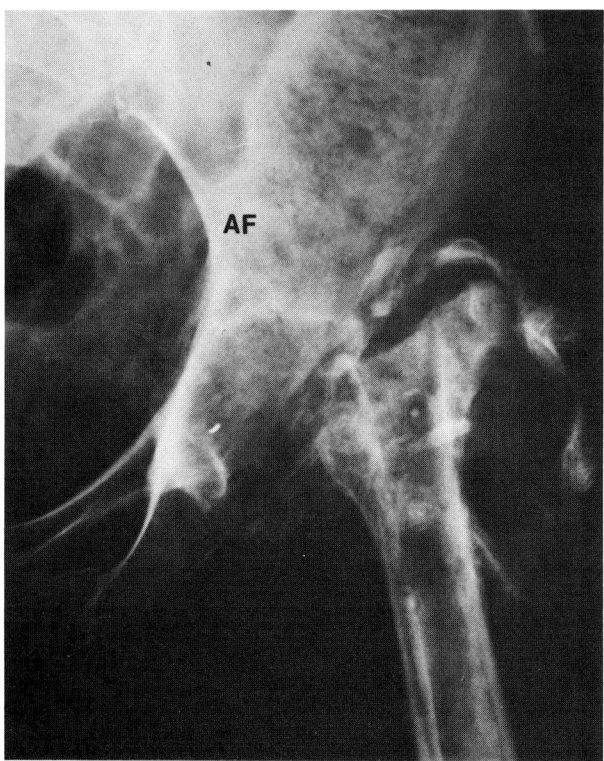

Figure 6-12A. This 53-year-old woman had a resection arthroplasty for a *Staphylococcus epidermidis* infection.

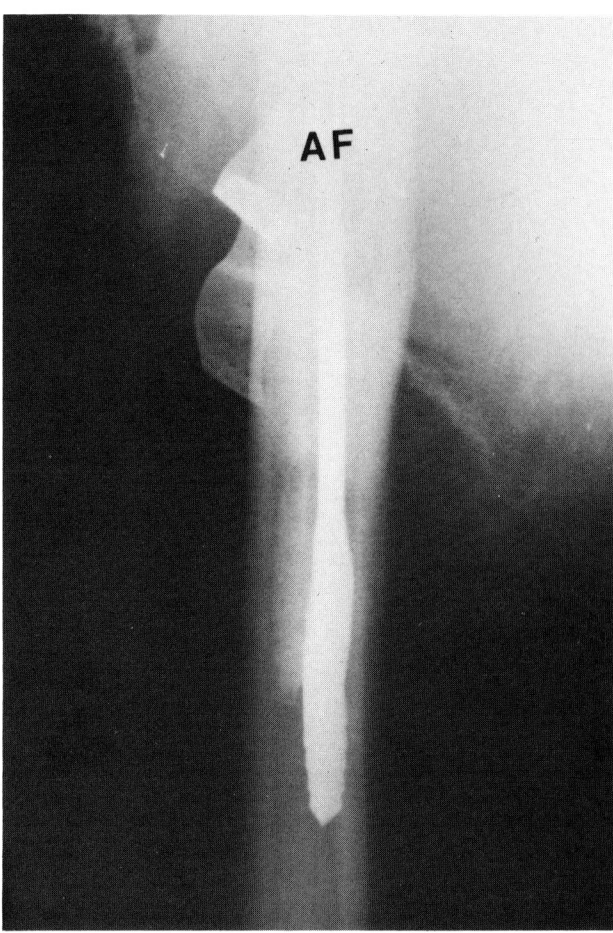

Figure 6-12B. The referring surgeon was aware that he had perforated the lateral cortex while removing the cement.

component. Two others had a fracture at the junction of an allograft proximal replacement and the patient's femur, making a total of six hips (14%) with femoral fractures. All were associated with a failed hip arthroplasty. One patient with a long stem custom uncemented Moore prosthesis sustained an intra-operative fracture. Three patients had cemented total hip replacement stems. Two of these patients fell and had fractures just distal to well-cemented stems that were not loose. One other patient had a loose cemented stem and sustained a fracture about the stem when he fell. Two other patients had stress fractures distal to uncemented stems following proximal femoral allograft replacement.

Review of Literature. The results of traction treatment for fractures related to total hip stems have not been favorable. There is a high incidence of nonunion, malunion and/or loosening of the component.[17] In addition to the poor results, most elderly patients cannot tolerate prolonged bed rest. With long oblique fractures, cerclage wires can theoretically be used, but without additional fixation they are not strong enough to allow mobilization of the patient and failure is likely. Plates have been used successfully,[18] but screw holes create stress risers and fractures can occur at the end of the plate.

The best immediate results have been reported with local

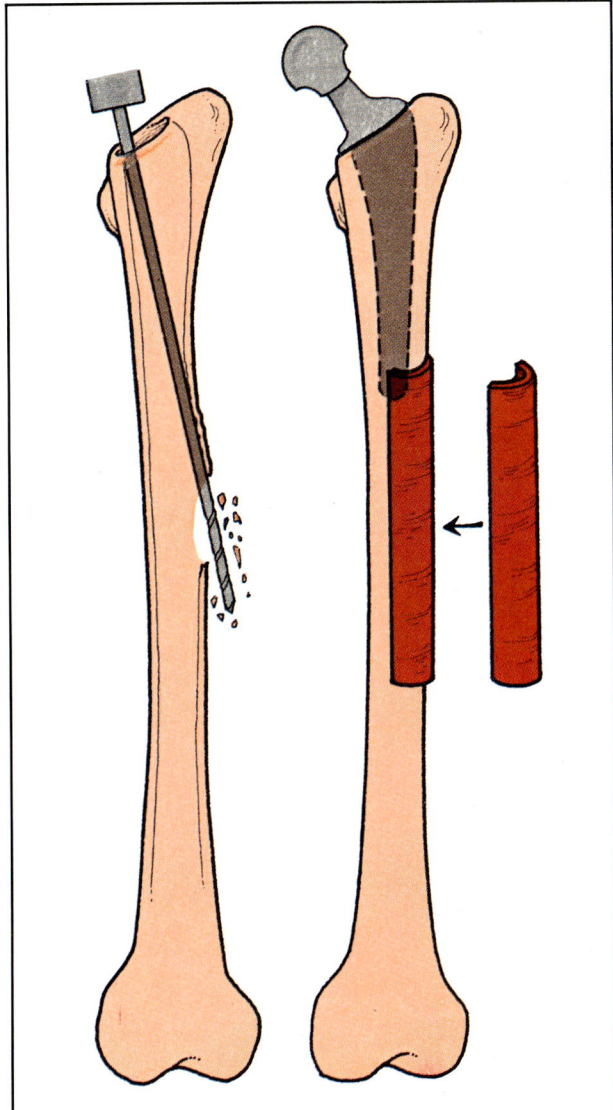

Figure 6-12C. The defect was grafted with autogenous strips of bone from the iliac crest and then the femur was protected by means of a large cortical allograft.

autografts used in conjunction with cemented long stems which extend well past the fracture;[19] however, this technique has several disadvantages. In order to insert the new long stem, the old component must be removed, even if it is not loose. Although cement per se does not prevent union of a fracture if bone contact is good, it can prevent healing if extrusion between the fracture fragments occurs. A stem that is cemented on either side of a fracture can theoretically cause a nonunion because the fracture fragments cannot impact (Figure 3-31). Finally, a cemented long stem component always produces cemented long stem disease if it is in place long enough.

Authors' Preferred Treatment. There are two types of femoral fractures associated with total hip replacement. The first is a fracture of the patient's femur with viable bone on both sides of the fracture. This may be simple and transversely oriented or a more complex, obliquely-ori-

ented spiral fracture. The second is a fracture at the junction of a nonrevascularized proximal femoral allograft replacement and the normal distal vascularized bone of the patients femur.

Fracture About or Below the Stem of a Femoral Component. Such fractures should heal in four to six months whether or not there is a component in place as long as fixation is adequate for that period of time. We prefer to treat the fracture by open reduction and by fixation with two massive femoral onlay cortical struts obtained from an allograft femur that is split into equal halves and that should extend at least 12cm. proximal and distal to the fracture. Combined they should cover at least two thirds of the circumference of the recipient femur. As with all onlay cortical struts, it is necessary to contour the inside of the struts to the outside of the patient's femur. Fixation of the two struts is accomplished by multiple Luque wires (Zimmer, Warsaw, IN). Although we have successfully used three separate tibial struts on a femur, we now feel that these struts are not strong enough and a fatigue fracture could theoretically occur before union occurs. The femoral struts should be placed medially and laterally to the anatomically reduced femoral shaft.

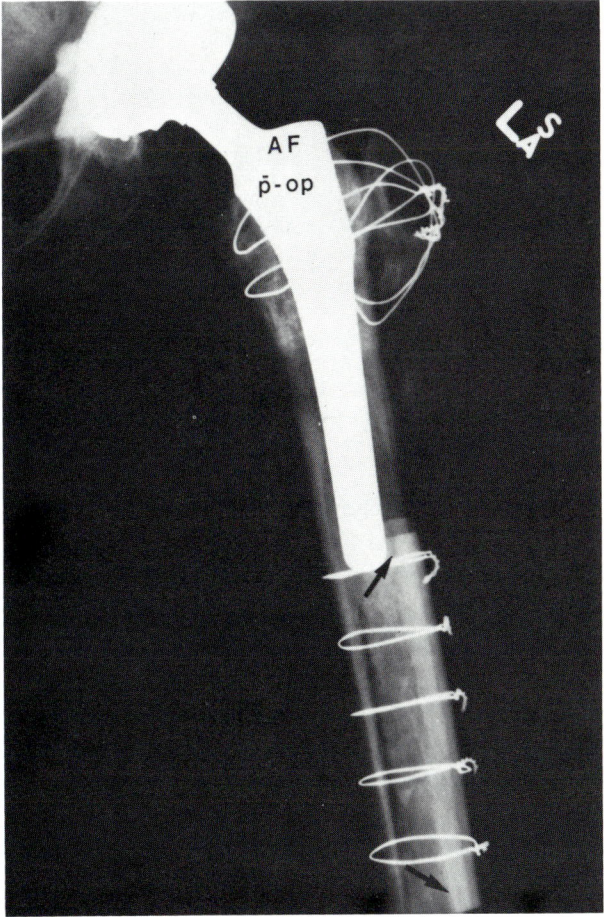

Figure 6-12D. X-rays just before discharge show the graft in place. Note the sharp ends of the graft. The tip of the standard length uncemented femoral component ends proximal to the defect.

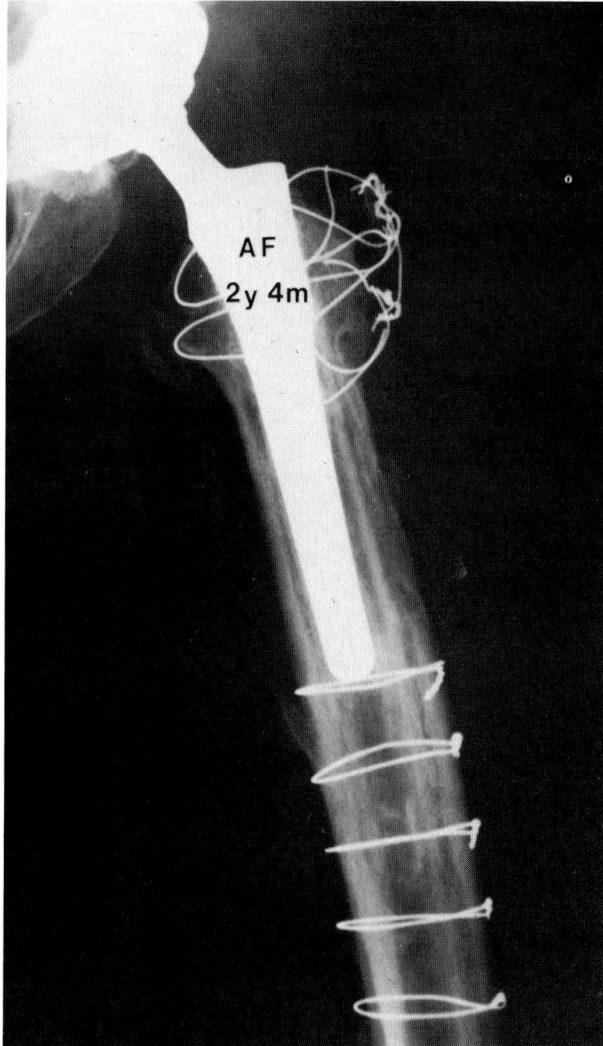

Figure 6-12E. X-rays at two years, four months show that the graft has united and the sharp ends of the graft now blend in with the cortex. Despite eight posterior dislocations which required closed reduction, the femur did not fracture. The patient has severe Parkinson's disease and must use a walker for balance. She has full motion and no pain but rates only 74 because of functional limitations imposed by Parkinson's disease.

If the old femoral component is not loose, it need not be disturbed. If it is loose, it should be changed. In this situation the fracture affords good distal exposure to remove the cement. Reduction and fixation of the fracture is performed and the surgeon's decision as to the length of the stem selected for revision should not be influenced by the fracture. We prefer to use an uncemented standard length stem for most revisions and do not feel that a long stem is usually necessary or desirable, even if used without cement.

These cortical onlay grafts are very strong because they are harvested from healthy, young donors, and the cortex is often ⅜ inch thick. The struts become weaker by four to six months, but by that time the fracture has united. Union of the fracture appears to occur very rapidly, probably because the struts have the same modulus as the patient's bone.

Although the function of the grafts is to splint the femur until union occurs, the grafts appear to unite to the femur as well.

In all four patients who had femoral shaft fractures, the hospital stay was under two weeks and the fractures have all healed. Although we used a cast brace in our first patient, we now feel that this is not necessary. In the three most recent cases, patients were allowed out of bed whenever they were comfortable (usually by the third postoperative day), and immediate partial weightbearing (30 to 60 lbs) was allowed, first with walkers and then with crutches. At eight weeks, patients progressed to canes as tolerated.

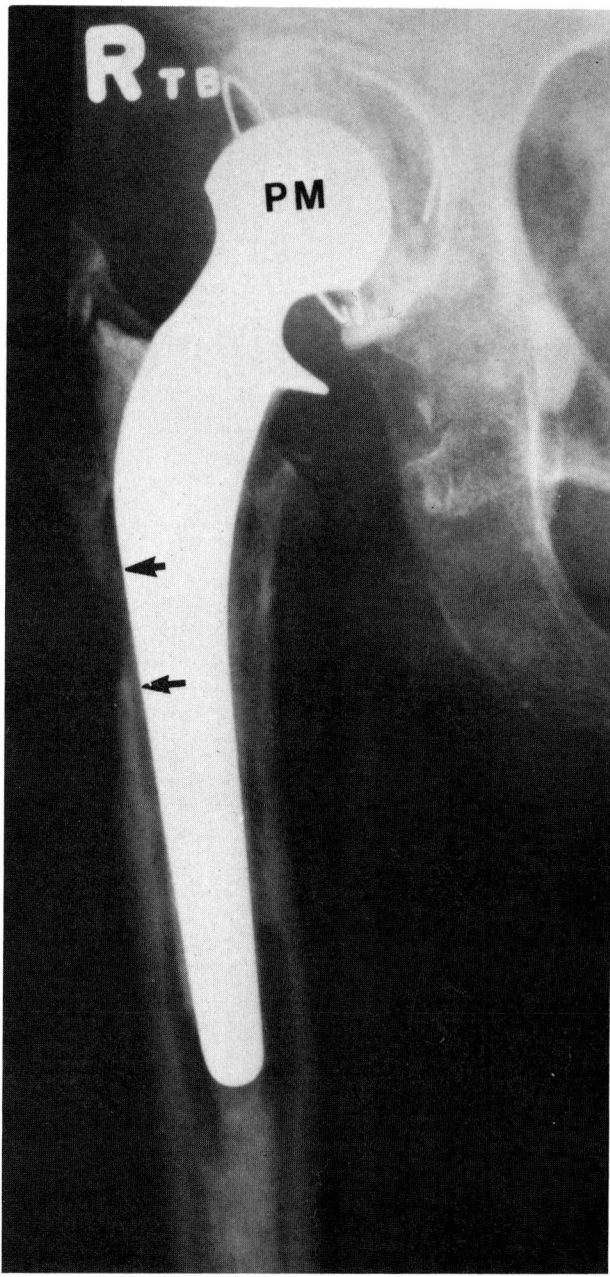

Figure 6-13A. This 76-year-old woman had an infected hip with a sinus extending to the large perforation just distal to the greater trochanter.

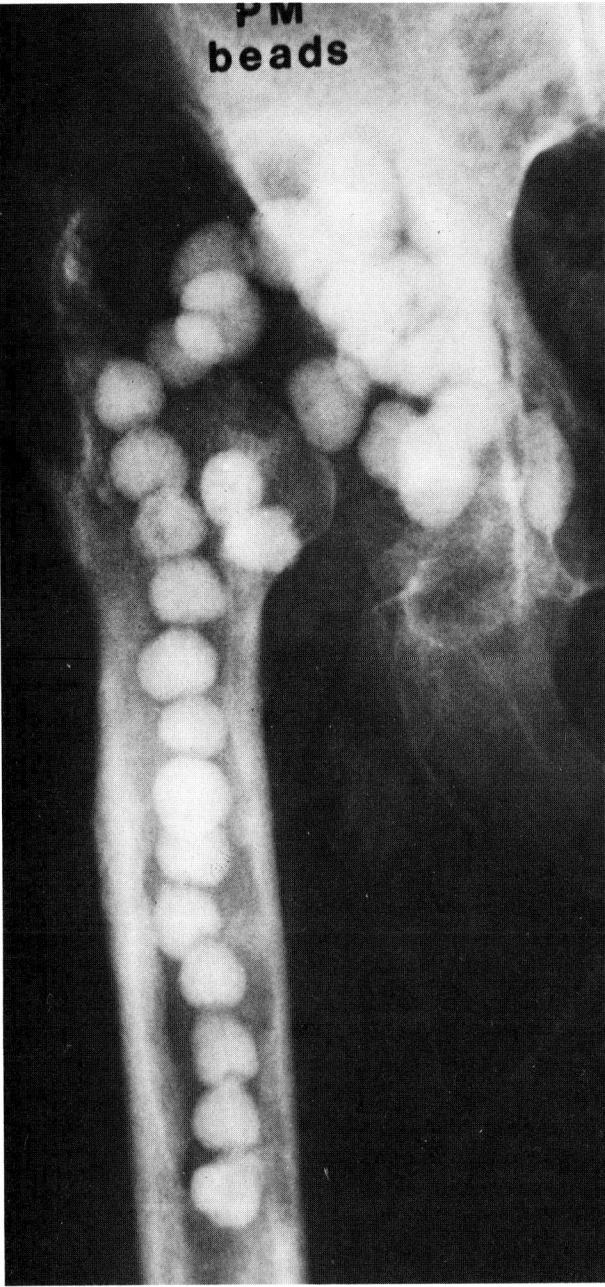

Figure 6-13B. An extensive debridement was performed. The arrows outline the original perforation. Unfortunately another 5cm.×1cm. perforation was created posterolaterally at the level of the distal end of the previous stem when the cement was removed. The patient was treated with tobramycin-impregnated beads and intravenous antibiotics for two months.

We feel that the use of onlay cortical allografts offers significant advantages over traction, the use of long stemmed implants, or metal plates and screws.

Clinical Examples

Case 1

The patient whose x-rays are seen in Figure 6-14A was 70 when she presented in 1982 with a fracture just distal to the tip of a cemented long stem prosthesis. Her initial

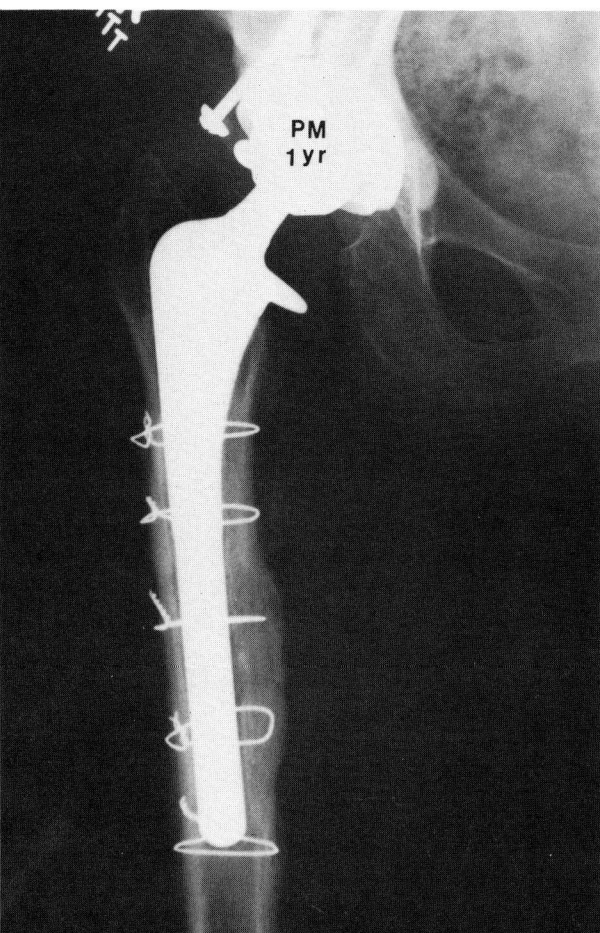

Figure 6-13C. A femoral head allograft was used to reconstruct the superior rim and superior intra-acetabular defect. All grafts appear to be doing well at one year. Neither component is cemented. The standard length femoral component extends just beyond the distal perforation. The patient uses a cane for balance and rates 96. Her sedimentation rate is 15.

problem was a base of neck fracture that went on to a nonunion. A conventional cemented total hip replacement failed because of femoral and acetabular loosening. At the time of revision of the femoral component to a long cemented stem in 1978, the femoral cortex was so thin that it could be deformed by manual pressure between the surgeon's thumb and index finger. When she fell four years later, the long stem component was still firmly fixed to the paper-thin proximal femur and could not have been removed without completely destroying the surrounding femur. The patient had multiple medical problems and did not tolerate bed rest and traction well. After one week in bed, it was obvious that she had to be mobilized because of her medical problems.

The trochanteric slide was used to approach the femur. A large allograft femur was split in half and the medullary surfaces were contoured to match the outer cortex of the patient's femur. The fracture was reduced and temporarily fixed with a cerclage wire and then the two cortical onlay femoral grafts were fixed with multiple cerclage wires (Fig-

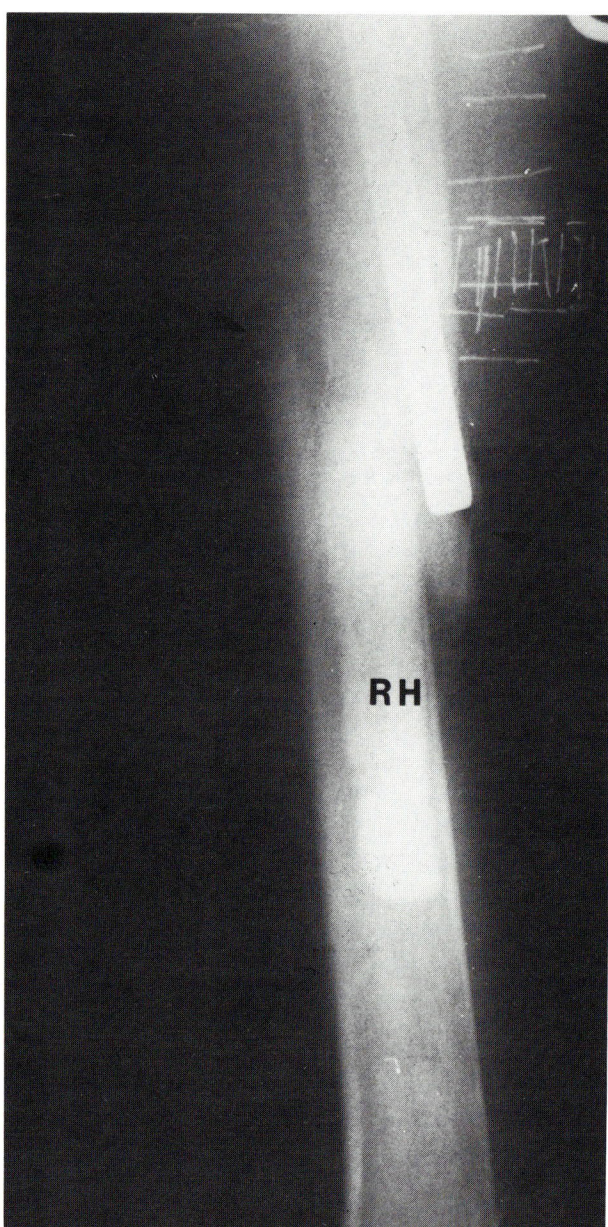

Figure 6-14A. This 70-year-old woman had a traumatic fracture just below the tip of a well-cemented long stem femoral component. The component could not have been removed from the proximal femur without destroying the bone.

ure 6-14B). The fracture and the junction between the allografts and the patient's femur were grafted with strips of autograft from the iliac crest. The patient was placed in a cast brace which she used for six weeks. She was able to get out of bed on the third postoperative day and was begun on partial weight bearing with a walker. The cast brace was removed at six weeks. In retrospect we feel that the brace was not necessary. The patient had no femoral pain after one week when she recovered from the surgical exposure. She used a walker permanently because of poor balance and a fear of falling, but she could bear full weight by eight weeks if someone accompanied her. X-rays at eight months suggest that the fracture has united (Figure 6-14C).

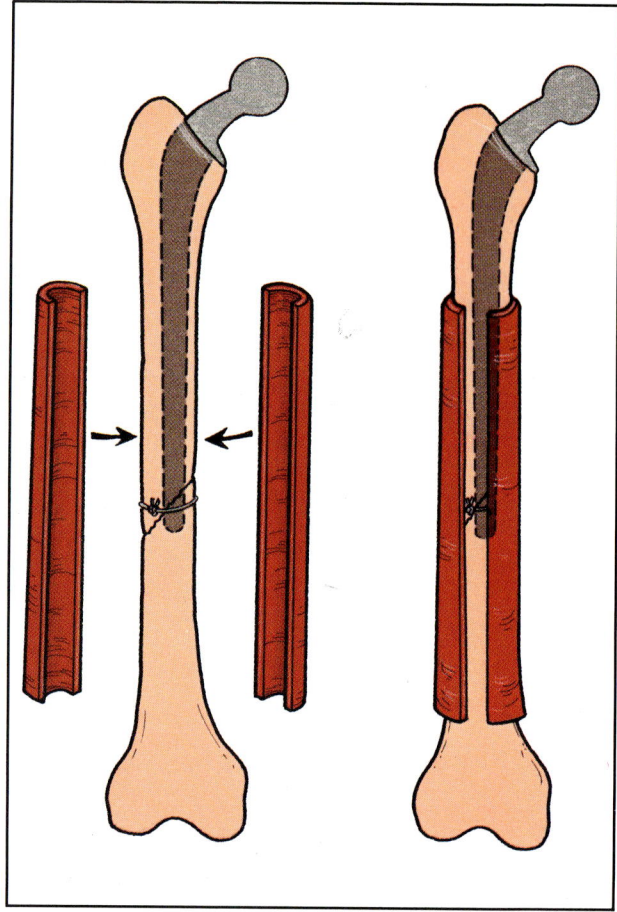

Figure 6-14B. An allograft femur was split in half. The medullary surfaces were contoured to fit the outside of the patient's femur and the two halves were used as an external splint. The fracture and the junction of the allografts with the patient's femur were grafted with strips of autograft from the ilium.

This patient died one year postoperatively of medical problems unrelated to her fracture or its treatment. Prior to her death, she did not have pain and had excellent motion; however, she had limited exercise tolerance because of unassociated medical problems and used a walker. She rated 75.

Case 2
The patient whose x-rays are seen in Figure 6-15A was 68 when she presented with a fracture distal to the stem of a well-fixed cemented total hip replacement. Her original total hip had been performed eight years previously. This was revised at four years because of femoral loosening. One year prior to admission she fell. From then on she had pain in her thigh and had to use crutches. She lived a distance away and her local physician obtained hip and knee x-rays which did not show the fracture. However, on examination she had a bowed femur and x-rays of the femur proved the diagnosis.

At surgery, the acetabular and femoral components were both well fixed. There was significant stress shielding of the calcar region of the femur and we elected to use an onlay

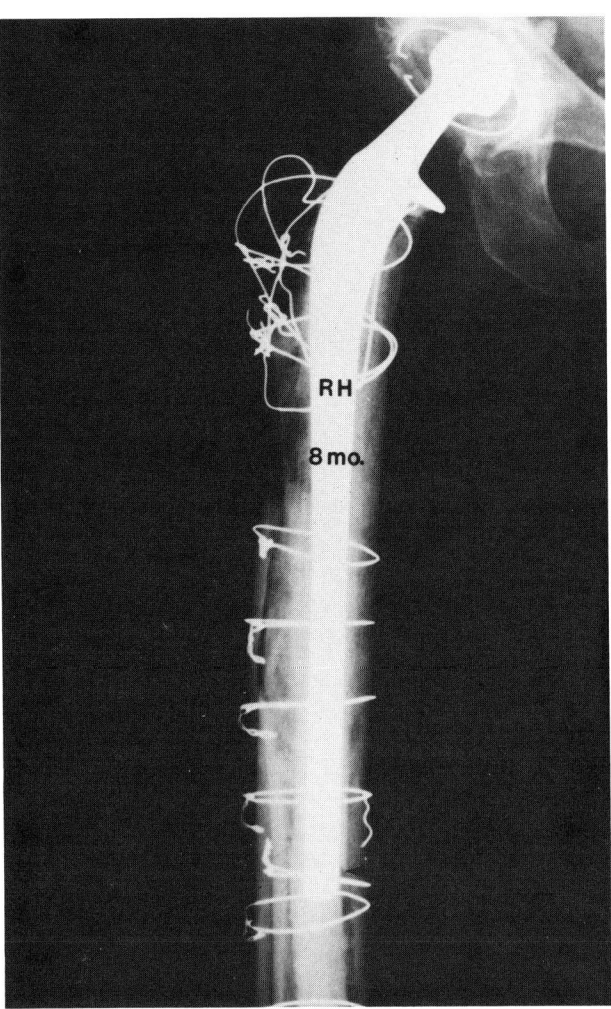

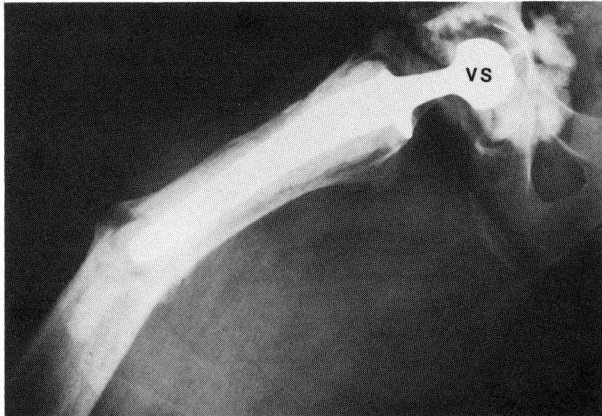

Figure 6-15A. This patient was 68 years old. By history the fracture occurred when she fell one year previously. She used crutches for that year but x-rays of her femur were not taken.

Figure 6-14C. X-rays at eight months suggest that the fracture had united. The patient had no pain and could bear weight but used a walker for balance. She rated 75.

allograft from a tibial plateau to reinforce this area. The rest of the tibia was cut into three equal struts. These allografts were placed laterally, anteriorly and medially and were held with cerclage wires (Figure 6-15B). Autogenous bone was used at the fracture site and at the junction of the onlay grafts and the patient's femur. The patient was up with crutches by the second postoperative day and was discharged to her home in seven days. She progressed to a cane at eight weeks. Because of an abductor lurch with unsupported walking, she required the cane for a total of six months but has not used support since. X-rays at six months suggest that the fracture had united (Figure 6-15C). X-rays at one year seven months appear unchanged except for the fact that the grafts appear to be remodeling and perhaps uniting to the patient's femur (Figure 6-15D). There may be slight bowing seen on the lateral view (Figure 6-15E). The patient rates 89.

Case 3

The patient whose x-rays are seen in Figure 6-16A was 58 when he presented to the emergency room after he had

fallen. He had a long history of hip problems starting with a fracture dislocation 22 years previously. An open reduction was performed. A cup arthroplasty was performed one year later. This was changed to a total hip replacement after ten years. Eleven years following the total hip he had obvious loosening of the femoral component and massive lysis of the proximal femur. He was scheduled for elective revision prior to his fracture (Figure 6-16B).

The vastus slide was used for exposure. The acetabular component was loose and was changed to a cementless component. The fracture of the femur allowed excellent exposure for cement removal. The fracture was reduced and temporarily held with two cerclage wires, then two femoral onlay grafts were used to reinforce the proximal femur. Autograft strips from the iliac crest were used to graft the fracture and the interfaces of the onlay allografts and the patient's femur. There was an associated calcar intramedullary defect that probably should have been grafted but the collar of the prosthesis appeared to be supported adequately by the remaining medial cortex (Figure 6-16C).

The patient initially did well and was discharged home on crutches at nine days. He was comfortable and was started on a cane at eight weeks. X-rays at nine months showed that the grafts seemed to be uniting and the fracture appeared healed but the uncemented femoral component had clearly subsided (Figure 6-16D). The patient had no pain but needed a cane to walk without an abductor lurch. Repeat x-rays at one year (Figure 6-16E) show little change. The patient still has no pain but requires a cane for walks of over one mile. He is ⅞ inch shorter and rates 93. The calcar deficiency clearly should have been grafted and a larger femoral component might also have prevented subsidence.

This patient is pleased with his result; however, he must be considered a failure, not of the bone graft for the fracture, but of an uncemented component. If he ever needs revision, he would be an ideal candidate for a combined calcar and medial strut calcar graft (Figure 6-5C).

Fatigue Fracture of an Allograft. Whereas fixation is usually only necessary for a few months with most femoral

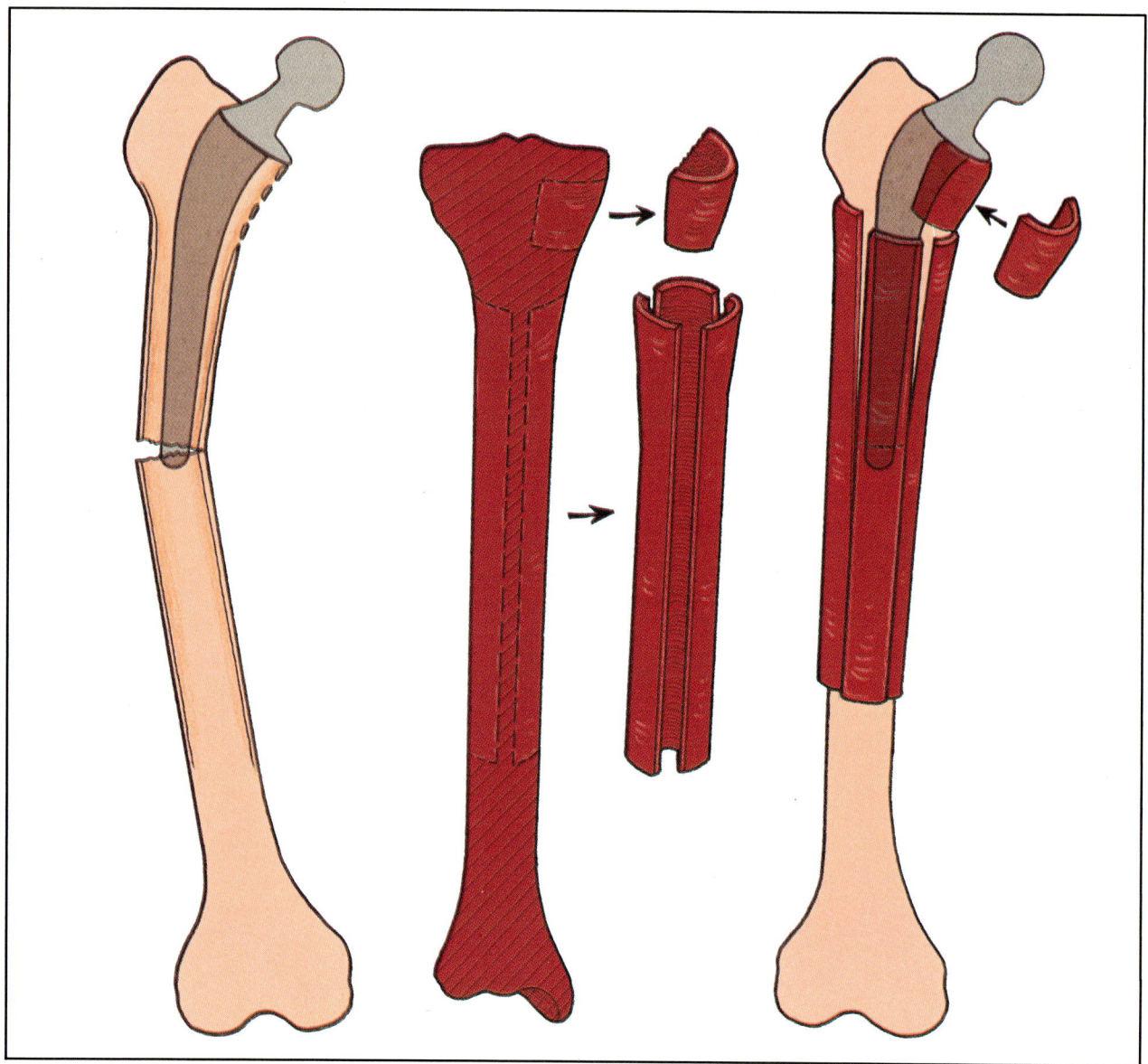

Figure 6-15B. An allograft tibia was split into three equal struts. One was placed laterally, the second anteriorly, and the third medially.

shaft fractures, the junction between a proximal femoral allograft and the recipient bone may take more than a year to unite. In our initial enthusiasm, we neglected to appreciate this obvious difference and have two patients who sustained a stress fracture at the interface between an allograft proximal replacement and the recipient bone. If the proximal allograft is short, it is supported by the stem of the femoral component, but if it extends below the femoral component, the stresses on the tension (lateral) side of the junction are too great for allograft struts to sustain. These grafts are strong enough initially but as they revascularize, they become weaker. Our two patients fractured at two and six months respectively.

Case 1

The patient whose x-rays are seen in Figure 6-17A was 70 when she presented with a fracture distal to a cemented long stem component. Reconstruction of her acetabular defect has been previously discussed (Figure 5-42). Her original diagnosis was degenerative arthritis of the right hip and she had her first total hip replacement performed eight years previously. This failed three years later and was revised using a long stem cemented prosthesis. Unfortunately an intra-operative fracture occurred and she required two axillary crutches for all steps following this procedure. Prior to her reconstruction, she had gross motion at the distal tip of the femoral component. X-rays showed a nonunion of the fracture and loss of the proximal two thirds of the femur.

The nonunion was verified at the time of revision. The proximal fragment was not adequate for reconstruction and the proximal two thirds of an allograft femur was used to replace this area of bone loss. The remaining medial strut of the patient's proximal femur measured 7 inches in length

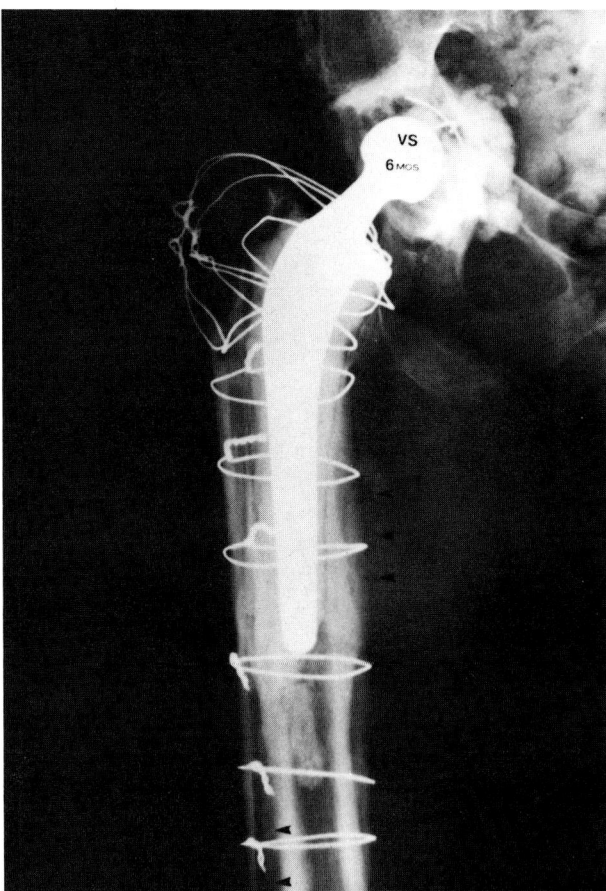

Figure 6-15C. At six months, the fracture appears to have united. The patient had no pain and discarded her cane.

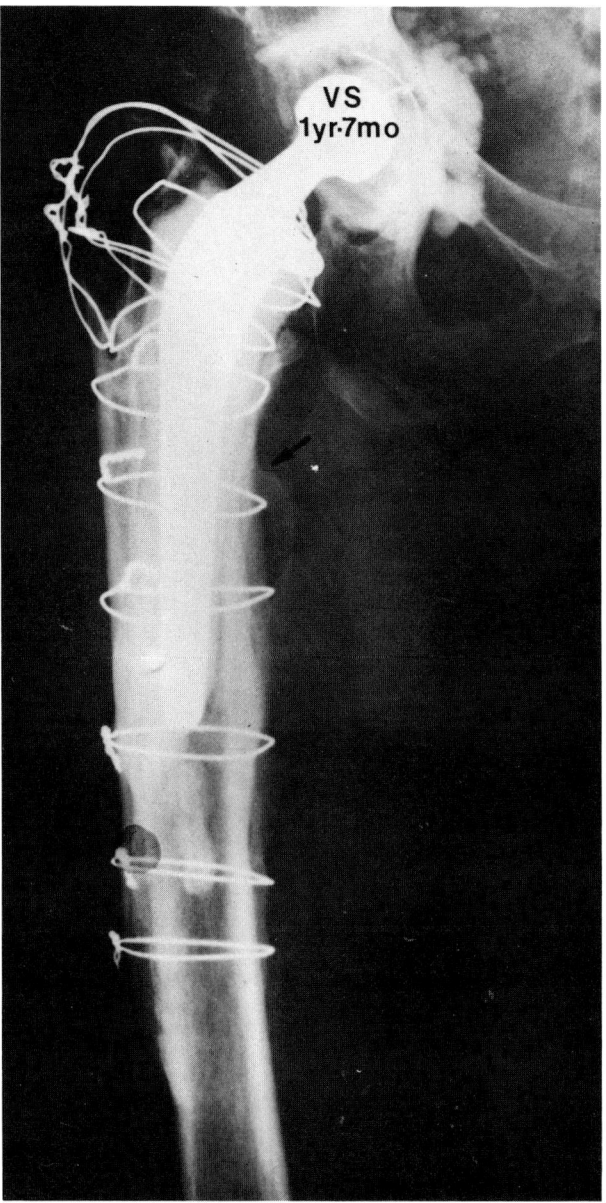

Figure 6-15D. X-rays at one year, seven months show little change except that the allografts appear to be uniting to the femur. Note that the distal end of the lateral femoral graft has rounded off and the interface between the graft and the femur that was obvious at six months can no longer be seen. There may be some bowing of the femur.

and was placed anteriorly over the junction of the allograft and the patient's distal femur. A side strut in continuity with the allograft femur bridged the junction of the allograft and the patient's femur laterally and a second allograft that was 4 ½ inches in length was placed medially (Figure 6-17B). All grafts were circumferentially wired.

The patient initially did well and at seven weeks could walk comfortably without support (Figure 6-17C). At eight weeks she had the sudden onset of pain and obvious varus bowing. X-rays showed that the side strut had fractured at the junction of the allograft and the patient's distal femur (Figure 6-17D). In retrospect, there were two errors in judgment in this case. The first was the fact that the medial graft was much too short (4 ½ inches). The second was that we tried to use a method that has worked well with fractures of a well-vascularized femur in a situation that was not comparable. In a normally vascularized femur, the fracture fragments are load sharing with the allograft struts and by two or three months, the fracture has started to heal and there is progressively less strain on the allograft struts. At the same time as the fracture is becoming stronger, the allografts are becoming weaker because they are starting the process of revascularization. However, union between an avascular proximal femoral allograft and the vascularized distal fragment may take years instead of months to become

strong while the allograft struts become progressively weaker in a matter of months. Without any other fixation at the fracture site, fatigue fracture of the struts should be anticipated. Using a longer stem without cement would not have helped because both the allograft and the patient's distal femur flare at this point and as with an intramedullary rod, fixation of a fracture in the distal third of the femur is not sound unless an interlocking device is used as well. For reasons mentioned previously, we are not enthusiastic about using a cemented long stem.

The logical choice for the original reconstruction would have been to use a supracondylar plate and a longer medial

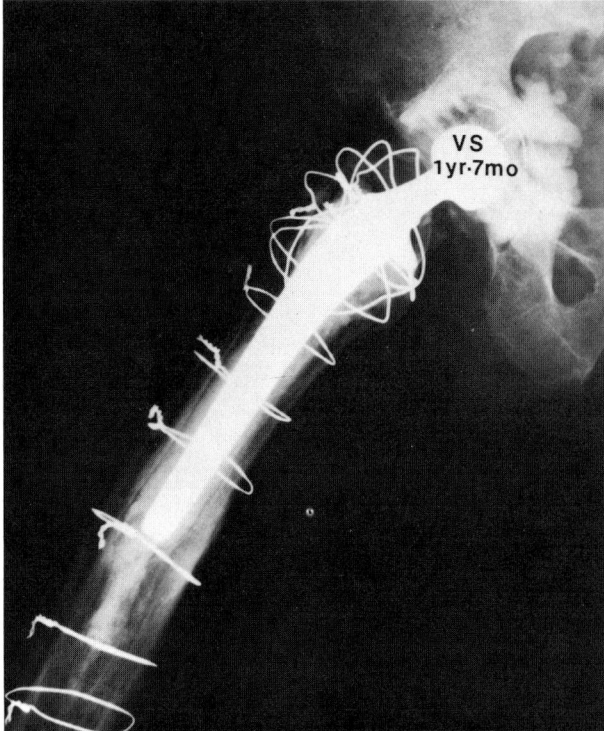

Figure 6-15E. There is also a suggestion of bowing seen on the lateral view. We now prefer to split a femur into two equal halves rather than to use thinner struts from the femur or tibia; however, this patient walks without support, has no pain and rates 89.

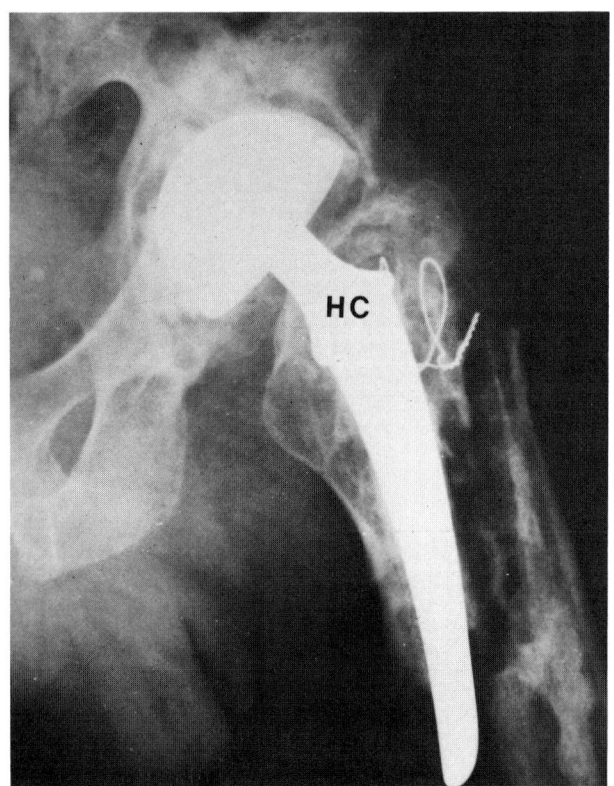

Figure 6-16A. This 58-year-old man fell and sustained this subtrochanteric fracture about the stem of a loose cemented femoral component.

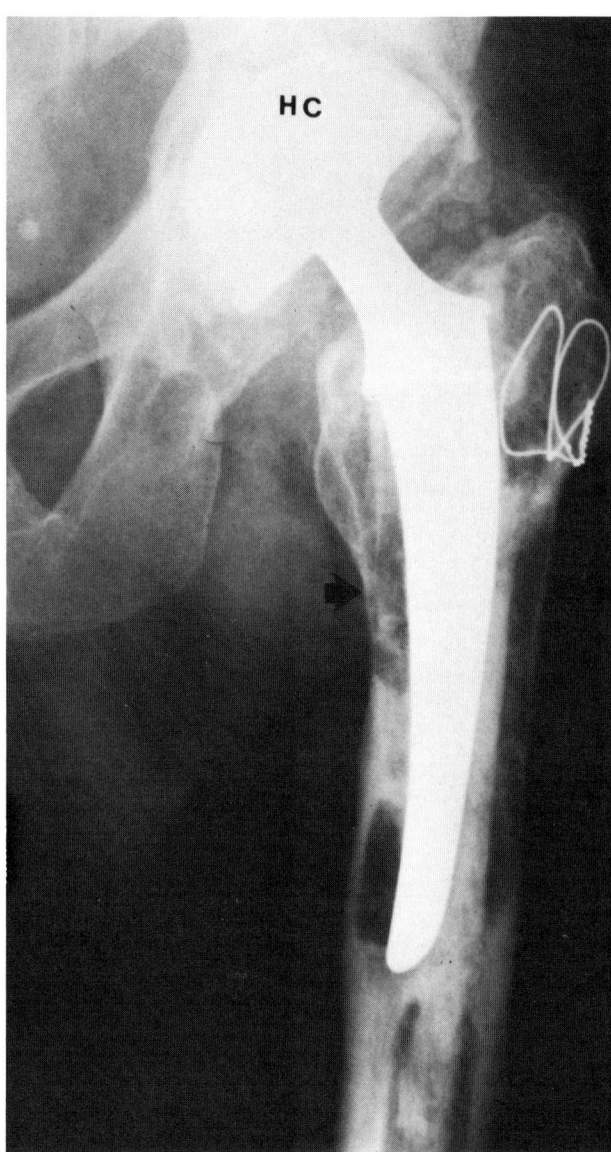

Figure 6-16B. The patient had a total hip replacement 11 years previously. He developed massive lysis and had a loose femoral component that had subsided. He was scheduled for revision before his fall.

strut. This was in fact the salvage reconstruction that was chosen. The previous lateral strut was used anteriorly and the autograft strut that had previously been used anteriorly was placed within the medullary canal. A new very large allograft strut was placed medially. The twelve-hole supracondylar (DCP) plate (Synthes, Ltd., Wayne, PA) had five screws in the allograft proximally and seven in the distal fragment (Figure 6-17E). Since the screw holes of a DCP plate are larger than the screws themselves, further compression can theoretically occur with partial weightbearing. Compression forces are therefore still transmitted to the butt joint between the graft and the patient's femur and tension forces are controlled by the supracondylar plate. There is excellent distal fixation in the relatively weak bone of the patient's distal femur because of the blade and excellent

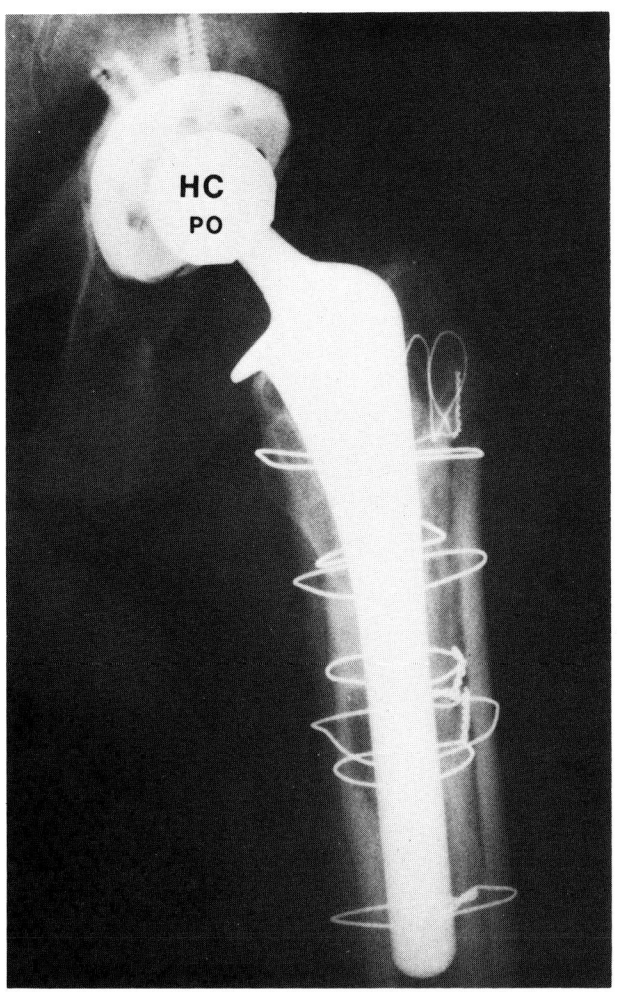

Figure 6-16C. The fracture was treated by means of medial and lateral onlay cortical grafts and an uncemented femoral component. In retrospect, the calcar intramedullary defect probably should have been grafted as well.

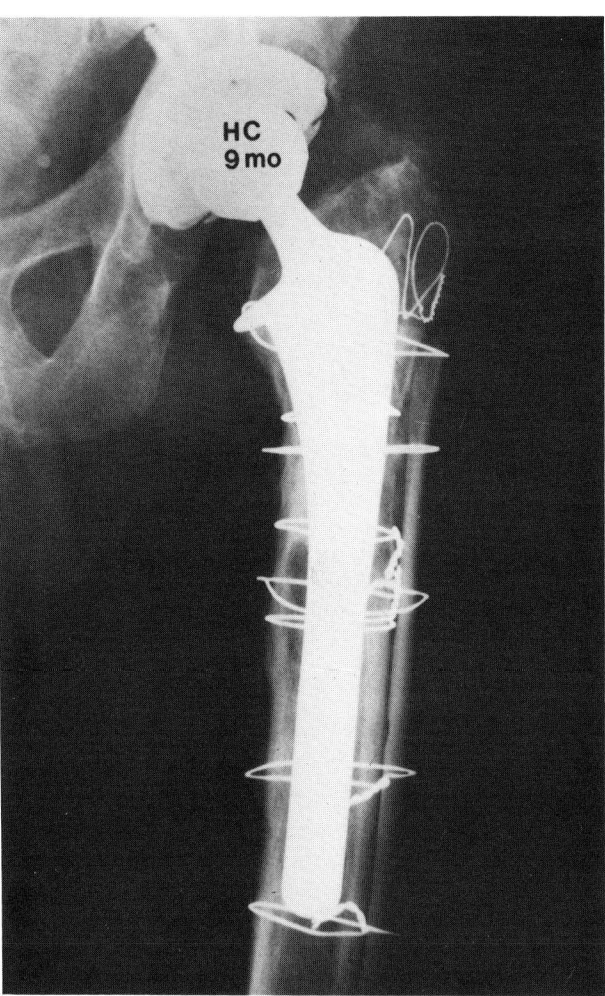

Figure 6-16D. At nine months, there was obvious subsidence of the femoral component. Compare the relationship of the calcar to the proximal wire with that immediately postoperative (Figure 6-16C).

proximal fixation by the screws in the very strong bone of the allograft femur.

At five months the second reconstruction appears to be doing well (Figure 6-17F). The patient has no pain and motion is excellent. She is able to walk unsupported for short distance without a limp; however, she is using crutches to protect the ipsilateral ankle, which has an unrelated injury. She rates 78.

Circumferential Deficiencies of the Metaphysis and Diaphysis

Deficiency of the entire proximal femur is seen with increasing frequency in revision total hip surgery. There is often sufficient bone available after the first failure of a total hip to allow reconstruction without major bone grafting, but subsequent revisions may require extensive bone grafting procedures, especially if cemented long stems have been used. In our series, there were 11 hips (26%) with circumferential proximal femoral deficiency.

The etiology was failed cemented total hip replacement in nine, a failed long stem uncemented Moore prosthesis in one and a subtrochanteric fracture below an arthrodesis in one.

Review of Literature. Proximal femoral replacement prostheses secured with cement have been used in reconstruction following tumor resection.[20] This same technique has been recommended in deficiency of the proximal femur for problems other than tumors.[21] Osteochondral allografts, and allografts in conjunction with prostheses have been used in reconstruction of the proximal femur after tumor resection.[22] McGann et al. reported a small series of patients with cemented long stem prostheses used in conjunction with proximal femoral allograft reconstruction for failed total hip replacement.[23] There are now several additional reports concerning such reconstructions in the literature.[24-26] The majority of authors have recommended long stemmed components with cement used in both the proximal and distal fragments. Head et al. have recently reported their experience with proximal femoral allografts

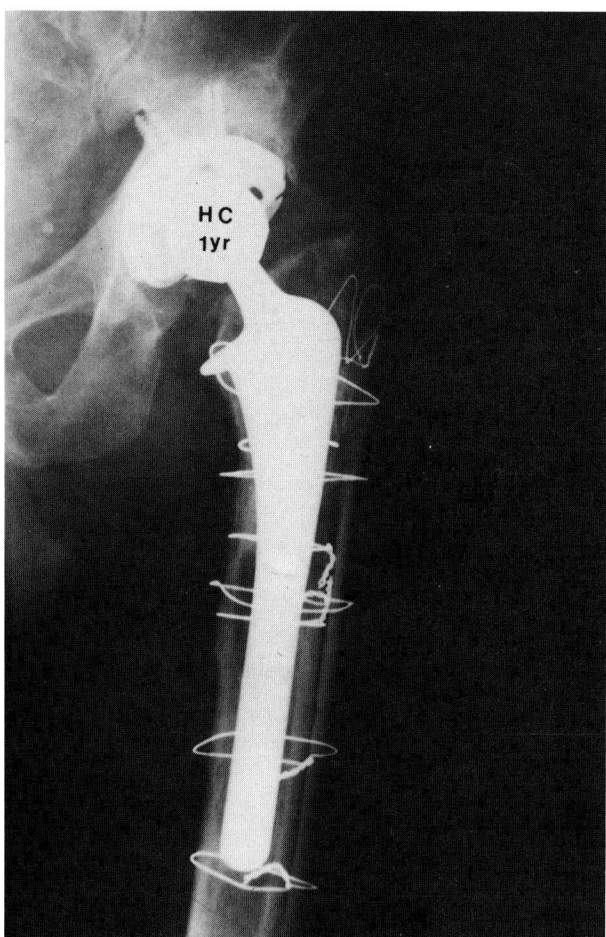

Figure 6-16E. X-rays at one year show no further change. The patient still requires a cane to walk smoothly but has no pain and is pleased with his hip. He rates 93. The grafts appear to be uniting to the patient's femur. Note the distal rounding of the lateral graft.

and long stem prostheses. They used cement in both the allograft and the patient's femur in eight patients, in just the patient's femur in two, and no cement in four.[27]

Authors' Preferred Treatment. There are two clinical patterns of proximal femoral deficiency. The first is loss of the metaphysis and trochanter with a thin shell of the proximal diaphysis remaining. The second is total deficiency of the proximal femur.

Deficiency of the Metaphysis and Trochanter With a Thin Shell of Proximal Diaphysis Remaining. In our series there were only two patients with this deficiency (5%). One was associated with a resection arthroplasty for a septic cemented total hip and the second with an uncemented custom long stem Moore prosthesis.

We prefer the trochanteric slide to approach the femur in these complex reconstructions because by definition the patient's trochanteric fragment is always in contact with nonviable allograft bone.

As in all major deficiencies, we feel that it is better to save as much of the patient's femur as possible and to use allografts to supplement whatever bone is left. The metaphyseal region of an ipsilateral allograft femur can be

hollowed out enough to allow the deficient but living thin diaphysis to be placed within this. A long lateral cortical strut from the allograft extends distally and allows both reinforcement of the patient's cortex and fixation of the allograft with cerclage wires. A medial allograft cortical strut can be used if the medial cortex is also deficient. Supplementary cortical and cancellous strips from the iliac crest are added to the junction of the allograft to the patient's bone. The remnant of the patient's greater trochanter is kept in continuity with the quadriceps (trochanteric slide) and is wired to the greater trochanter of the allograft. Standard length uncemented femoral components are used. The sintered surfaces of the femoral components are in contact with viable bone of the patient's deficient proximal femur which in turn is reinforced with the allograft.

Clinical Examples

Case 1

The patient whose x-rays are seen in Figure 6-18A was 24 when he presented with a resection arthroplasty. Ten years previously, he sustained a fracture dislocation of his hip that required open reduction. He then had an attempt at arthrodesis prior to his first total hip replacement. Three subsequent revision arthroplasties were performed. The last involved an acetabular reconstruction using a femoral allograft that was converted to a resection arthroplasty because of a major *Staphylococcus aureus* infection. He had deficiency of the metaphysis and trochanters and a very thin shell of proximal cortex. There were several perforations laterally in the proximal shaft (Figure 6-18B). He was 5″ short. His complex acetabular reconstruction has been previously described (Figure 5-49).

The metaphysis of a larger ipsilateral allograft femur was cleared of cancellous bone using the Midas Rex (Midas Rex Institute, Fort Worth, TX) so that the diaphysis of the patient's femur could be placed within it. A large lateral cortical strut from the allograft reinforced the deficient lateral cortex (Figure 6-18C). Autogenous strips from the iliac crest were placed at the junction of the allograft and the patient's femur. A trochanteric slide was used for exposure and the remaining wafer of the patient's greater trochanter was wired to the allograft greater trochanter.

X-rays in the immediate postoperative period appeared satisfactory (Figure 6-18D). At six and a half weeks the patient began to use a cane and with its use had no pain and walked smoothly. Unfortunately he had three posterior dislocations that required reduction and at least six subluxations during his third and fourth month. He has not dislocated since then but his acetabular component has shifted position within the proximal tibial allograft (Figure 5-49D). At 11 months the grafts appeared to be doing well (Figure 6-18E) but the patient was disappointed because he was still three inches short. Because of this shortening, a simultaneous shortening of the right feumr by 1⅜ inch and lengthening of the left femur by ⅞ inch was performed,

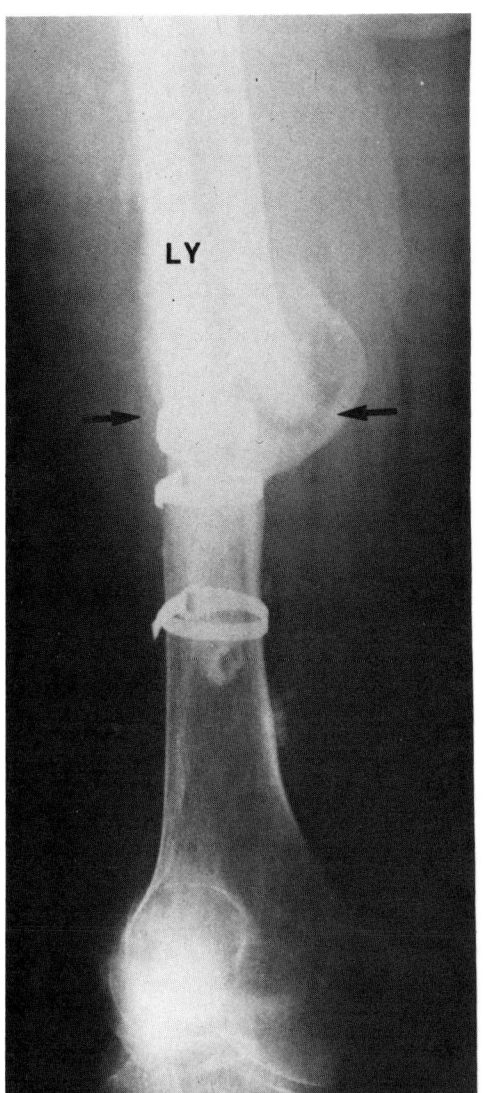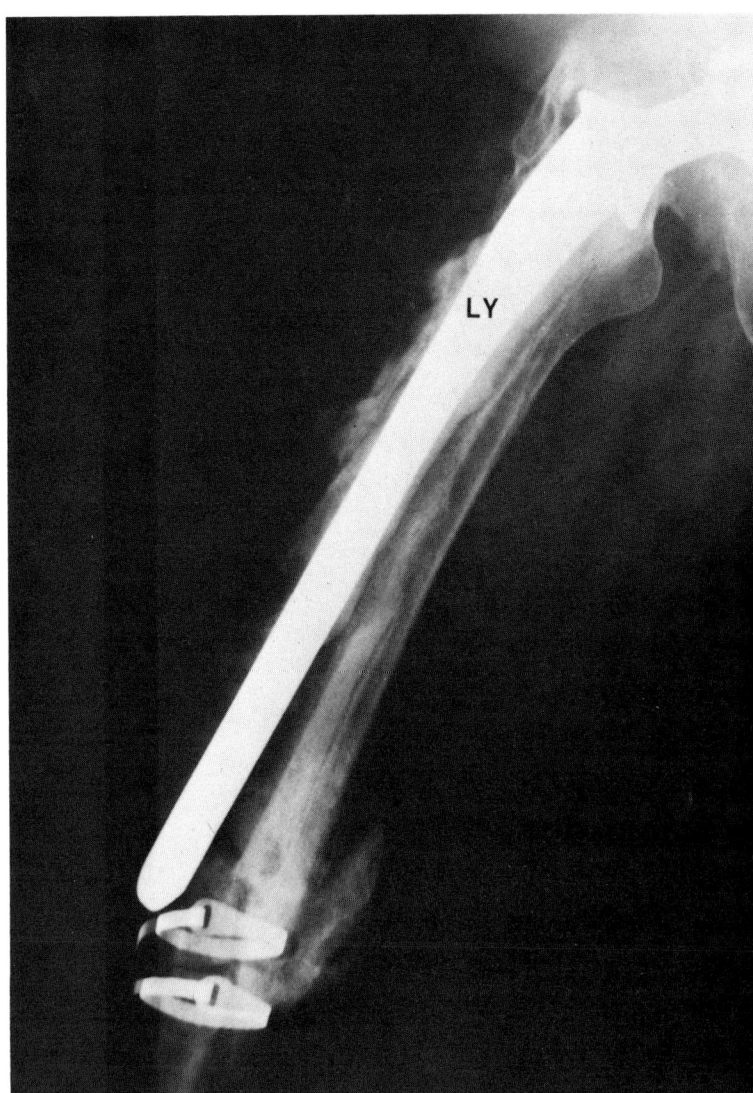

Figure 6-17A. This 70-year-old woman sustained this fracture during her second revision five years prior to admission. She required two crutches for all steps since that revision and had gross motion at the fracture site (outlined by arrows). There was not enough proximal bone to permit reconstruction with an onlay graft.

using bone from the right femur, 14 months after the initial reconstruction.

The right femur united uneventfully and x-rays of the lengthened femur were initially satisfactory (Figure 6-18F) but fixation was lost at five weeks when the proximal screws of the supracondylar plate pulled out of the soft bone (Figure 6-18G). These proximal screws were removed and replaced by cerclage wires. A large medial cortical onlay allograft was used to reinforce the compression side of the femur (Figure 6-18H) and held in place by the cerclage wires. The original onlay lateral strut was biopsied at the time of this procedure. It bled freely and clinically had united to the shaft of the patient's femur. The biopsy showed many persistent empty lacunae but woven bone was present at the periphery (Figure 6-18I). X-rays one year, seven months following the original proximal femoral reconstruction show union of the original allograft but the acetabulum has shifted into more abduction (Figure 6-18J). X-rays at

one year, nine months from the original reconstruction, and six months from the distal medial onlay graft, show that the lengthening osteotomy appears to have healed and the medial onlay graft is incorporating (Figures 6-18K and 6-18L). The patient has no femoral pain or tenderness but does have groin pain from his loose acetabular component and uses a cane. He rates 67 and is scheduled for revision of his acetabular component.

Case 2

The patient whose x-rays are seen in Figure 6-19A was 62 when she presented with a complex deficiency involving both the acetabulum and femur. She had the original diagnosis of slipped capital femoral epiphysis which was treated with a Smith-Petersen nail. She had two other childhood operations and then four cup arthroplasties. There was significant bone loss prior to the insertion of this uncemented custom long stem Moore prosthesis (Figure 5-47B).

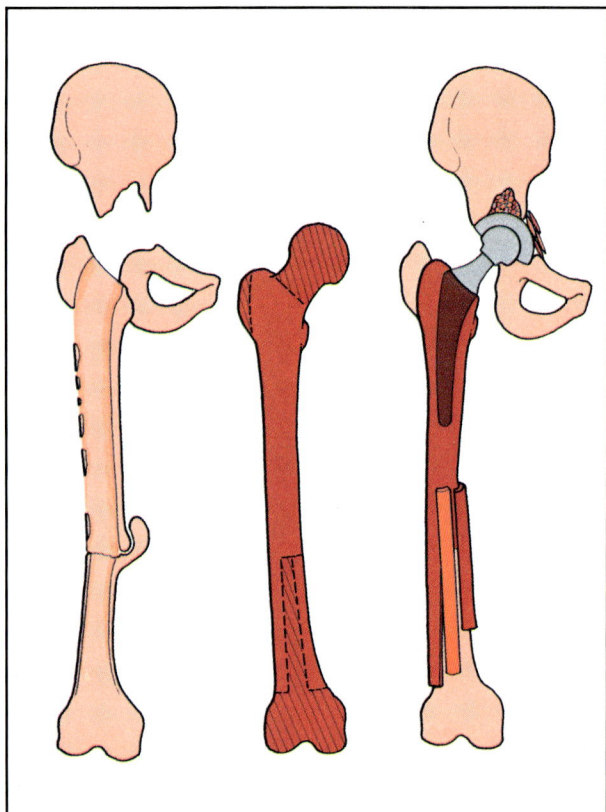

Figure 6-17B. A proximal femoral allograft was used with a long side strut, a short medial allograft strut and an anterior autograft strut. An uncemented femoral component was used as a press fit.

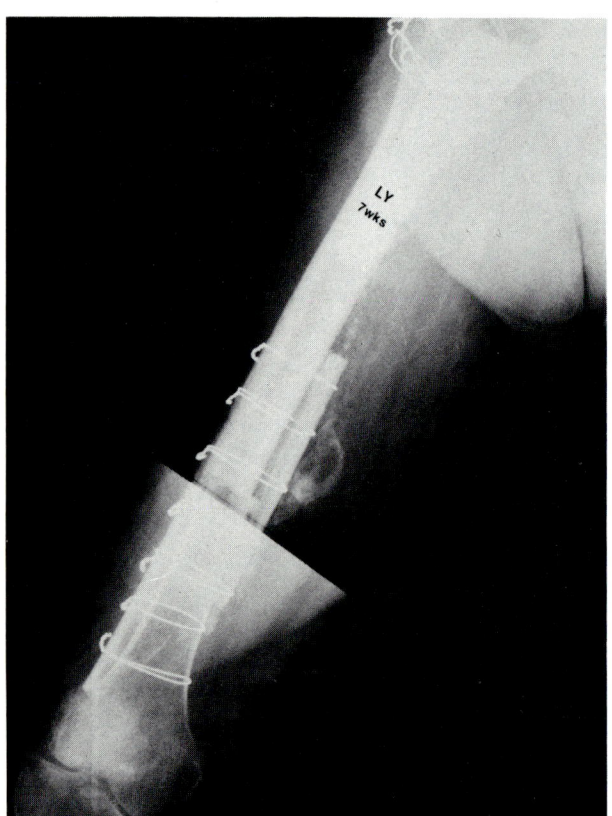

Figure 6-17C. The patient was doing well at seven weeks.

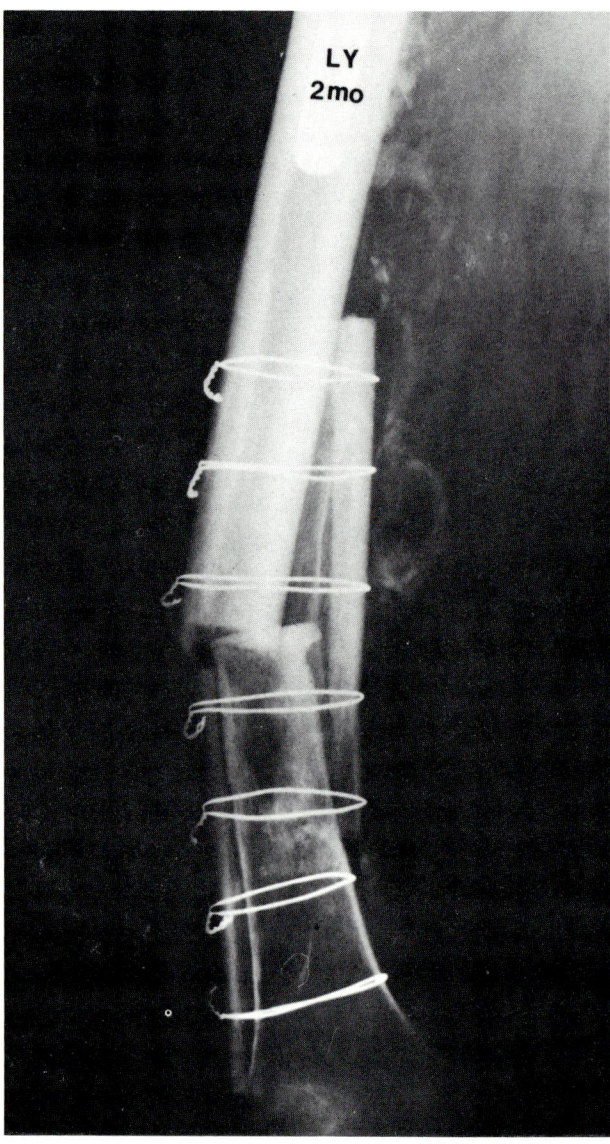

Figure 6-17D. Unfortunately a fatigue fracture occurred at two months. In retrospect this should have been anticipated as the medial strut is too short and since union between an allograft and the patient's femur may take years instead of months to unite, the lateral allograft strut is subjected to excessive tensile stresses.

She required two axillary crutches for all ambulation during the 22 years that this prosthesis was in place. There was dramatic femoral cortical resorption. The prosthesis protruded anteriorly just above the patella (Figure 6-19B). Her complex acetabular reconstruction has been previously discussed (Figure 5-47).

In the presence of this severe femoral deficiency, with loss of the metaphysis and trochanter and with only a paper thin shell of diaphysis, we anticipated a fracture when the prosthesis was removed because the femoral cortex was so thin that it could be deformed by the pressure of the surgeon's thumb and index finger. When the proximal femur was reamed, the expected fracture did occur at the distal end of the femoral rasp (Figure 6-19C). An ipsilateral femoral allograft, larger than the patient's femoral diameter was

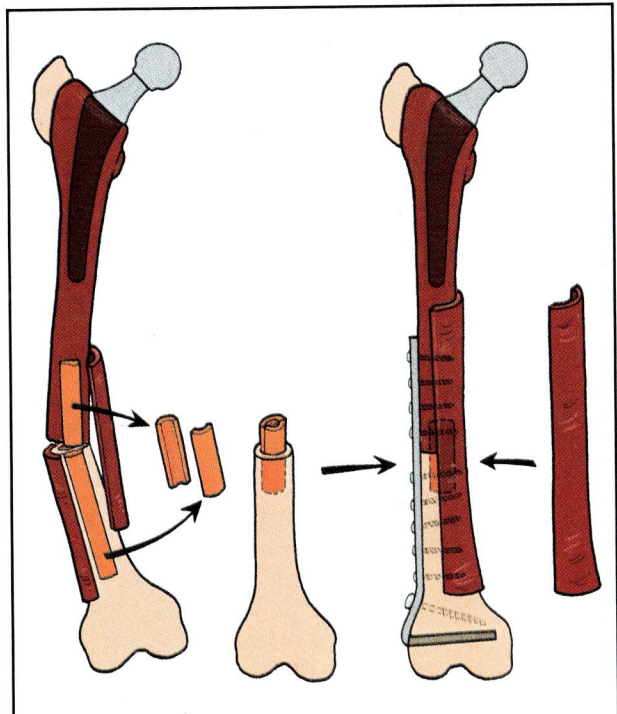

Figure 6-17E. A 12 hole DCP supracondylar A-0 plate (Synthes, Ltd., Wayne, PA) served as a tension band to provide resistance to varus stresses while the butt joint theoretically is allowed compression forces because of the large screw holes in the plate. A new very large medial allograft strut was fashioned in the usual way and the old lateral strut was placed anteriorly. The old autograft strut was placed within the medullary canal.

hollowed out and the thin shell of the patient's femur was placed within this. The sintered surfaces of the uncemented femoral component were in contact with living bone. The allograft provided a calcar and both trochanters. A long side strut to the knee reinforced the thinned and fractured femur. Two other allograft struts from the same allograft femur were used to stabilize the femoral fracture which was at the tip of the standard length prosthesis. One was placed anteriorly and one medially. The anterior perforation at the distal femur was filled with an additional allograft (Figure 6-19D). cortical and cancellous strips from the iliac crest were used to graft the interfaces. The trochanteric slide was used for the exposure and the thin wafer of the patient's greater trochanter was wired to the allograft greater trochanter.

This patient used two axillary crutches for eight weeks. She then began to use a single crutch. She has had no pain since discharge. Since the fracture has never been visible on any postoperative x-rays, it is hard to tell when this united. At six months, there was x-ray evidence of some incorporation of the onlay grafts (Figure 6-19E).

At one year three months, further incorporation has occurred (Figures 6-19F through 6-19I). The patient walks short distances at home without support but despite steady improvement in abductor strength she still has an abductor lurch. She walks normally with a cane but because of carpal

tunnel syndrome, she prefers an axillary crutch to a cane. With a crutch she can walk one half mile and is limited from walking further by arthritis of her contralateral knee. She has full motion, no pain and rates 82. X-Rays at one year ten months are satisfactory (Figure 6-19H).

Total Deficiency of the Proximal Femur. In our series, there were nine patients (21%) with total deficiency of the proximal femur. Five had failed cemented long stem total hip replacement prostheses; two had failed conventional total hip replacements; one had a custom proximal femoral replacement long stem cemented prosthesis; and one had a subtrochanteric fracture below a fused hip.

Treatment. The trochanteric slide provides excellent exposure for dealing with proximal femoral deficiencies and is the approach of choice as the patient's greater trochanter or abductors must be reattached to the nonviable allograft greater trochanters.

We feel that it is important to save as much of the patient's bone as possible and to use an ipsilateral proximal femoral replacement allograft with a butt joint between the graft and the distal recipient femur in conjunction with a

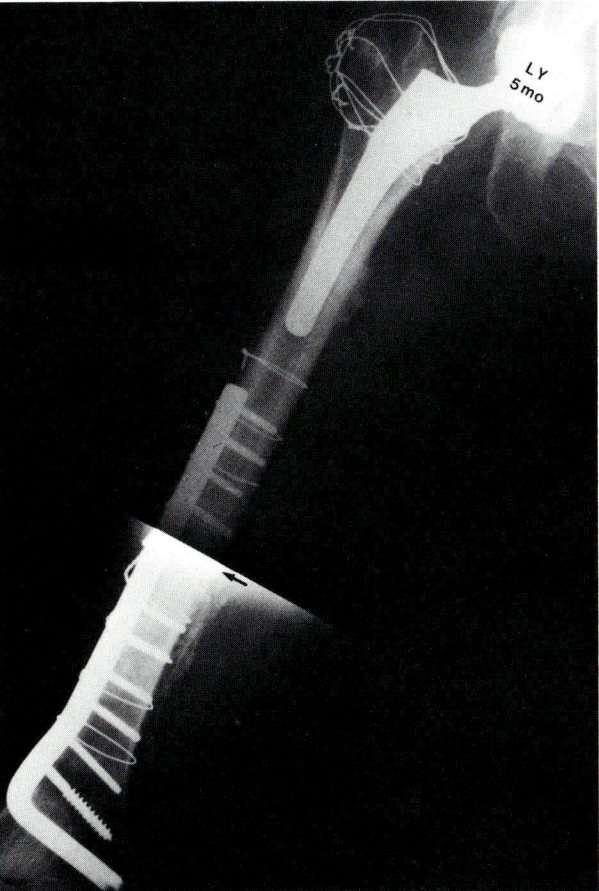

Figure 6-17F. X-rays at five months after the second reconstruction appear quite satisfactory. The arrow points to the junction of the allograft and the patient's femur. The patient has no pain and has excellent motion. She can bear full weight without pain and without limp for short distances, but is still using two crutches because of an unrelated ipsilateral ankle injury. She rates 78.

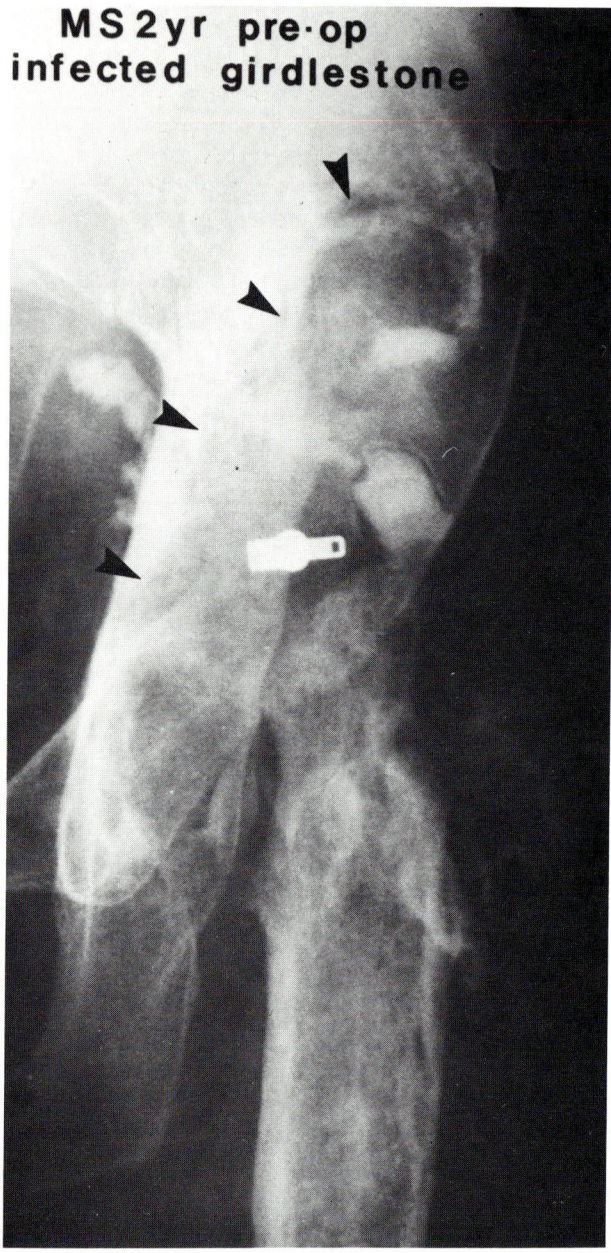

MS 2yr pre·op infected girdlestone

Figure 6-18A. This 24-year-old man initially had an open reduction of a posterior fracture dislocation of his hip. He then had an attempt at arthrodesis which was unsuccessful and was converted to a cemented total hip replacement. After his third revision, he became septic with *Staphylococcus aureus* and had a resection arthroplasty. The metaphysis and the lesser and greater trochanter are absent. He was 5″ shorter. The lateral cortex of the femur was very thin and had several perforations.

distal cortical strut from the allograft. This distal strut is used for fixation and also helps to reinforce the recipient femur. A medial cortical allograft is usually necessary as well. Onlay grafts should be held with cerclage wires.

Although we used cemented long stem prostheses early in our series, we now do not feel that cement is indicated in proximal femoral deficiencies. Even if the sintered surfaces of an uncemented prosthesis are entirely in contact with nonviable allograft bone, a very accurate press fit of the

prosthesis can be obtained within the allograft. Fixation is likely to remain secure, even if bony ingrowth never occurs. Standard-length prostheses are adequate in the majority of cases but if the junction of the allograft to the host coincides with the distal tip of the prosthesis, it may be necessary to use a mid-length component to extend beyond this junction by 6 to 7cm. to avoid a stress riser. There is no advantage in using a stem that extends beyond the junction of the middle and distal third of the recipient femur because an uncemented stem affords no fixation in this area of the femur. At this level a lateral blade plate used as a tension band is preferable (Figures 6-17E and 6-17F). If a tension band plate is used over an area of the femur that has a stem within it, cerclage wires about the plate and the femur are preferable to screws that are placed about the stem.

Clinical Examples

Case 1

The patient whose x-rays are seen in Figure 6-20A was a 44-year-old man who presented to us in December of 1983 with a loose custom 75mm. acetabular component and a

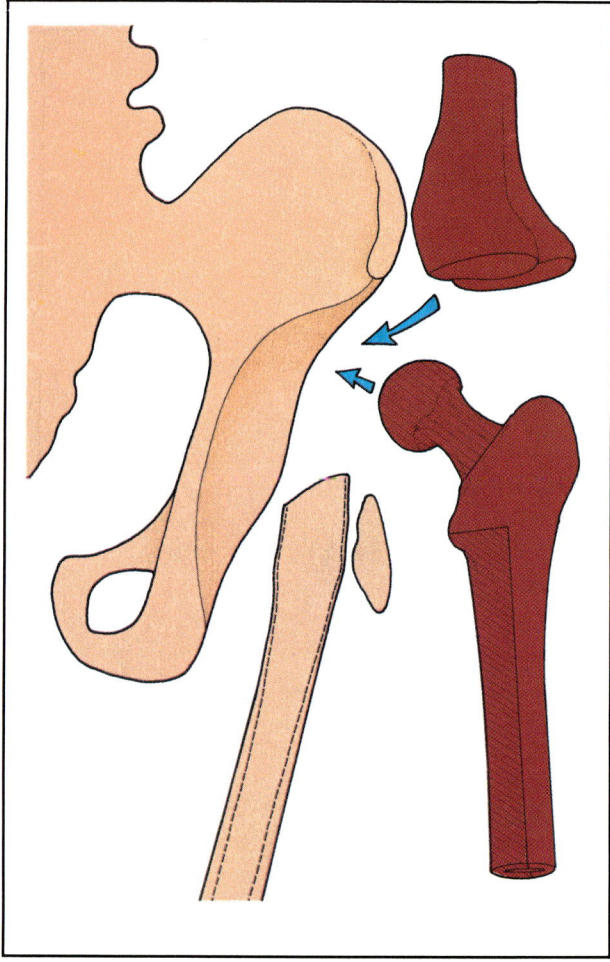

Figure 6-18B. A proximal tibial allograft was used to reconstruct the acetabulum. An ipsilateral allograft femur, larger than the patient's femur was used to reconstruct the femur.

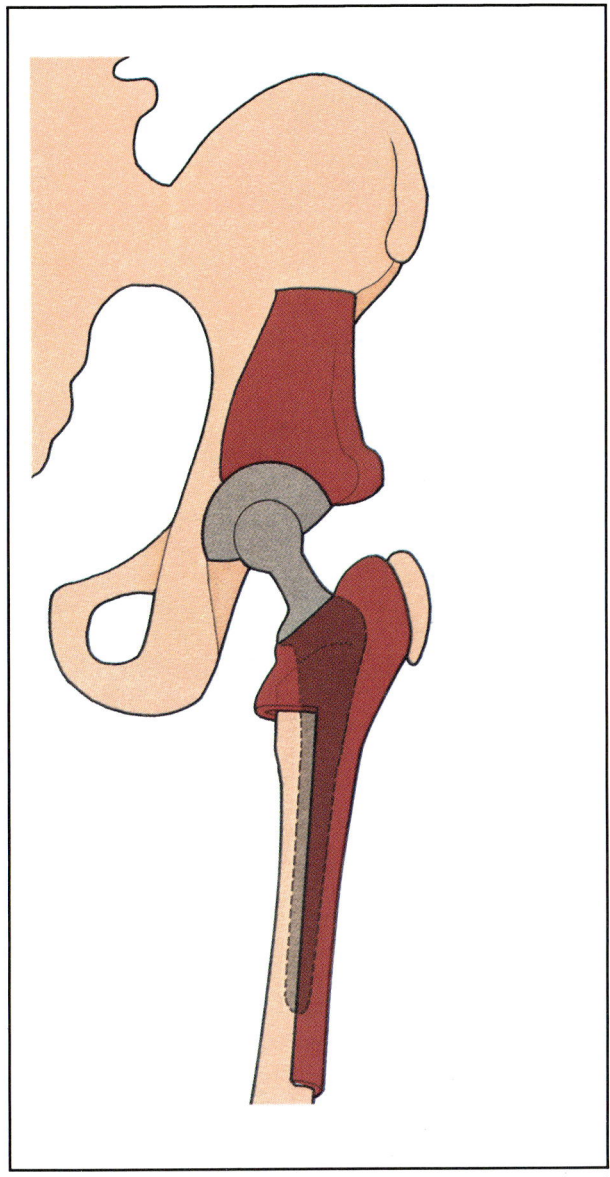

Figure 6-18C. The metaphysis of the allograft femur was hollowed out and the thin shell of the patient's diaphysis was placed within this. An uncemented femoral component had its sintered surfaces partially in contact with the patient's living bone. A large lateral strut from the allograft, reinforced the thin lateral cortex of the patient's femur.

proximally loose but distally fixed cemented long stem prosthesis. His original diagnosis was Legg-Calves-Perthes disease. He had two cup arthroplasties and then a total hip replacement, which was revised two years prior to admission. A cemented long stem was used. After the revision, the trochanteric wires were removed without relief of pain. Reconstruction of this patient's complex right acetabular defect (Figure 5-46) and femoral defect (Figure 6-8) has been previously described.

On the left hip, a trochanteric slide was used for exposure. The acetabular deficiency was treated by means of a distal femoral allograft. The left femoral component was grossly loose proximally but distal to the isthmus, the

cement was firmly attached to the stem and could not pass through the isthmus (cemented long stem disease). Inadvertant vigorous attempts at extraction of the femoral component resulted in a markedly comminuted fracture of the stress-shielded proximal femur (Figure 6-20B). A proximal femoral allograft was required. A step cut was made distally and two onlay allografta were used to reinforce the junction between the allograft and the patient's distal femur. The remnants of the patient's proximal femur were left attached to the adjacent muscles and were approximated to the allograft by means of cerclage wires (Figsures 6-20C and 6-20D).

This procedure was very difficult and was lengthy because of intra-operative difficulties. However, the patient did well and was discharged on the twelfth postoperative day on two crutches. He returned for his first followup appointment at six weeks and was using a cane. The grafts appear to be uniting at two years, ten months (Figures 6-20E

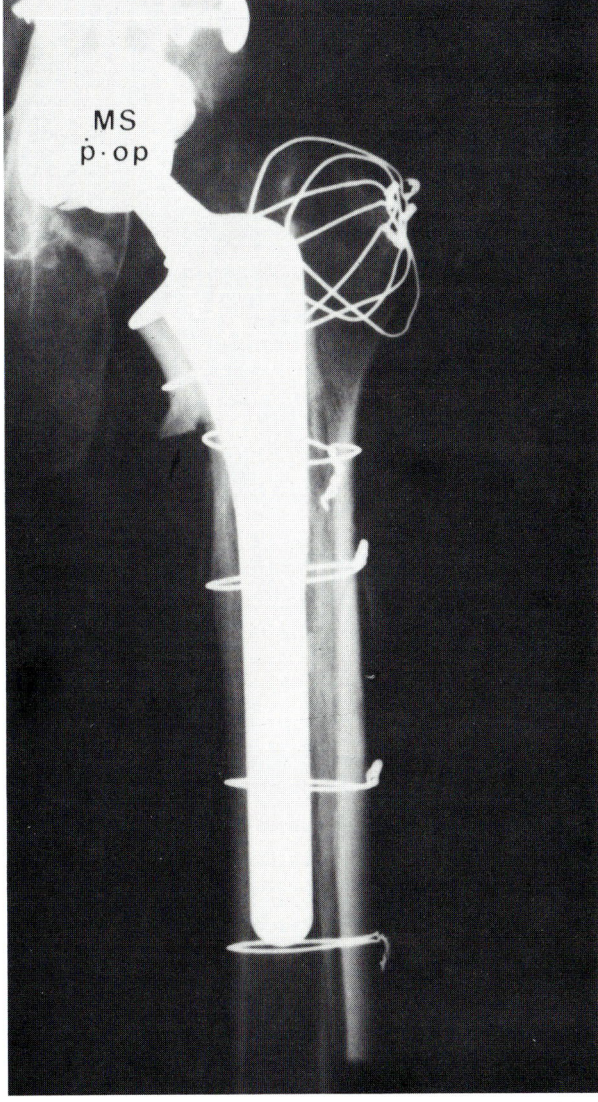

Figure 6-18D. X-rays immediately postoperatively appear satisfactory. The patient left the hospital at 12 days using crutches.

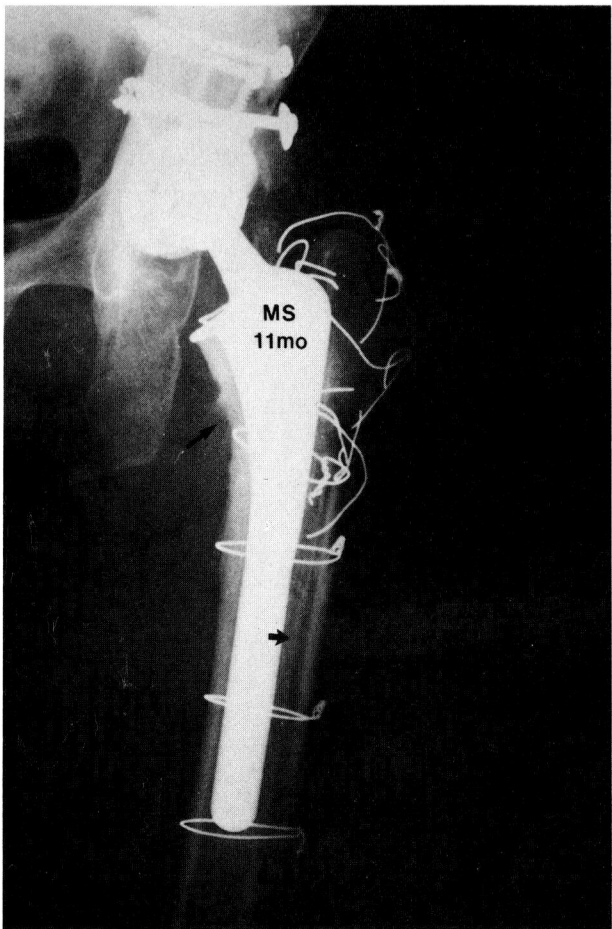

Figure 6-18E. At 11 months, the lateral strut has rounded off distally and appears to be uniting to the patient's femur. The medial metaphysis is remodeling (arrows), but the patient was disappointed because he was 3" short.

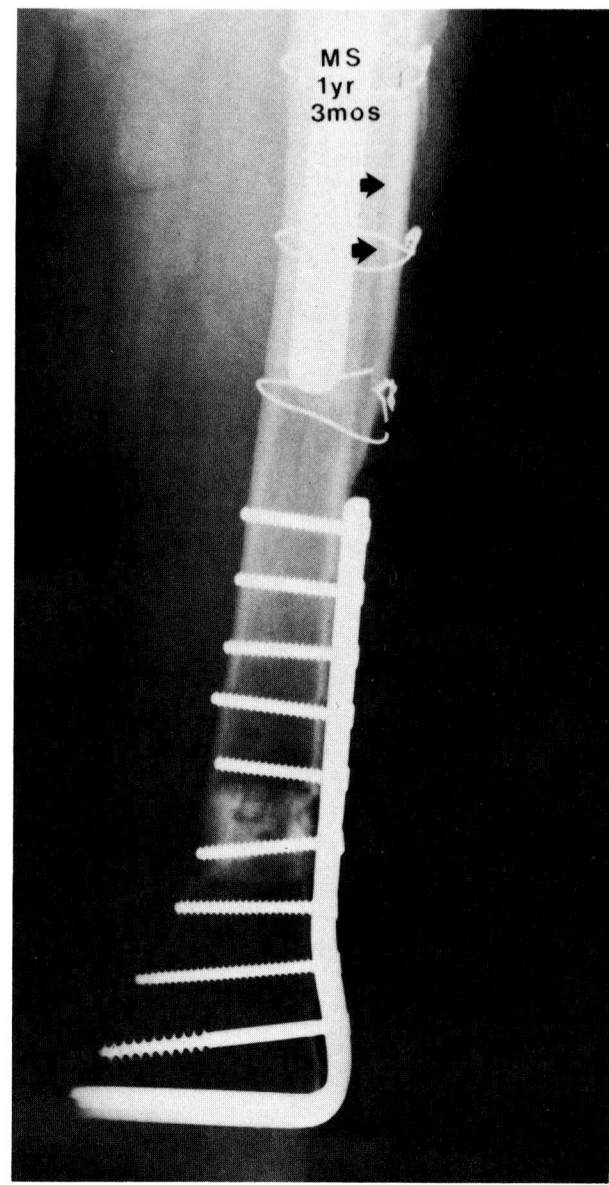

Figure 6-18F. One and three-eighths inches was taken out of the right femur and seven-eighths of an inch of this bone was simultaneously placed in the lengthened left femur. The right femur was fixed with a plate and united without difficulty and without a quadriceps lag. Immediate postoperative x-rays of the left femur appear satisfactory. The graft from the right femur can be seen in the supracondylar area and has increased density compared to the disuse osteopenia of the left femur.

and 6-20F). At three and one half years the patient is pleased with his hip and rates 89.

Faced with the same problem, we now would have windowed the distal femur anteriorly in order to remove cement distal to the isthmus and would have used a conventional length uncemented femoral component after the window was reinforced with a femoral onlay graft.

Case 2

The patient whose x-rays are seen in Figure 6-21A was 38 when she presented with a painful left hip. At three years of age she had polio that primarily involved her left leg. She had significant weakness of this extremity and at age 13 had an arthrodesis of her left hip. At age 21 she had a subtrochanteric fracture of this hip. She had an infection after the first attempt at repairing the fracture. Six additional procedures were done in the hope of attaining union but all failed. The proximal fragment was then excised, leaving her with a resection arthroplasty. Five years prior to admission, she had her first total hip replacement using a cemented acetabular component and a cemented custom long stem proximal femoral replacement component. The hip became

infected and required debridement and antibiotics. Because of recurrent dislocation, the acetabulum was revised on two more occasions. Following one of her total hip procedures she developed sciatic distribution pain and complete loss of all remaining motor power in the left lower extremity. The hip spontaneously dislocated and was reduced by the patient on numerous occasions. She had intractable pain in her hip and anterior thigh as well as severe sciatic distribution pain which radiated to her foot. She had been addicted to various narcotics and at one time was taking over 75 Percodan a week. At the time of admission she was taking

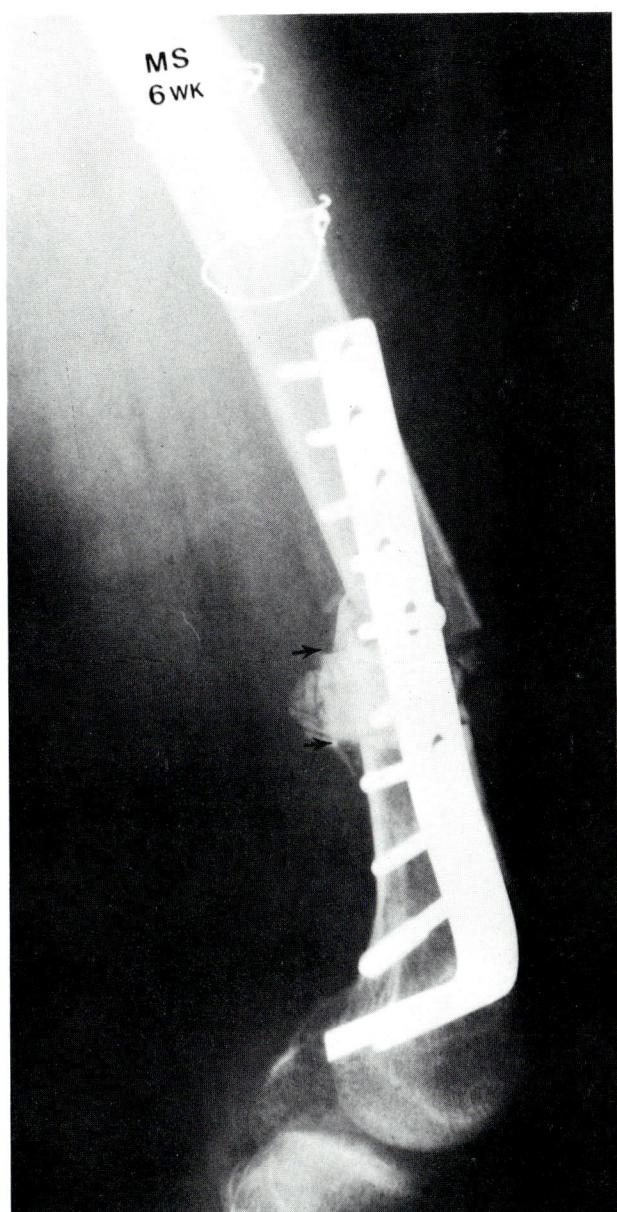

Figure 6-18G. Unfortunately fixation was lost at five weeks when the screws in the proximal fragment pulled out of the soft bone.

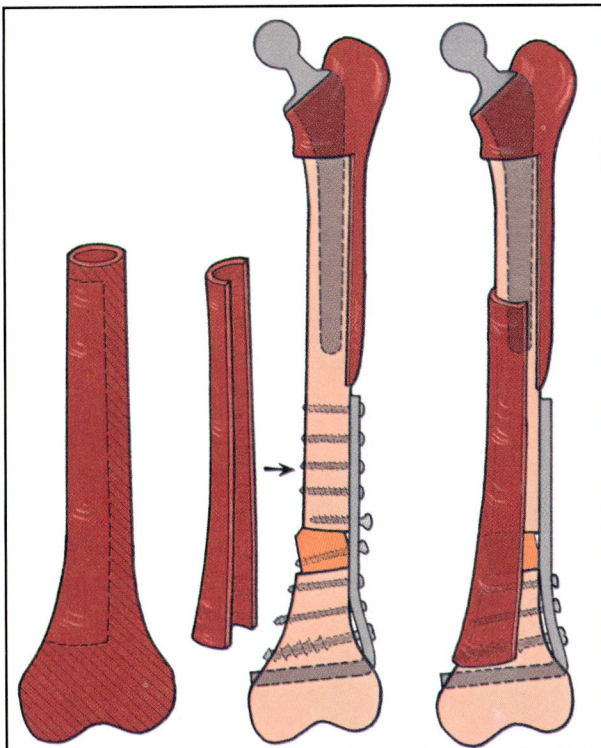

Figure 6-18H. A large medial cortical onlay graft was used to reinforce the anteromedial aspect of the lengthening osteotomy site and the proximal screws of the supracondylar tension band, plate were replaced with cerclage wires.

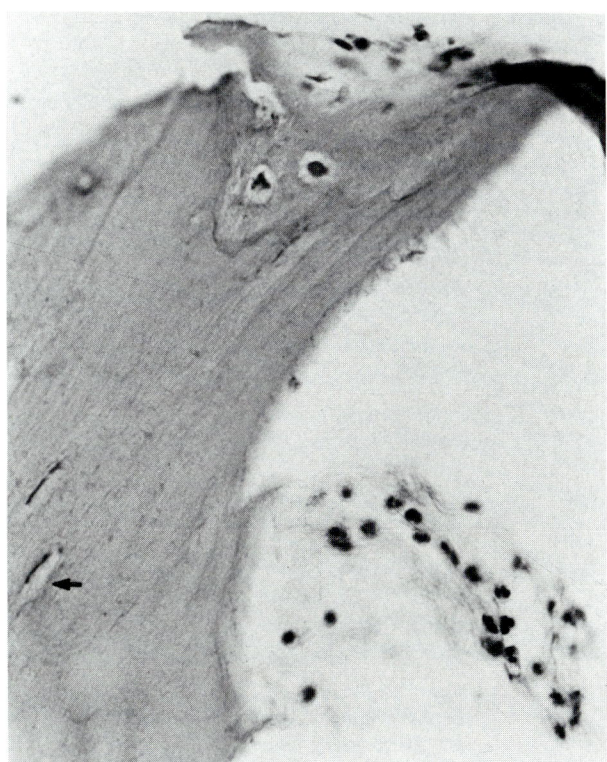

Figure 6-18I. At one year, three months, the proximal femoral side strut bled freely and appeared united to the patient's femur. A biopsy showed persistent empty lacunae (arrow) but woven bone was present at the periphery.

12 60mg. codeine tablets each day. She required crutches for all steps. Her sedimentation rate was 125 and joint fluid obtained from hip aspiration grew out alpha streptococcus.

A resection arthroplasty was carried out using the trochanteric slide (Figures 6-21B and 6-21C). The patient was treated in skeletal traction with tobramycin-impregnated beads and systemic antibiotics for six weeks and then a revision was done. Her complex acetabular reconstruction has been previously described (Figures 5-48C, 5-48D, and 5-48E). A femoral allograft was used to replace the absent proximal femur. A long lateral strut was left in continuity with the proximal allograft femur and extended to the knee. This strut aided in fixation of the graft as well as reinforced the thin and perforated distal lateral cortex. A second onlay cortical allograft strut was used medially to reinforce the

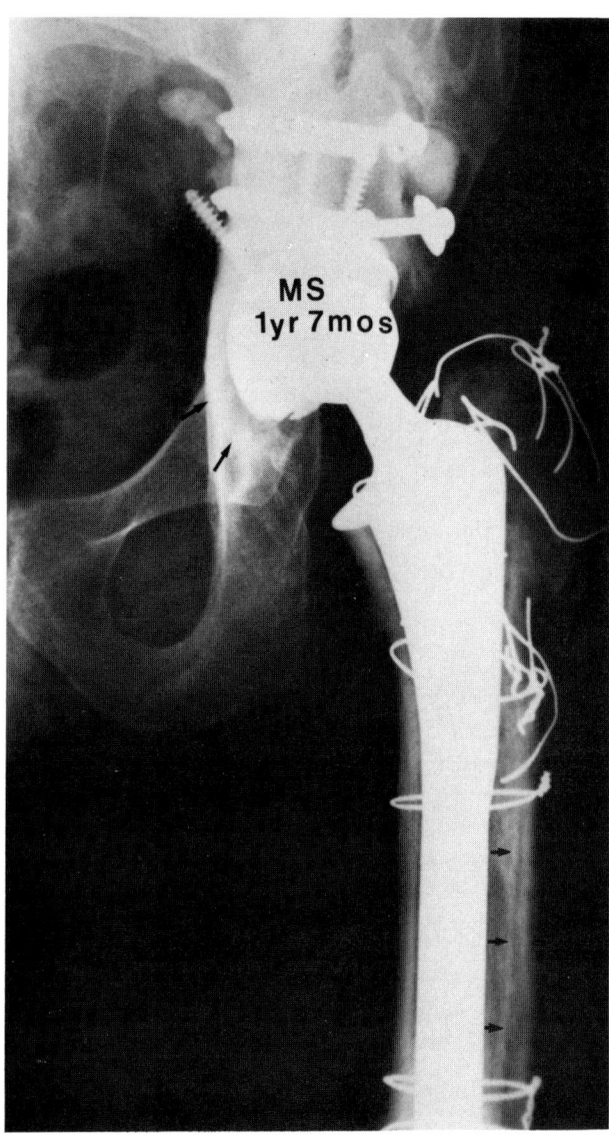

Figure 6-18J. X-rays one year, seven months from the original proximal femoral reconstruction show that the lateral strut has united. There has been a superolateral shift of the acetabular component.

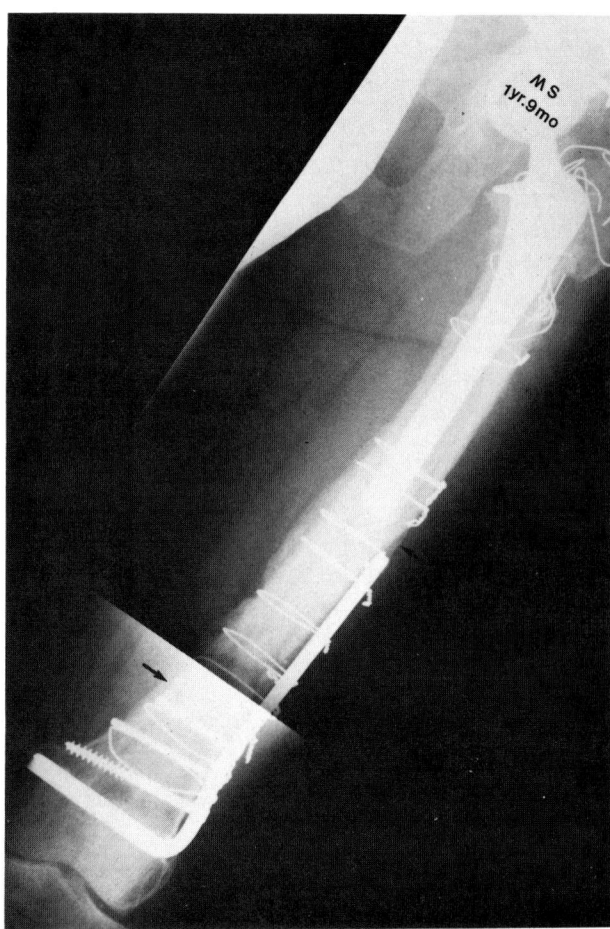

Figure 6-18K. X-rays one year, nine months from the original proximal femoral reconstruction and six months since the onlay graft for the distal lengthening osteotomy appear satisfactory.

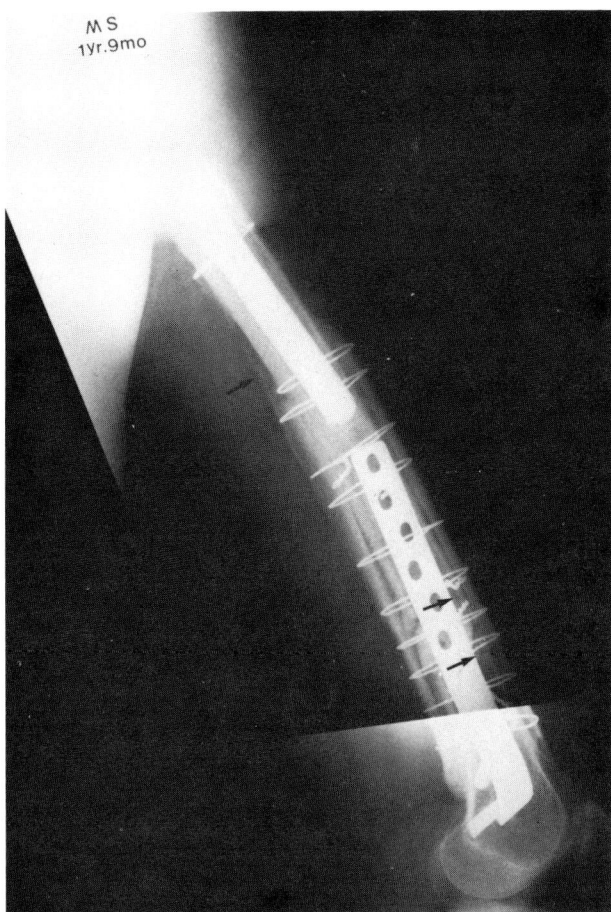

Figure 6-18L. X-rays one year, nine months since the proximal femoral reconstruction and six months since the distal reconstruction show that the medial side strut, which was used to reinforce the lengthening osteotomy site, appears to be uniting to the patient's femur. The two lower arrows outline the autograft used for the lengthening procedure.

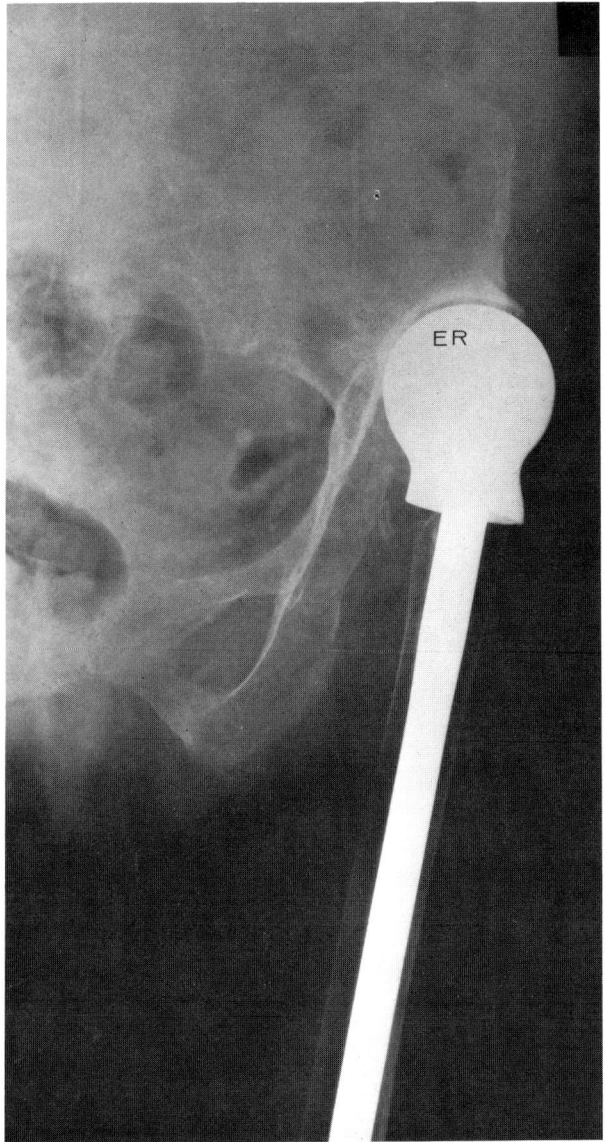

Figure 6-19A. This 62-year-old woman presented with this complex acetabular and femoral deficiency. She had undergone multiple previous operations. The last was placement of this custom, uncemented long stem Moore prosthesis. She required two axillary crutches for all steps for the 22 years that this prosthesis was in place. Note the dramatic bone loss of the femoral shaft.

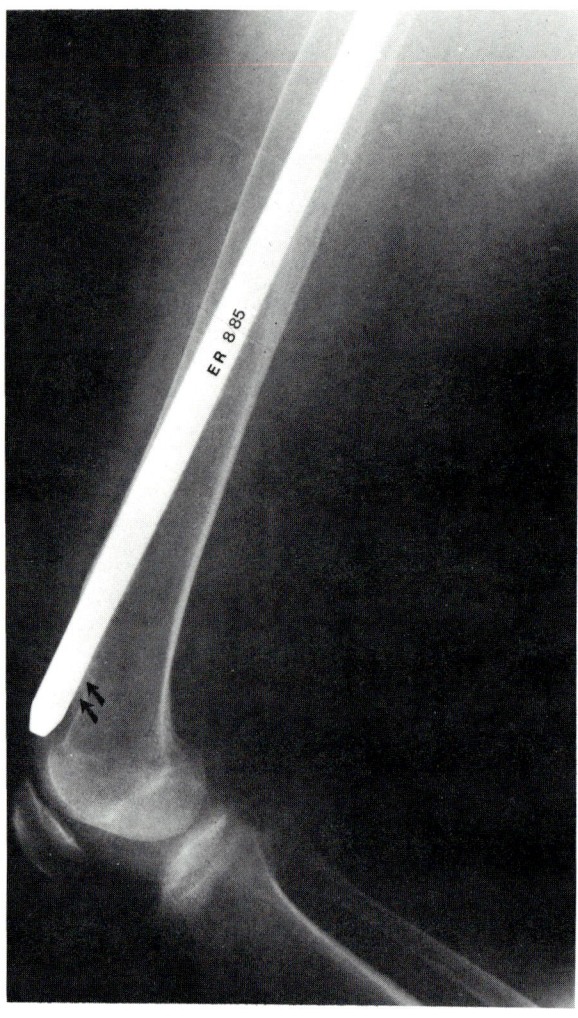

Figure 6-19B. The tip of the prosthesis protruded through the anterior femur close to the superior pole of the patella.

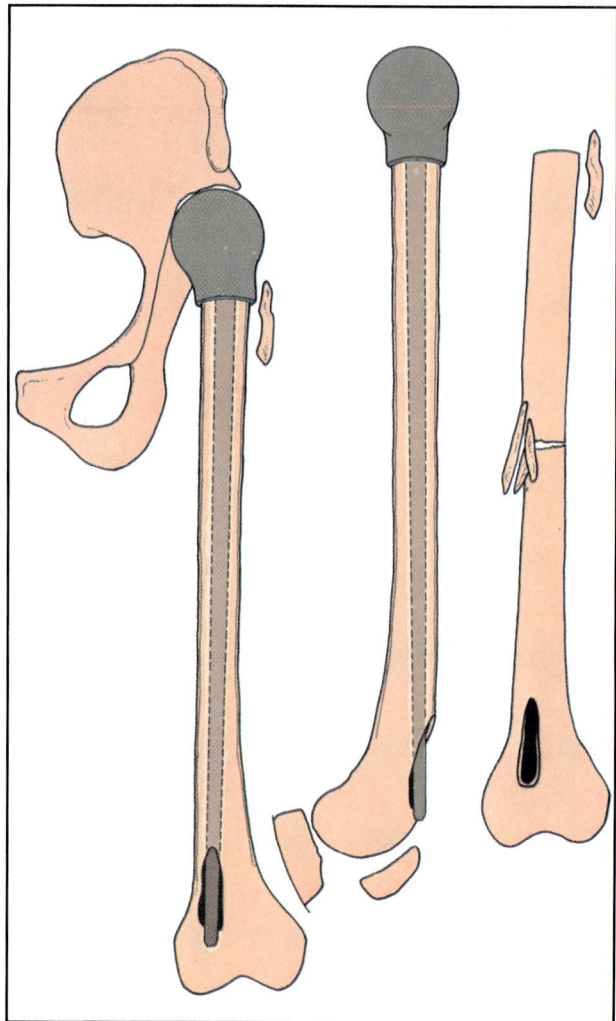

Figure 6-19C. The proximal diametaphyseal bone is absent. The distal tip of the prosthesis protruded through the anterior cortex. A fracture through the paper thin cortices of the femur occurred at the distal end of the femoral rasp during surgery.

junction between the allograft and the patient's femur and also to provide reinforcement of the thin distal shell of the patient's femoral cortex (Figure 6-21D). Autograft strips from the iliac crest were used at the junction of the allografts and the patient's femur. There was no trochanteric fragment but the abductor and the quadriceps were left in continuity (trochanteric slide) and were placed over the allograft greater trochanter.

Intravenous antibiotics were continued for two weeks and then the patient was discharged on oral antibiotics, which she took for four more months. She used two axillary crutches with 30 lbs of weight on the leg. The grafts appeared to be doing well at ten months (Figure 6-21E).

Unfortunately she fell and dislocated her hip at 12 months (Figure 6-21F). The hip was reduced by closed means (Figure 6-21G) and she was placed in an abduction brace which she wore for six weeks. At followup of one year, five months, she has not dislocated again. She still uses two axillary crutches because of her flail extremity. She

has no groin or thigh pain but still takes 20 tablets of codeine 30mg monthly because of persistent sciatic distribution pain in the sole of her foot. She rates 74.

We now feel that when the stem of the prosthesis ends at or proximal to the junction of the allograft to the patient's femur, either a longer uncemented stem that bypasses the junction by 6cm. or a long supracondylar tension band plate that extends at least 10cm. proximal to the junction should be used. Whenever the lateral plate overlies the intramedullary stem, cerclage wires can be used instead of screws (Figures 6-18K and 6-18L).

Because, by necessity, this patient has to protect her flail extremity permanently with crutches, the side strut did not sustain a fatigue fracture (Figure 6-17D). In this particular case a longer stem would not have provided further support and we now would have used a long supracondylar plate.

Case 3

The patient whose x-rays are seen in Figures 6-22A and

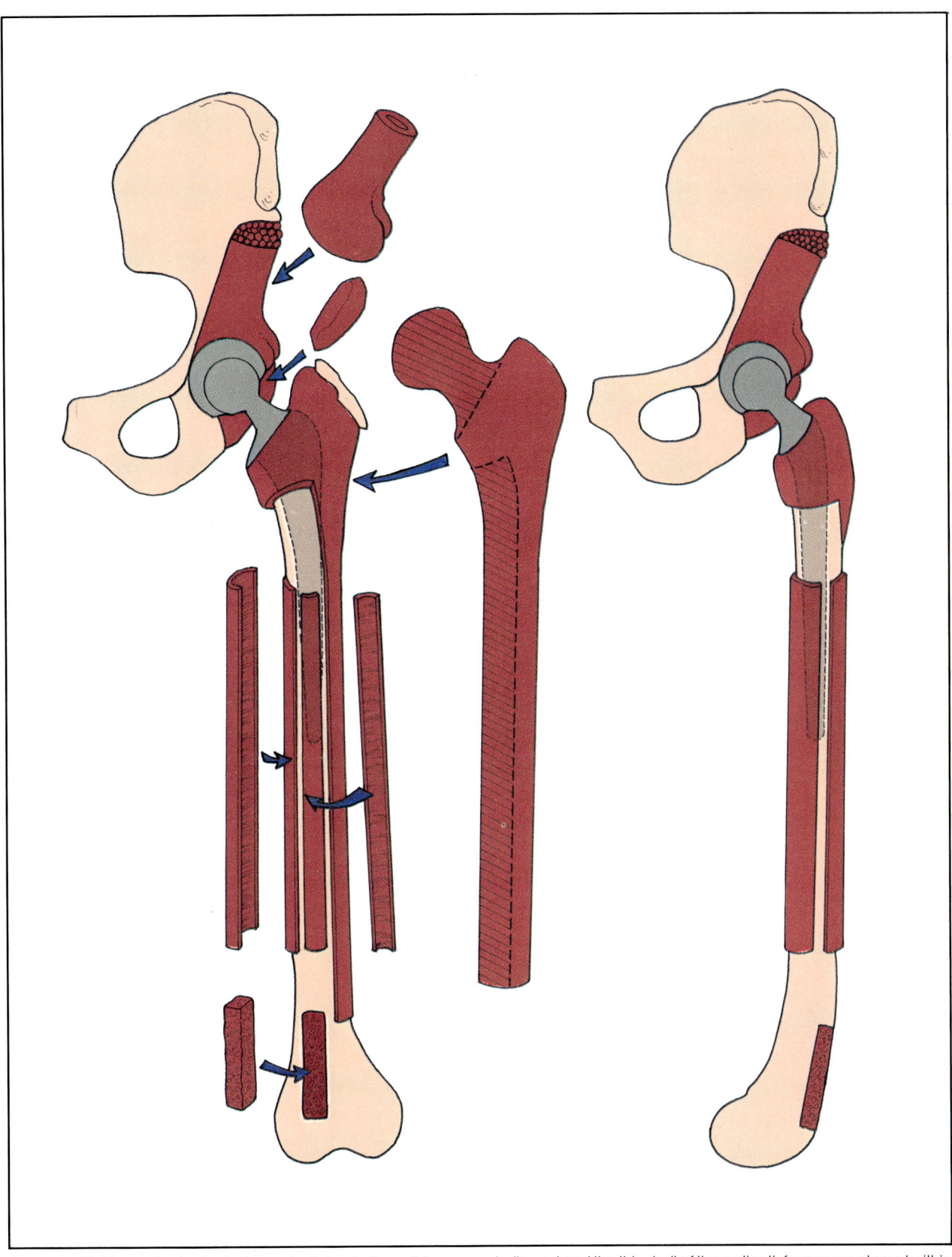

Figure 6-19D. The metaphysis of a larger ipsilateral allograft femur was hollowed and the thin shell of the patient's femur was placed within it. The sintered surfaces of a standard length uncemented femoral prosthesis were partially in contact with living bone. The long side strut extended to the supracondylar area and reinforced the thin lateral femur. It also helped in fixation of the fracture. Two other struts from the allograft femur were used to help stabilize the fracture at the distal tip of the prosthesis. Another allograft was placed in the supracondylar defect. Cortical strips from the iliac crest were used at the graft-host interfaces.

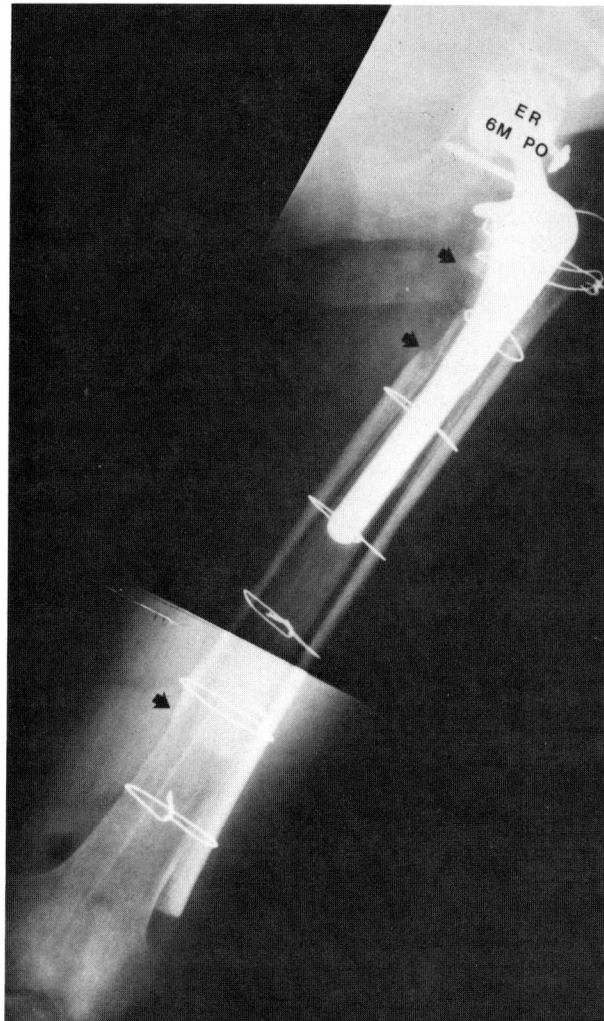

Figure 6-19E. At six months there is some evidence of incorporation of the onlay grafts. The two proximal medial arrows outline the area of the patient's proximal femur that was not covered by allograft.

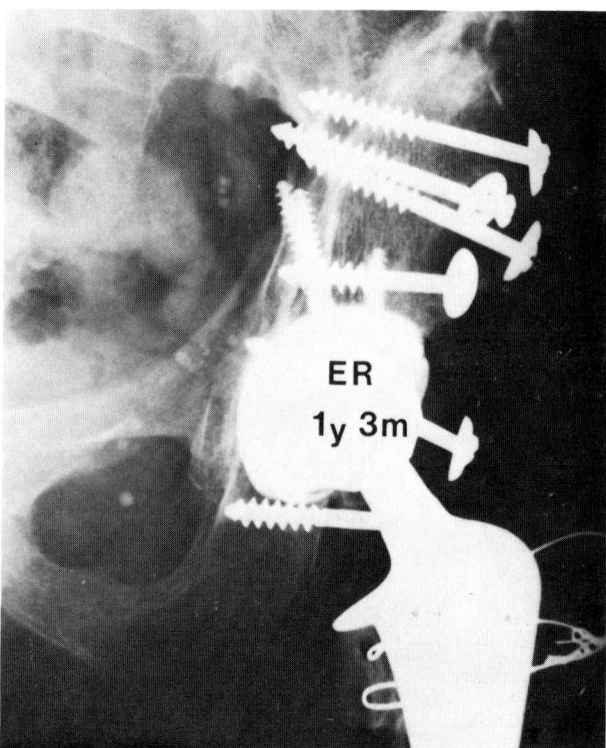

Figure 6-19F. The grafts appear to be doing well at one year, three months. The prosthesis has not subsided and the collar rests on the calcar of the allograft.

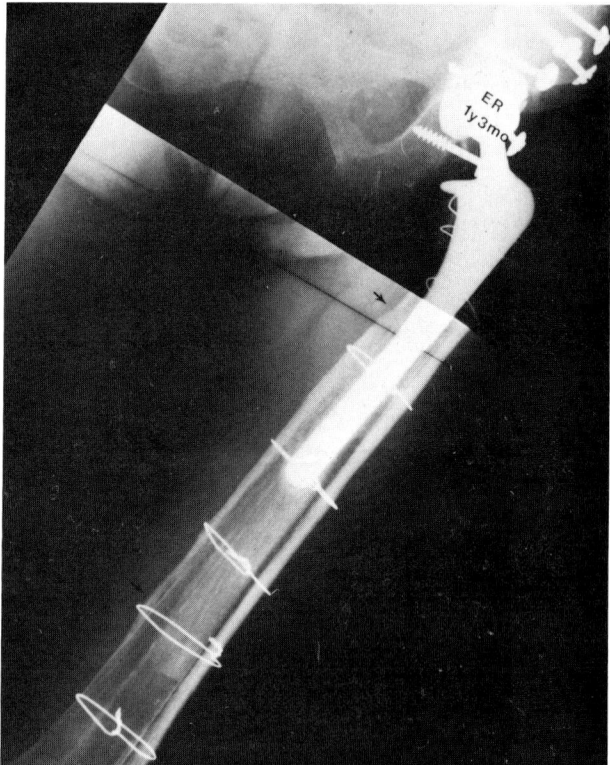

Figure 6-19G. The distal onlay grafts appear to be uniting at one year, three months. There is some scalloping of the medial (compression) strut. The patient rates 82 and walks one half mile with a single crutch. Her exercise tolerance is limited by arthritis of her contralateral knee.

6-22B was 58 when she presented with a loose acetabular and femoral component. Her original diagnosis was degenerative arthritis. She had undergone three cup arthroplasties, a total hip replacement, an exploration and finally a revision nine years previously. She had an uncomplicated total hip on the right side, but at the time of admission for reconstruction of the left hip she was grossly obese and was carrying at least one hundred pounds more than her ideal body weight. She was incapacitated by pain and required two axillary crutches for all walking.

There was a superior intra-acetabular defect and a medial wall perforation. Strips from the iliac crest were used for the medial defect, and a mixture of autograft and allograft morsellized bone was placed in the superior intra-acetabular defect. An uncemented acetabular component was used.

We had initially hoped to use a trochanteric and lateral cortical onlay graft to reconstruct the femur but there was no proximal bone left except for a thin medial strut of cortex (Figures 6-22C and 6-22D).

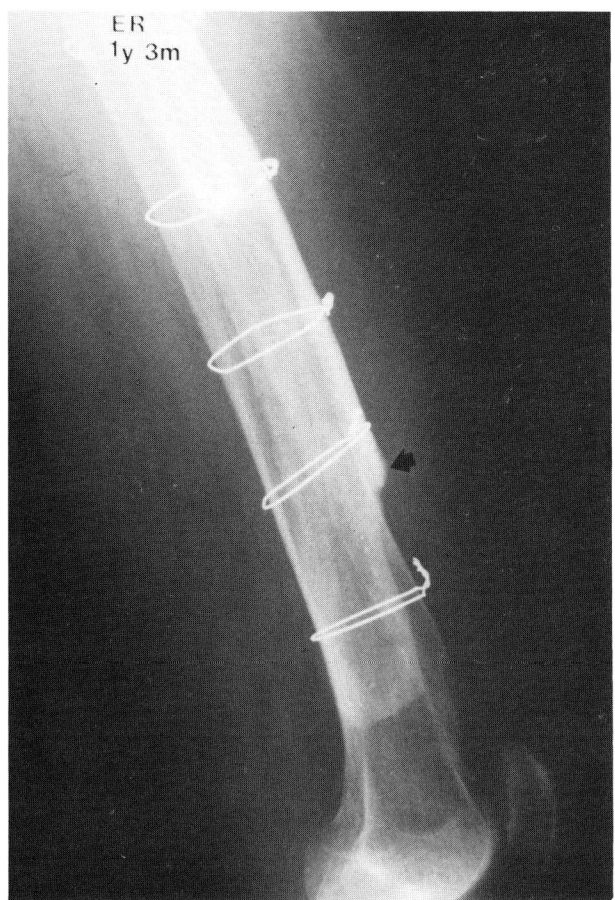

Figure 6-19H. A lateral of the distal femur shows remodeling of the anterior strut. The inlay graft in the suprapatellar area has probably united.

A circumferential proximal femoral allograft was used to reconstruct the metaphysis and trochanters of the proximal femur. A long lateral cortical strut from the allograft extended distally from the butt joint and was used both for fixation and for reinforcement of the very thin lateral femur (Figure 6-22E). Autogenous strips were used at the junction of the graft and host bone.

The grafts appear to be doing well at six months (Figure 6-22F). At short followup of nine months, the patient does not have groin or anterior thigh pain but complains of back, buttock, and posterior thigh pain in the sciatic distribution. This pain is improving but she still uses crutches for most walking and rates only 72.

This reconstruction is typical of our current concepts of proximal allograft replacement. Because the standard length stem bypasses the butt joint by at least 6cm. and fits tightly within the medullary canal, a longer stem or a tension band side plate is not necessary. The distal strut reinforces the deficient cortex and aids in fixation. Cement is not necessary or desirable.

Case 4

The patient whose x-rays are seen in Figures 6-23A and 6-23B was 39 when he presented with loose acetabular and femoral components. His initial diagnosis was a congenitally dislocated hip (Figure 6-23C). Fourteen years prior to admission he had his initial total hip replacement. This was revised after one year. At the time of his second revision, four years prior to presentation, a cemented long stem component was used. The acetabulum had a medial wall perforation, combined with superior intra-acetabular and superior rim defects. The femur had cemented long stem disease with proximal stress shielding and distal cement fixation. There were also several anterior perforations of the femur.

The trochanteric slide was used to approach the hip. The medial acetabular perforation was grafted with strips of autograft bone from the iliac crest. The superior intra-

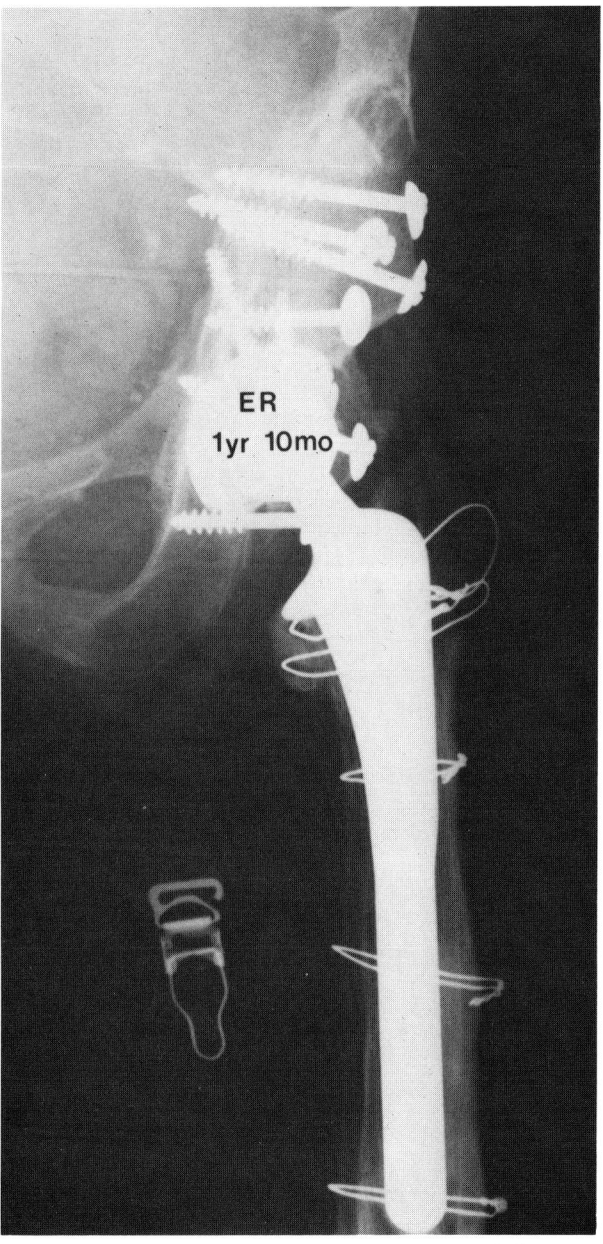

Figure 6-19I. At one year, ten months, there has been further remodeling of the femoral grafts.

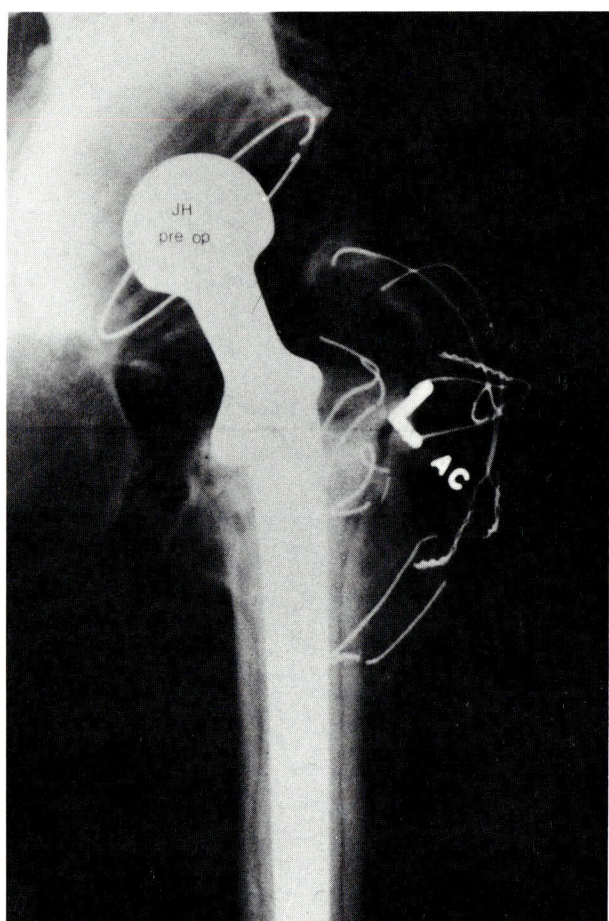

Figure 6-20A. This 44-year-old man presented with a loose 75mm. custom acetabular component. After only two years the cemented long stem femoral component was grossly loose proximally but the distal cement was firmly fixed to the stem and could not pass through the isthmus (cemented long stem disease).

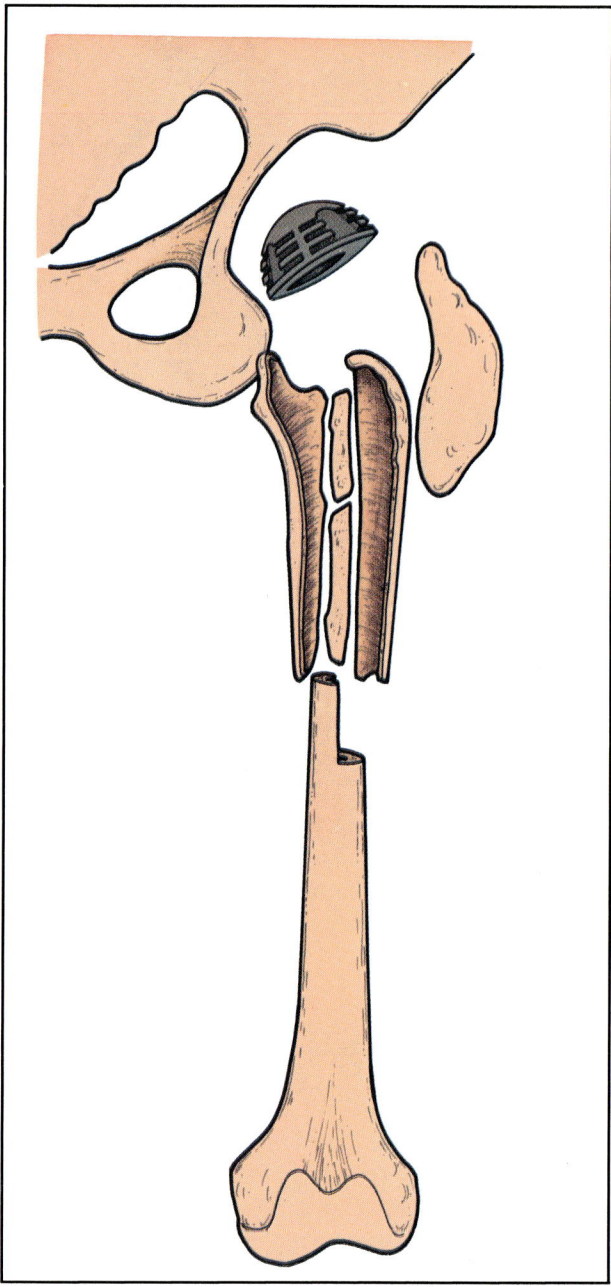

Figure 6-20B. The proximal femur was shattered when the prosthesis was removed. Under similar circumstances we would now window the distal femur (Figure 6-4C) to remove this cement.

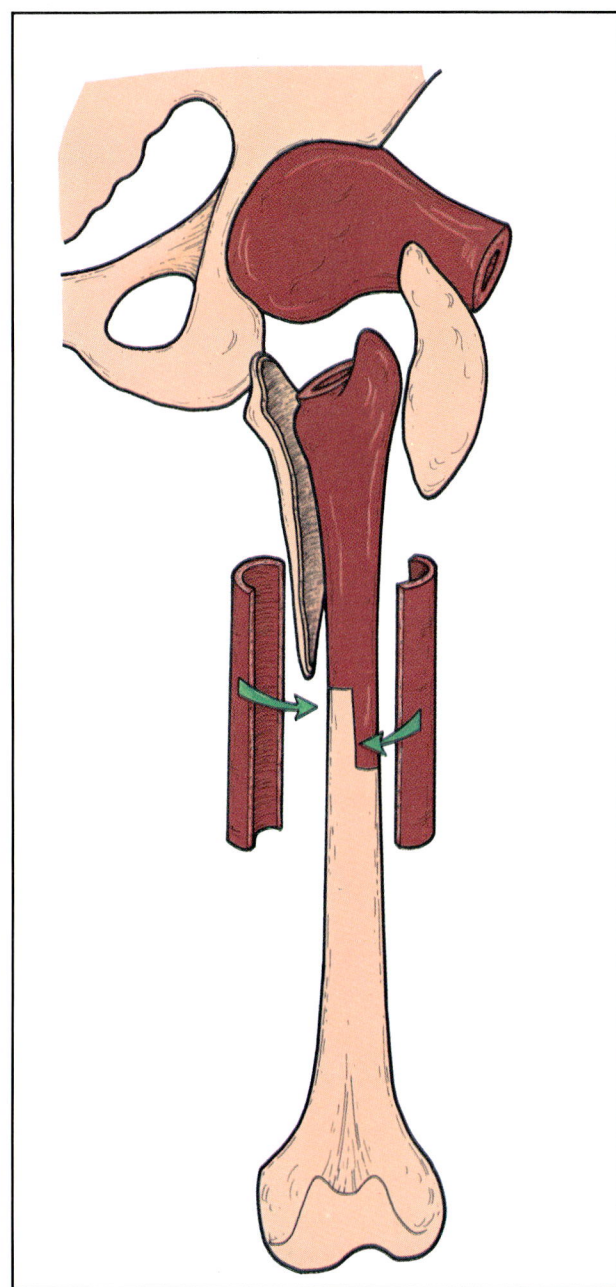

Figure 6-20C. A proximal femoral allograft was necessary. A distal step cut increased stability and provided a larger surface area to enhance healing. Two onlay femoral allograft struts were used to reinforce the junction of the allograft to the patient's femur. A trochanteric slide provided the necessary exposure and provided a blood supply to the patient's greater trochanter which was in contact with the allograft femur.

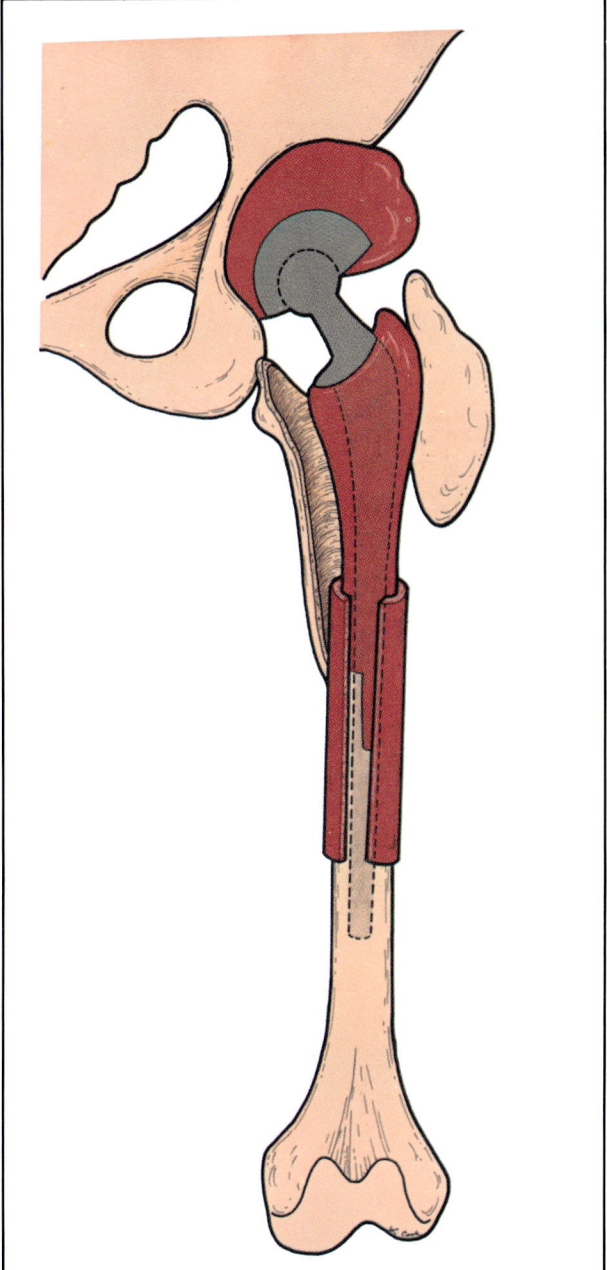

Figure 6-20D. The remnants of the patient's proximal femur were approximated to the allograft. A cemented long stem component was used in this case but we now would use an uncemented mid-length stem, bypassing the allograft-host junction by 6cm.

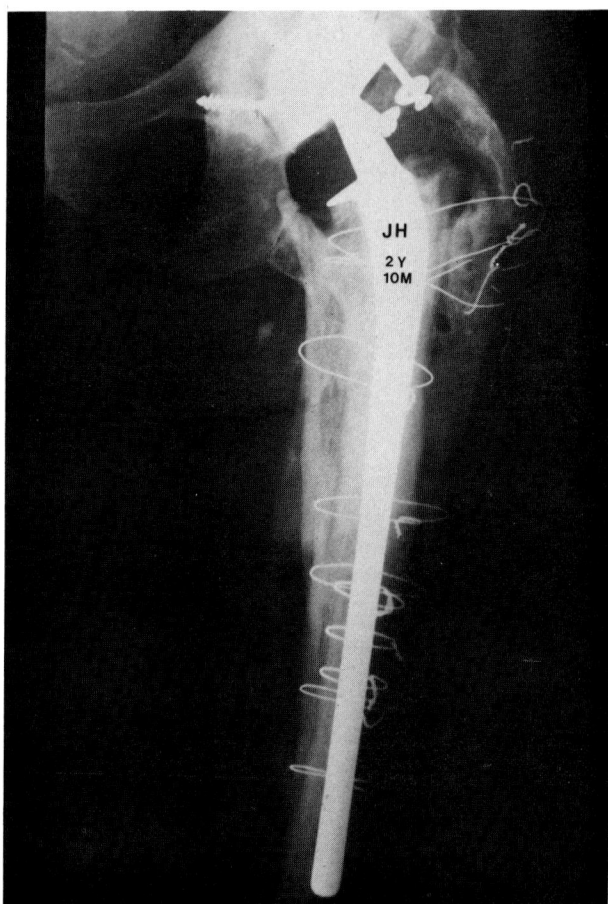

Figure 6-20E. The grafts appear to have united at two years, ten months. The patient is pleased with his hip and rates 89.

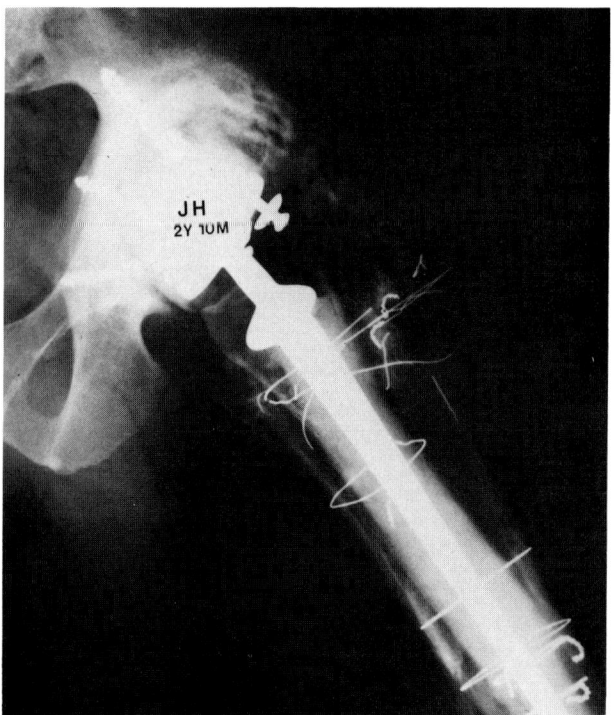

Figure 6-20F. The grafts appear to be doing well on the frog lateral view.

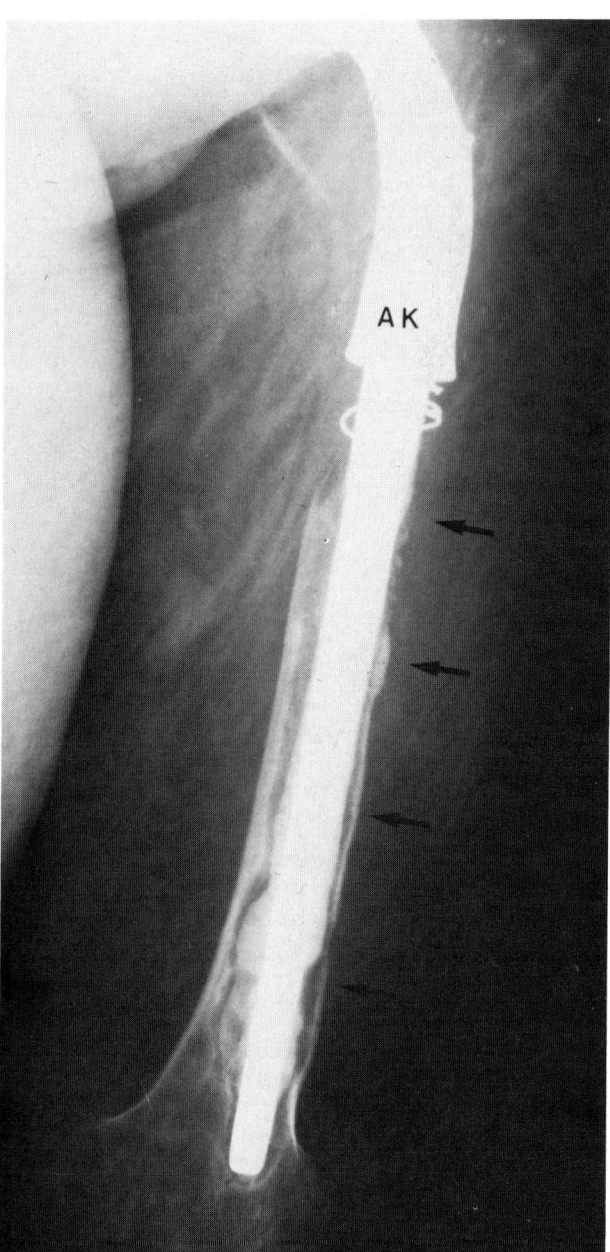

Figure 6-21A. This 38-year-old woman had polio as a child and had residual weakness of the left lower extremity. After 12 operations, she presented with this loose acetabular component and loose custom proximal femoral replacement prosthesis. The distal femur was very thin and had several perforations. During one of her previous acetabular reconstructions, she had a sciatic injury with severe sciatic nerve distribution pain and her weak extremity became completely flail. She took 12 60mg codeine tablets a day because of intractable pain. She was infected with alpha streptococcus.

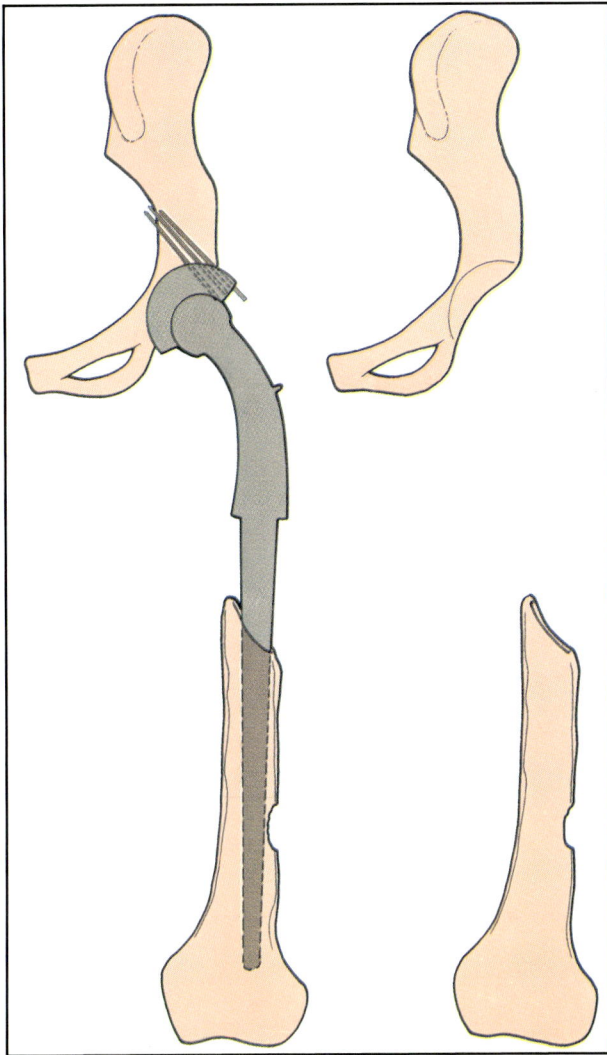

Figure 6-21B. A cemented custom long stem proximal femoral replacement component was used. Stress shielding caused further bone loss of the remaining femur. There were several large perforations of the distal lateral femoral cortex.

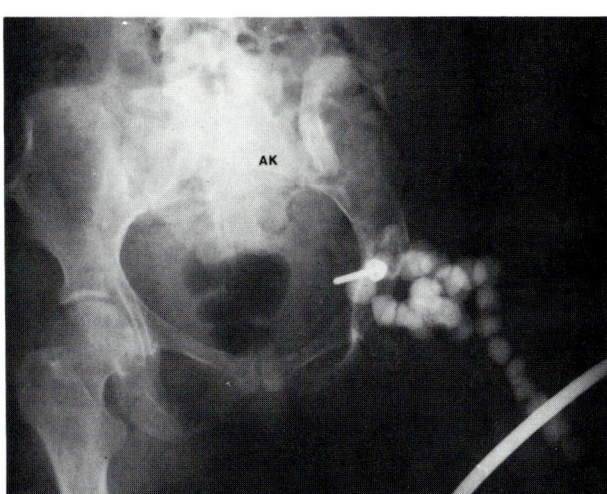

Figure 6-21C. A resection arthroplasty was performed. After extensive debridement, antibiotic impregnated beads were inserted and the patient was treated with antibiotics for six weeks.

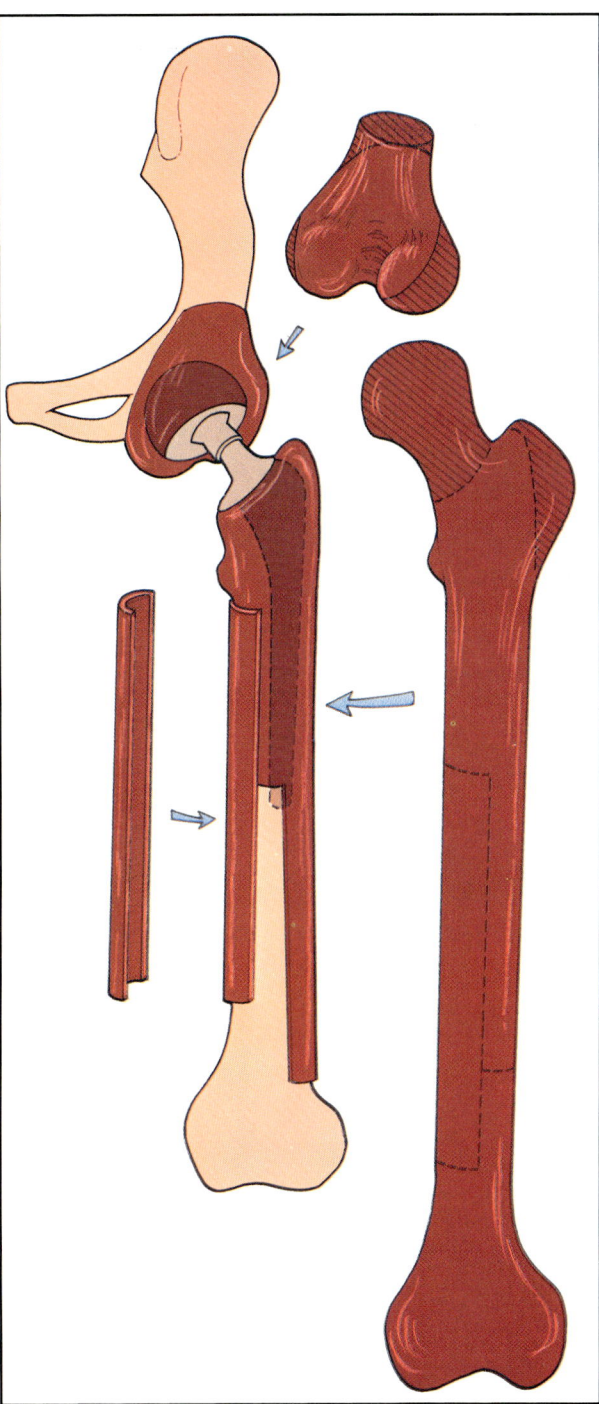

Figure 6-21D. A distal femur was used to reconstruct her global acetabular deficiency. A proximal femoral allograft was used to replace the absent proximal femur. A long lateral strut was left in continuity with the proximal allograft femur and extended to the knee. This strut aided in fixation of the graft and reinforced the thin and perforated distal lateral cortex. A second medial onlay cortical allograft strut reinforced the junction between the allograft and the patient's femur and provided reinforcement of the thin distal shell of the patient's femoral cortex.

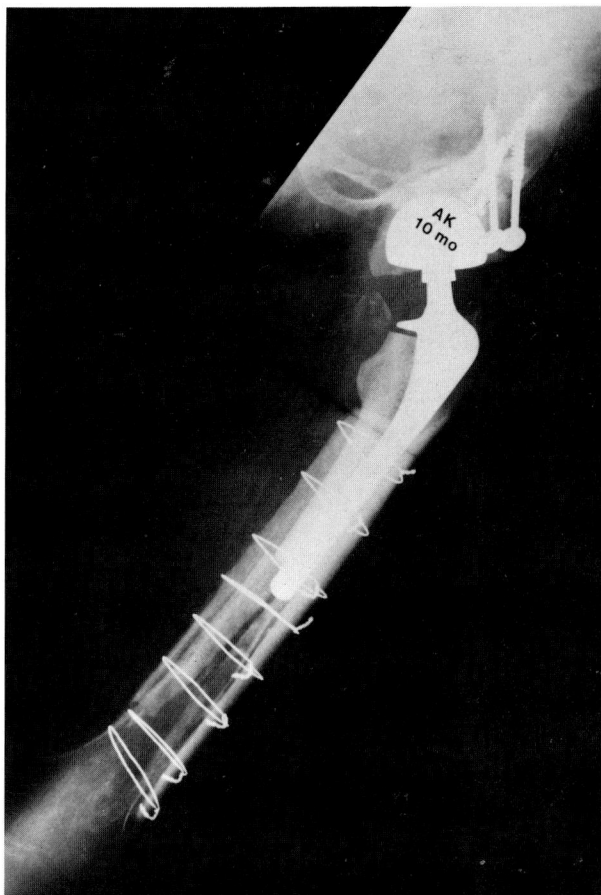

Figure 6-21E. The grafts appear to be incorporating at ten months. The sedimentation rate was 10 and the patient's hip pain was completely relieved. She still took 20 tablets of codeine 30mg per month because of residual sciatic pain in her foot. She will always require two axillary crutches because of her weakness.

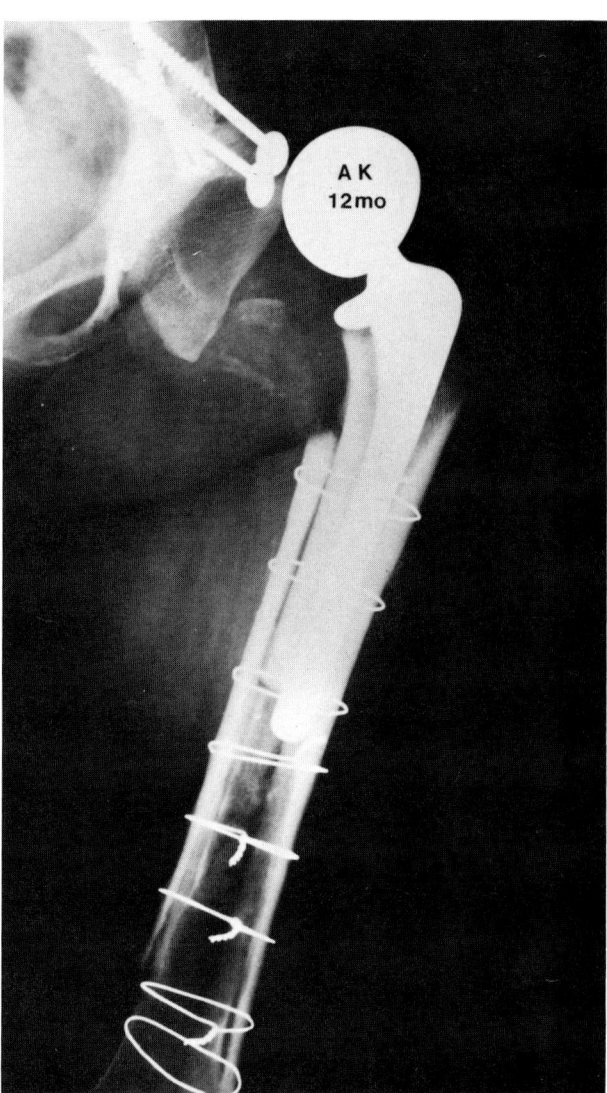

Figure 6-21F. At one year the patient fell and sustained an anterior dislocation. The grafts appear to be doing well. She was reduced by closed manipulation and was placed in an abduction brace for six weeks.

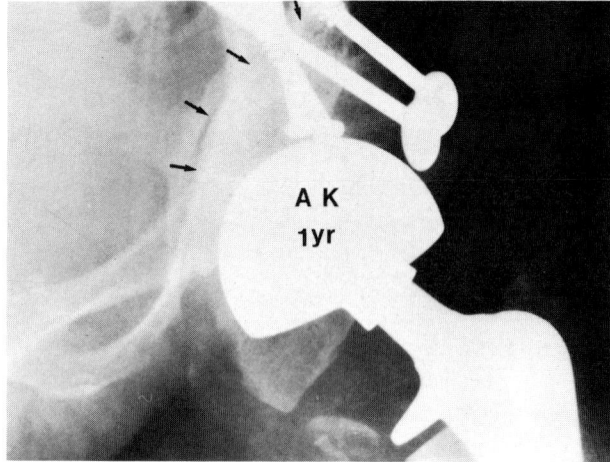

Figure 6-21G. The hip was reduced by closed methods and has not dislocated again. The arrows outline the graft-host interface. The patient rates 74.

acetabular defects were packed with a mixture of autograft and allograft morsellized bone and then a solid allograft was taken from the allograft femoral head and was used to reconstruct the superior intra-acetabular and superior rim defects. An uncemented acetabular component was used.

The proximal femur was absent except for the greater trochanter (which was kept in continuity with the vastus lateralis) (Figure 6-23D). A proximal femoral replacement allograft was butted against the patient's remaining femur and since the major cortical thinning and the perforations were anterior, a long anterior cortical strut, which extended to the knee, was left attached to the allograft and was used both for fixation and to reinforce the anterior cortex. Two other long allograft struts were placed anterior and posterior to the linea aspera (Figure 6-23E). An uncemented standard length femoral component was used and extended at least 6cm. past the butt joint of the allograft and the patient's femur.

The patient was discharged at 12 days on crutches. X-rays at eight weeks appeared quite satisfactory (Figures 6-23F and 6-23G) and the patient began to use a cane. At five months the patient was doing well and used a cane only

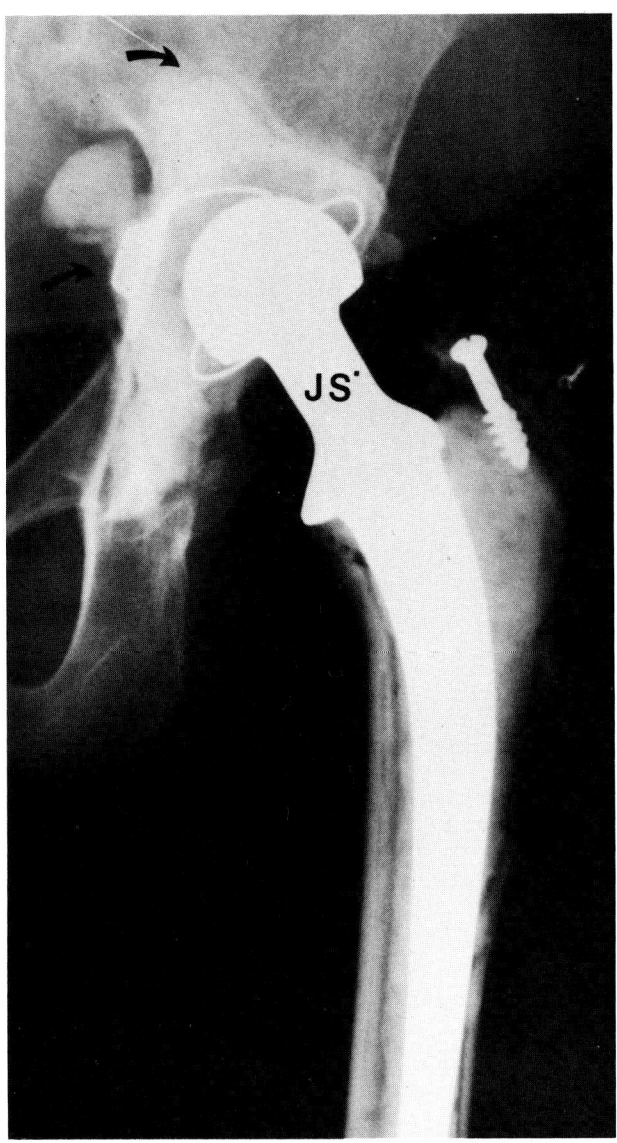

Figure 6-22A. This 58-year-old woman had multiple previous operations and presented with loose acetabular and femoral components. She was 100 pounds overweight, had severe pain, and required two axillary crutches for all steps. Except for the medial cortex, there was essentially no proximal femoral bone remaining.

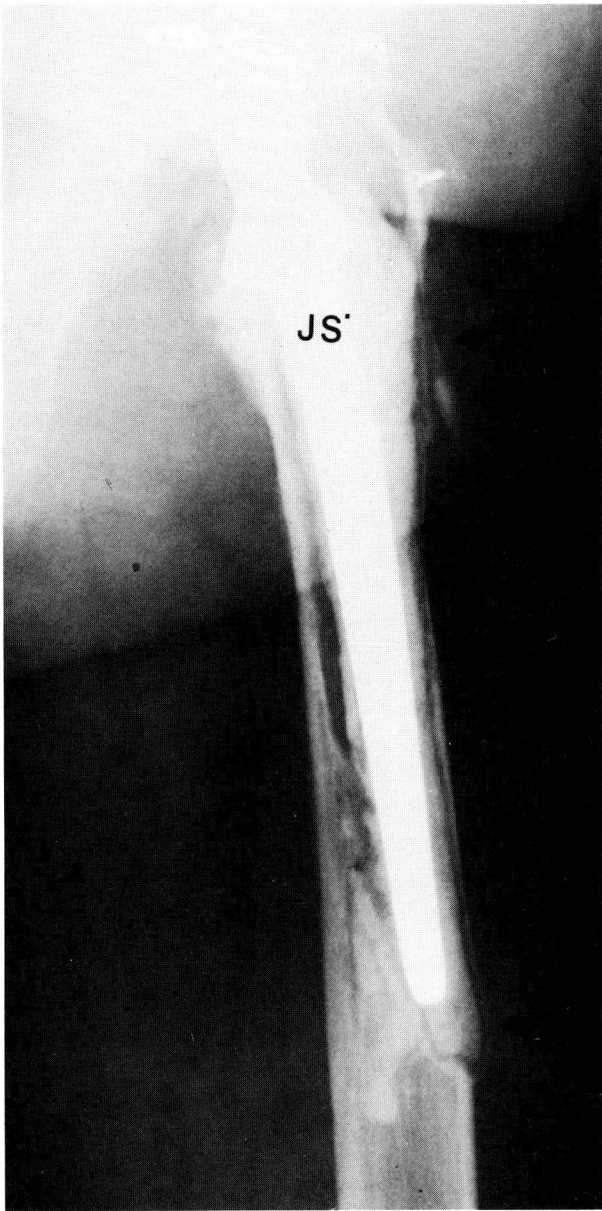

Figure 6-22B. There was marked thinning of the anterolateral cortex.

for long walks (Figure 6-23H). He rated 89. There was no trauma but at seven months he had the abrupt onset of supracondylar pain which increased over the next three days to a degree that required two axillary crutches. X-rays were initially unchanged but repeat x-rays one month later were suggestive of a healing supracondylar stress fracture (Figure 6-23I). Although the patient was subjectively much improved and was walking with a cane at the time these x-rays were taken, he was advised to go back on crutches. Six weeks after its onset, the pain disappeared and at ten months the patient uses a cane only for long walks and rates 89.

Case 5

The patient whose x-rays are seen in Figure 6-24A was 57 when he presented with a painful total hip replacement.

His hip problems started in 1960 with avascular necrosis, probably related to excessive alcohol intake. His first operation was probably a Moore prosthesis. This was revised to a Charnley-Muller total hip replacement in 1975 because of protrusio.

In 1980, the femoral component was revised because of loosening. An intra-operative fracture occurred and was treated by means of a cemented long stem component. The patient required two axillary crutches for all steps following that procedure and had increasing thigh pain and progressive shortening of the extremity in the year prior to presentation. He was 3cm. shorter on the involved side.

He had a loose acetabular component with a medial wall perforation and a superior intra-acetabular defect. The medial perforation was filled with strips of autogenous bone

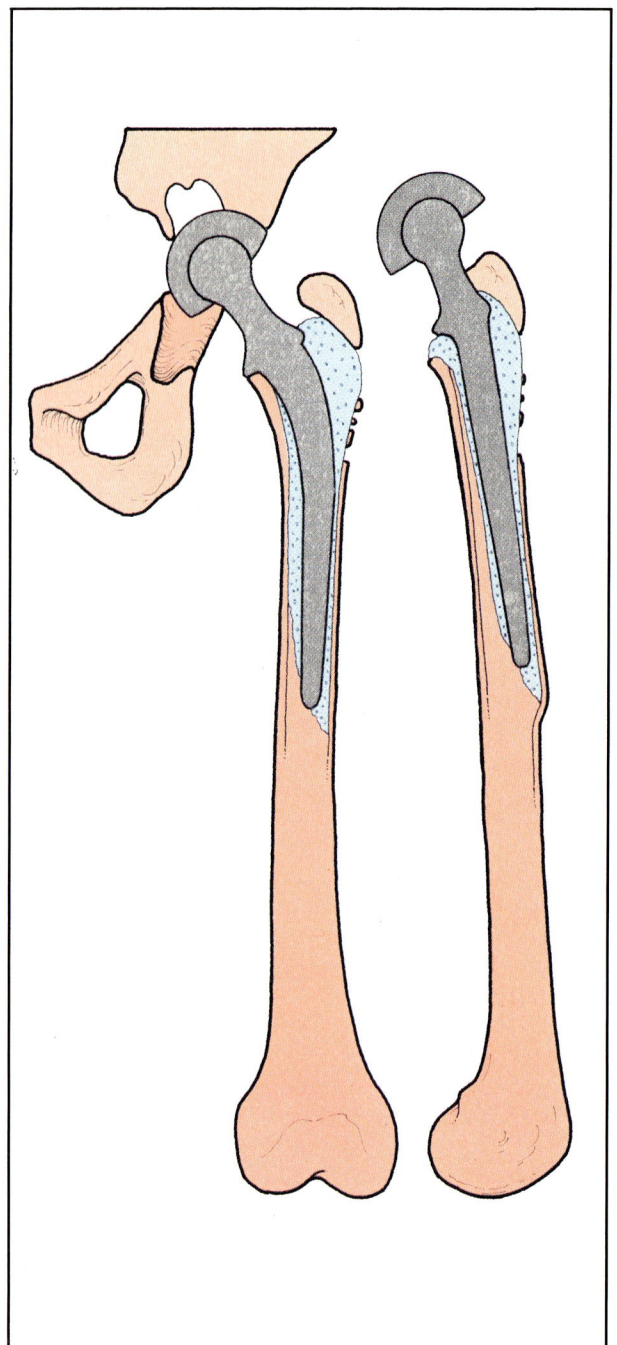

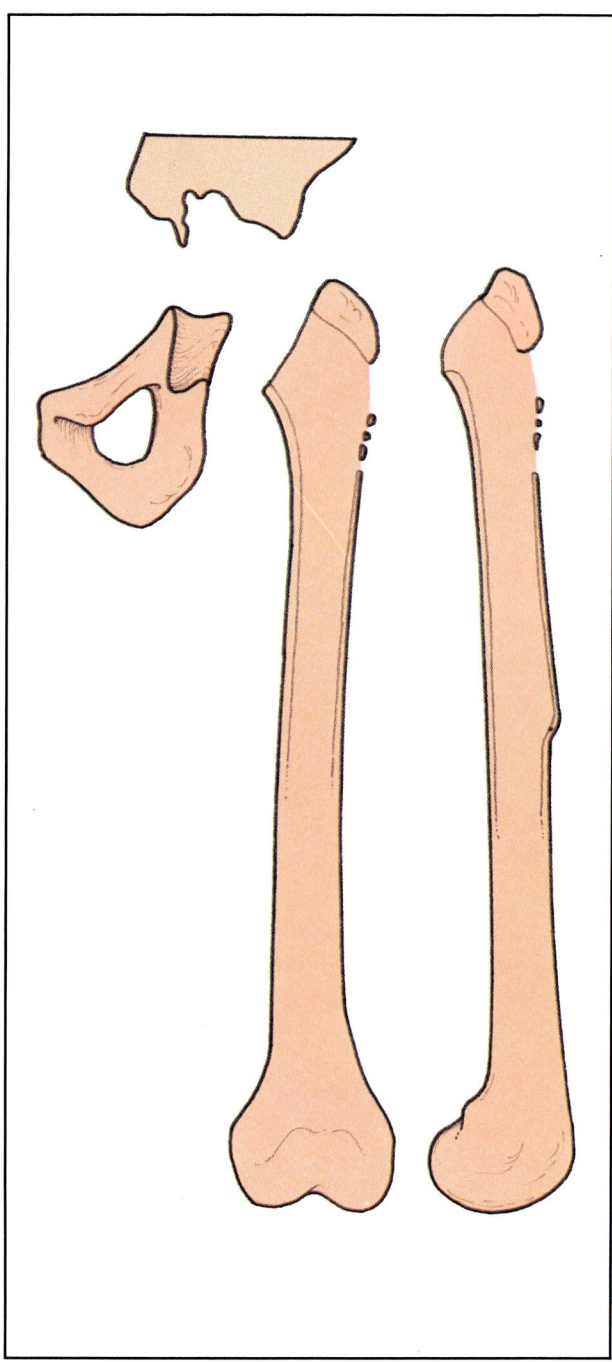

Figure 6-22C. The greater trochanter had no contact with bone and except for a thin medial strut, the prosthesis was supported only by cement.

Figure 6-22D. There was a medial acetabular perforation and a superior intra-acetabular defect as well as loss of the anterior, posterior, and lateral cortices of the proximal femur.

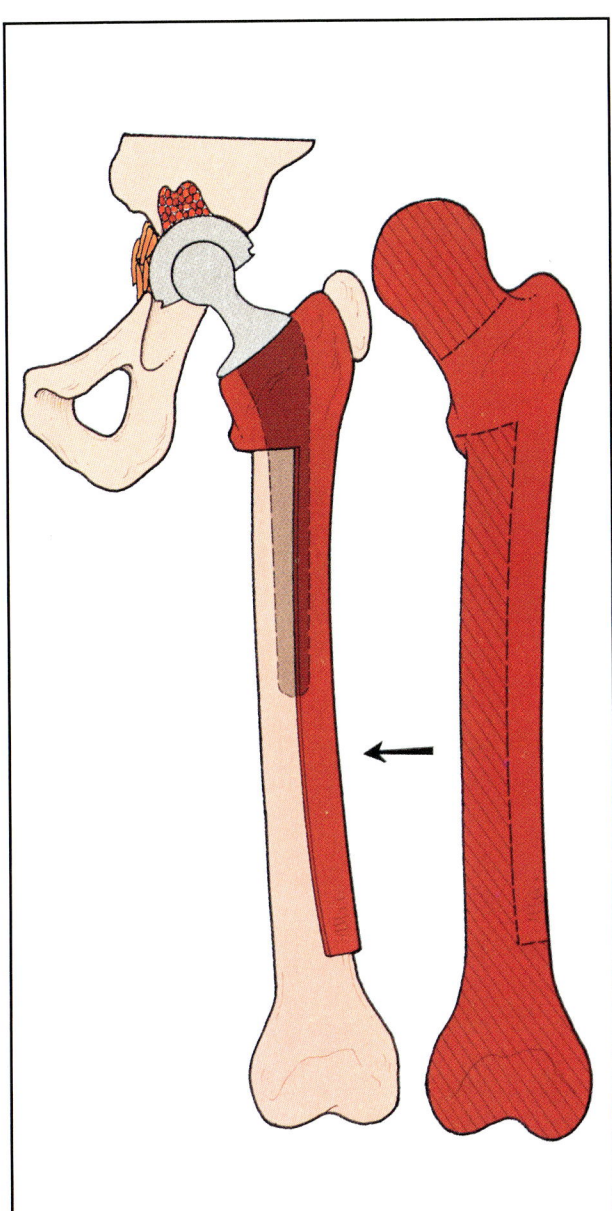

Figure 6-22E. The medial acetabular perforation was grafted with strips from the iliac crest and the superior intra-acetabular defect was grafted with a mixture of autograft and allograft morsellized bone. An uncemented acetabular component was used. A proximal femoral allograft was butted against the remaining cortex of the patient's femur and a long lateral side strut was used for fixation and to reinforce the lateral femoral cortex. A standard length uncemented femoral component was used.

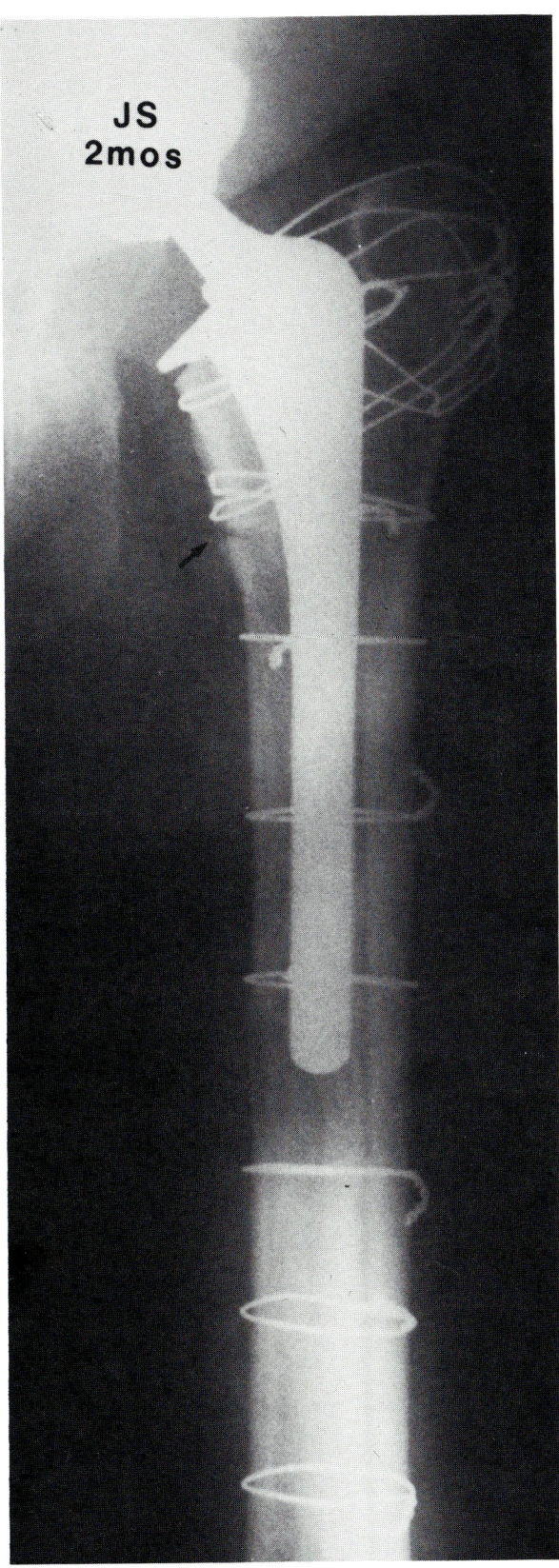

Figure 6-22F. X-rays at six months appear satisfactory. The arrow points to the butt joint. At followup of ten months, the patient has no groin or anterior thigh pain but does complain of back, buttock and posterior thigh pain in the sciatic distribution. Although this pain is subsiding she still uses two crutches for most steps and rates only 72.

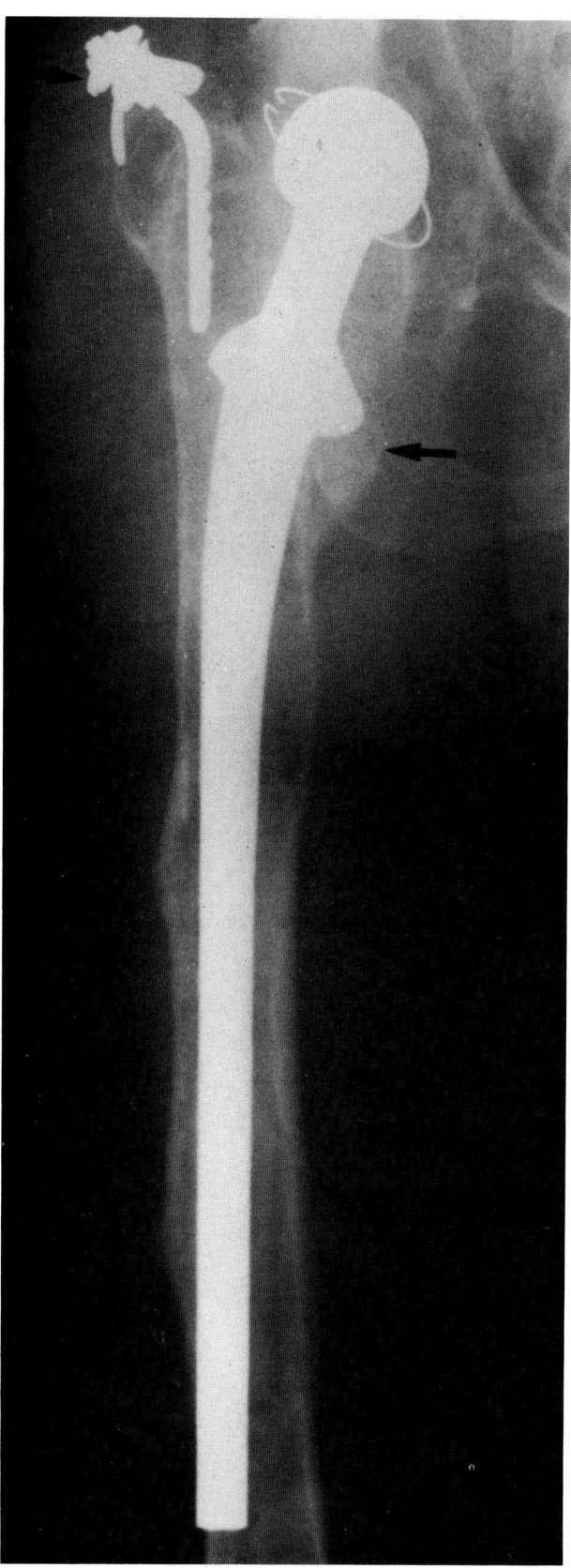

Figure 6-23A. This 39-year-old man presented with a loose acetabular component as well as a loose cemented long stem femoral component that had subsided. Nonradio opaque cement was used. Note the cemented long stem disease with thin stress shielded proximal cortices. The patient was 1½ inches shorter.

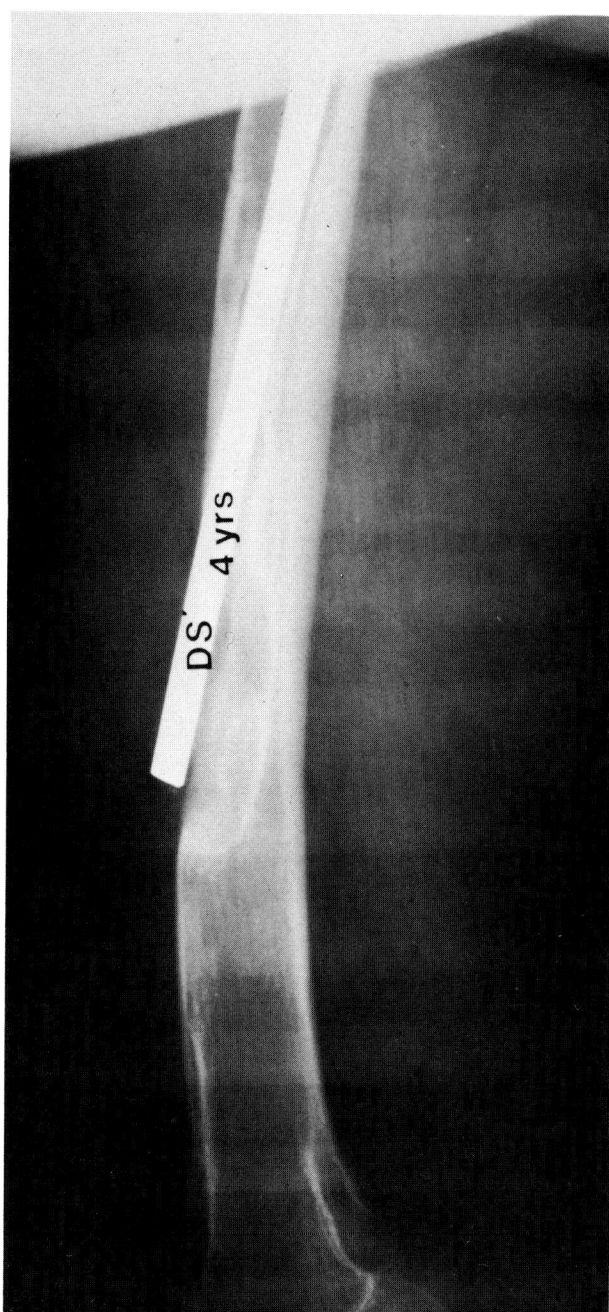

Figure 6-23B. There was a significant anterior bow of the femur. X-rays four years after this cemented long stem component had been inserted show that there was a perforation of the anterior femoral cortex.

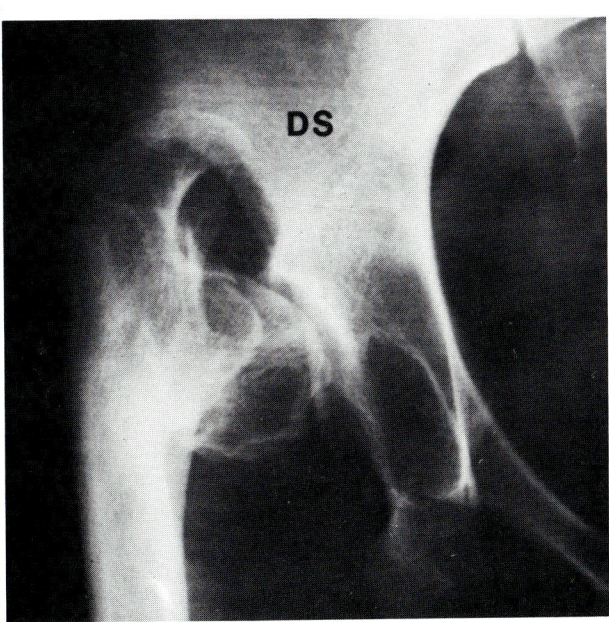

Figure 6-23C. His initial diagnosis was a congenitally dislocated hip.

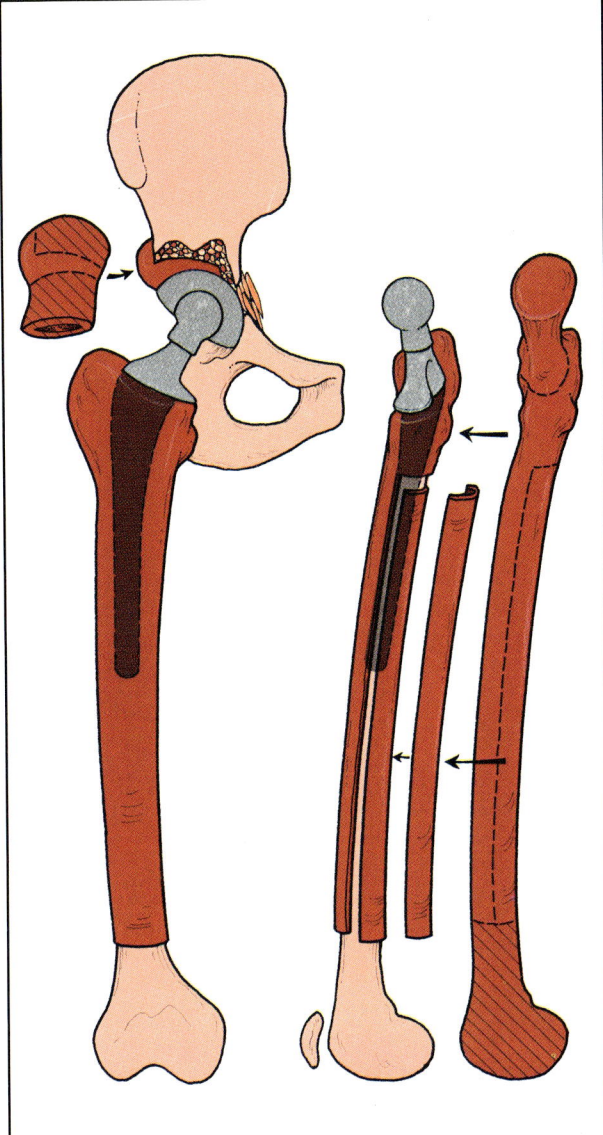

Figure 6-23E. The medial acetabular defect was grafted with autogenous strips from the iliac crest. The superior intra-acetabular defect was grafted with a mixture of autograft and allograft morsellized bone. The major superior intra-acetabular and superior rim defects were reconstructed by a single graft from the allograft femoral head. An uncemented acetabular component was used. A proximal femoral allograft was butted against the patient's remaining femur. A long anterior cortical strut extended to the knee and served to reinforce the thin and perforated anterior cortex. Two other long allograft struts from the same femur were used as well. One was placed medially and the other laterally to the linea aspera. A standard length uncemented femoral component was used.

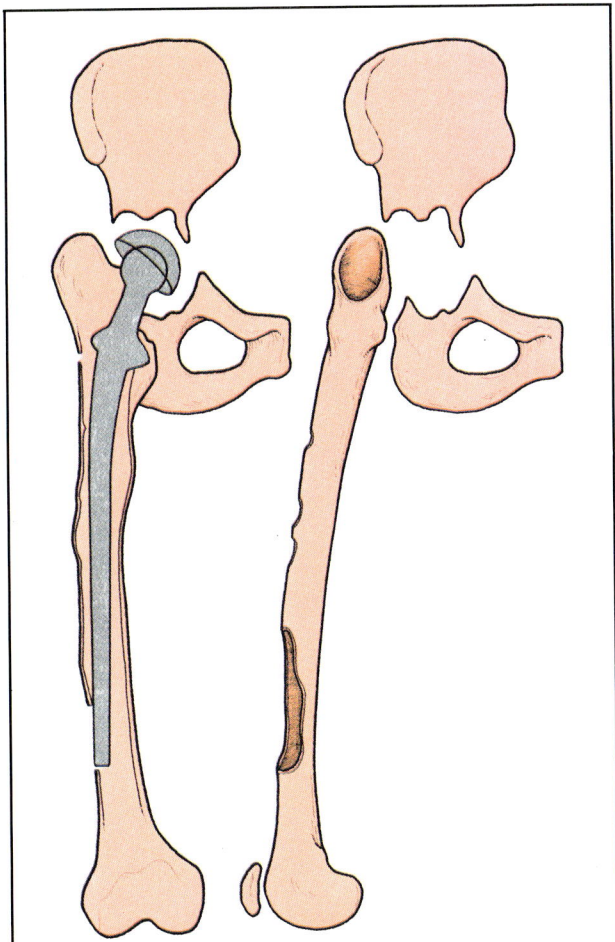

Figure 6-23D. The acetabular defect was extensive and consisted of a combined medial wall, superior intra-acetabular, and superior rim defect. The femur had very thin cortices and several anterior perforations.

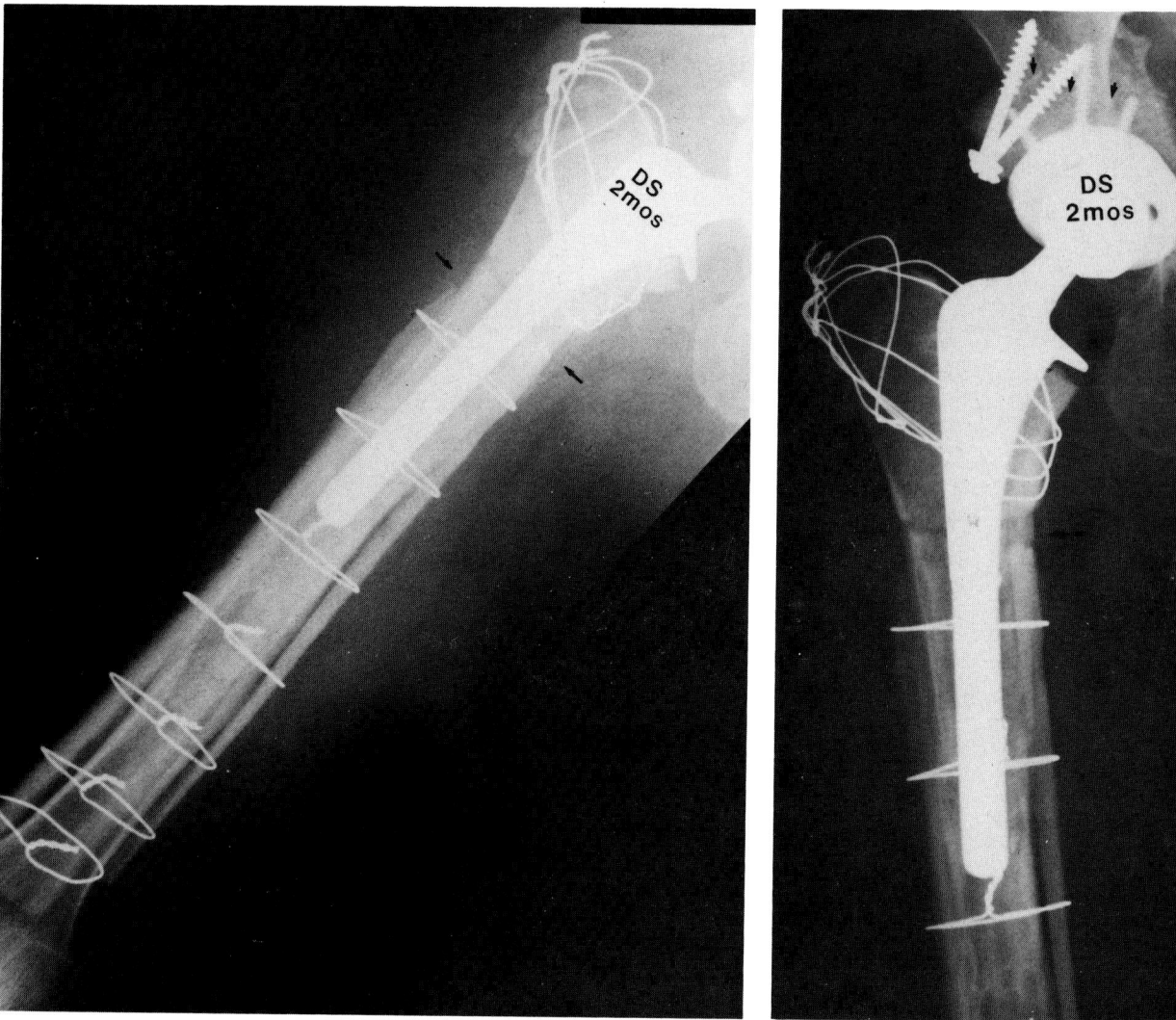

Figure 6-23F. X-rays at two months are satisfactory. The small arrows on the femur point to the butt joint of the allograft and the recipient femur. The arrows on the acetabulum outline the solid superior intra-acetabular and superior rim graft. The patient began to use a cane. He had no pain.

and a disc of allograft bone was placed intra-pelvically. The superior intra-acetabular defect was filled with a mixture of morsellized autogenous and allograft bone and an uncemented acetabular component was used (Figure 6-24B).

Except for the greater trochanter, the proximal 12cm. of the femur were essentially absent secondary to cemented long stem disease and to the fracture. The remaining femur had a major anterior defect and because of the malunion and bone loss, had a medullary canal that would have required a prosthesis with a stem diameter of greater than 26mm. An uncemented #4 PCA standard stem (Howmedica, Rutherford, NJ) was placed within a smaller proximal femoral allograft that in turn was placed within the excessively large medullary canal of the patient's femur. The allograft was shaped with the Midas Rex (Midas Rex Institute, Fort Worth, TX) to fit within the patient's femur and a ridge of bone was left anteriorly to fill the slot of the recipient femur and provided rotational stability. Two additional onlay allograft femoral struts were used to reinforce the junction

between the patient's femur and the allograft and autogenous strips from the iliac crest were used at the junction of the allografts and the remnants of the patient's femur. A trochanteric slide was used for the approach and the patient's greater trochanter was wired to the allograft greater trochanter.

At short followup of seven months, x-rays show that the grafts appear to be doing quite well (Figure 6-24C). The patient has minimal hip discomfort but takes two Darvocet capsules a day for an unrelated shoulder problem and requires a cane only for long outside walks. He is pleased with his function and rates 87.

Summary of Authors' Preferred Treatment for Femoral Defects

Although we prefer to use autograft bone whenever possible, it is rare that there is enough autograft bone

wire tightener and are twisted rather than tied. Transverse screws are undesirable because they can potentially prevent the grafts from impacting to a position of stability.

The exception may be a DCP type of supracondylar lateral plate (Synthes, Ltd., Wayne, PA) used as a tension band to reinforce an allograft that is subjected to varus bending loads. If resorption of the graft-host junction does occur, the screws can theoretically slide within the holes and allow further impaction to occur with weightbearing.

Although there is a place for cemented regular length stems in elderly patients with primary total hips, we feel that uncemented components should be used in most revision situations because the smooth eburnated bone resists cement intrusion and loosening often occurs more quickly than after a primary hip. There is never an indication for a long stem component that is cemented to the patient's femur except in palliative surgery in the terminal patient with a pathological fracture who has a life span of less than a year because such stems will routinely cause cemented long stem disease and the next reconstruction will be much more complex. There may be a place for a long stem that is cemented into a proximal allograft femur but is used as a press fit distally. However, we feel that a press fit, even in the proximal fragment is as satisfactory. Uncemented long stems may be necessary in some circumstances but also can cause stress shielding; whenever possible, we prefer to use standard length uncemented stems with proximal sintering. Distally sintered long stems are almost impossible to extract if bone ingrowth occurs and also cause stress shielding. We feel that such devices should not be used.

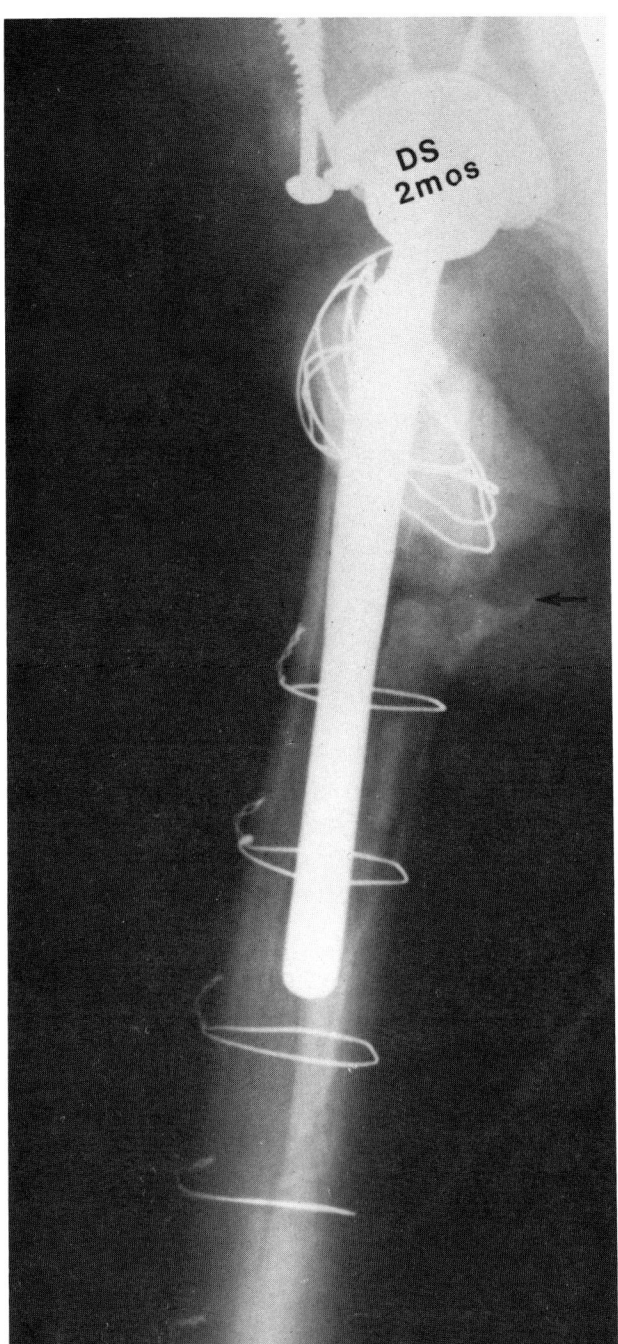

Figure 6-23G. The long anterior strut can be seen on this frog lateral view. The arrow points to the butt joint between the allograft and the patient's femur.

available to provide structural support for major femoral deficiencies. Allograft bone is therefore almost always necessary. However, we feel that all allografts should be supplemented with autograft strips from the iliac crest and/or morsellized bone from the femoral head or particulate bone from acetabular reamers if available.

Femoral grafts should be buttressed against the patient's bone if subjected to weight-bearing forces. If additional fixation is necessary, we prefer circumferential #16 Luque wires (Zimmer, Warsaw, IN) which are tightened with a

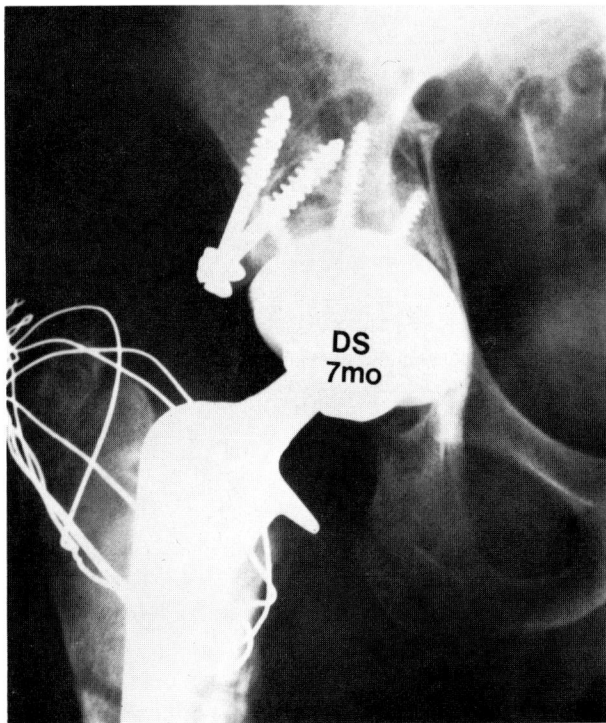

Figure 6-23H. At seven months the acetabular reconstruction appears to be doing well.

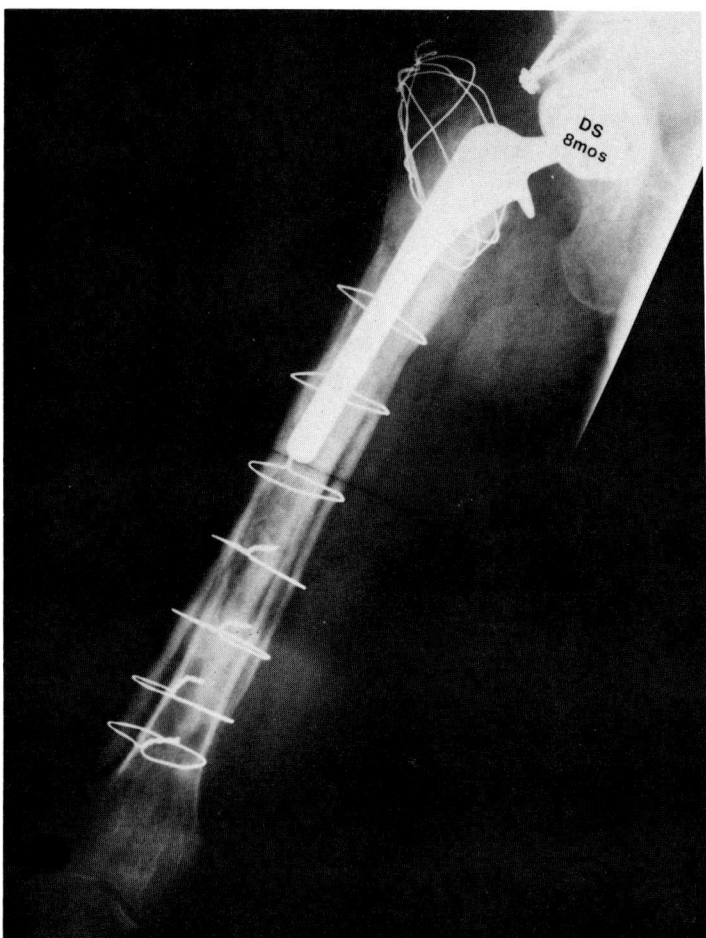 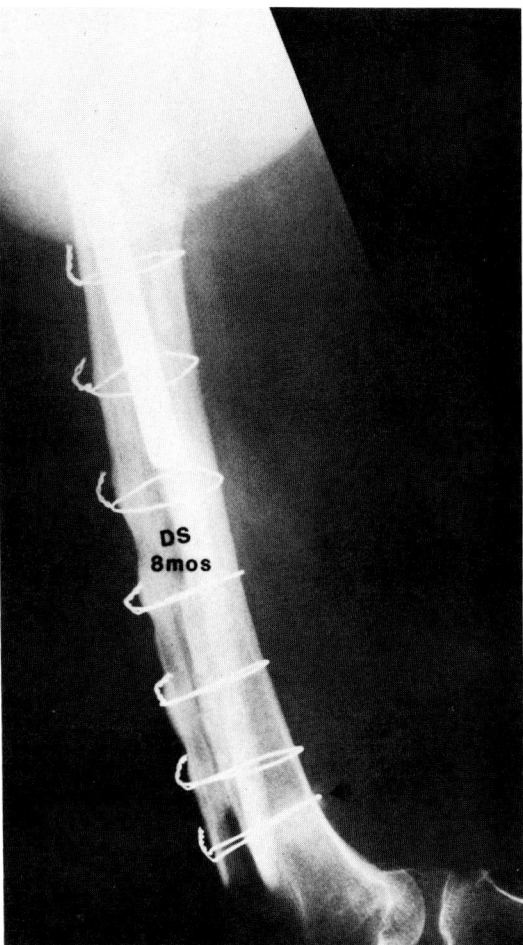

Figure 6-23I. There was no trauma but at seven months the onset of supracondylar pain that increased over the next three days to a degree requiring the patient to use two axillary crutches. X-rays were initially unremarkable but repeat x-rays one month later suggest a healing supracondylar stress fracture (see arrows). His pain disappeared six weeks after its onset and at ten months he rates 89 and uses a can only for long walks.

Calcar Deficiency

Calcar intramedullary defects with an intact calcar rim can be treated with a femoral neck and head, shaped like a cylinder and impacted within the medullary canal. Small defects secondary to a failed Moore prosthesis can be managed by a full thickness iliac crest graft used in the same fashion. Complete loss of the calcar is best managed by an allograft calcar and distal strut from an ipsilateral allograft femur.

Trochanteric Deficiency

Isolated greater trochanteric deficiency can be reconstructed with a femoral head and neck that is split in half and shaped to fit the recipient femur. Combined cortical and trochanteric deficiency may require an allograft replacement from an ipsilateral allograft femur which includes the trochanter and the missing cortex. Supplemental autogenous strips from the iliac crest should be added at the junction of the graft to the recipient femur.

Cortical Thinning and Perforation

Both can be managed by a strip of contoured allograft cortical bone that covers at least one third and preferably one half the circumference of the recipient femur and extends at least 8cm. proximal and distal to the area in question. It is easier, but not essential, to use a strut from the same area of an ipsilateral femur. Supplemental autogenous strips from the iliac crest are routinely added. It is not necessary for the stem of the femoral component to extend past the defect.

Femoral Fractures About or Below the Stem of a Femoral Component

A fracture that occurs below a stem of a vascularized femur can be stabilized by massive medial and lateral allograft struts (preferably from an allograft femur split in half) contoured to fit the outer surface of the recipient femur and that extend at least 12cm. proximal and distal to the fracture. Supplemental autologous strips from the iliac crest

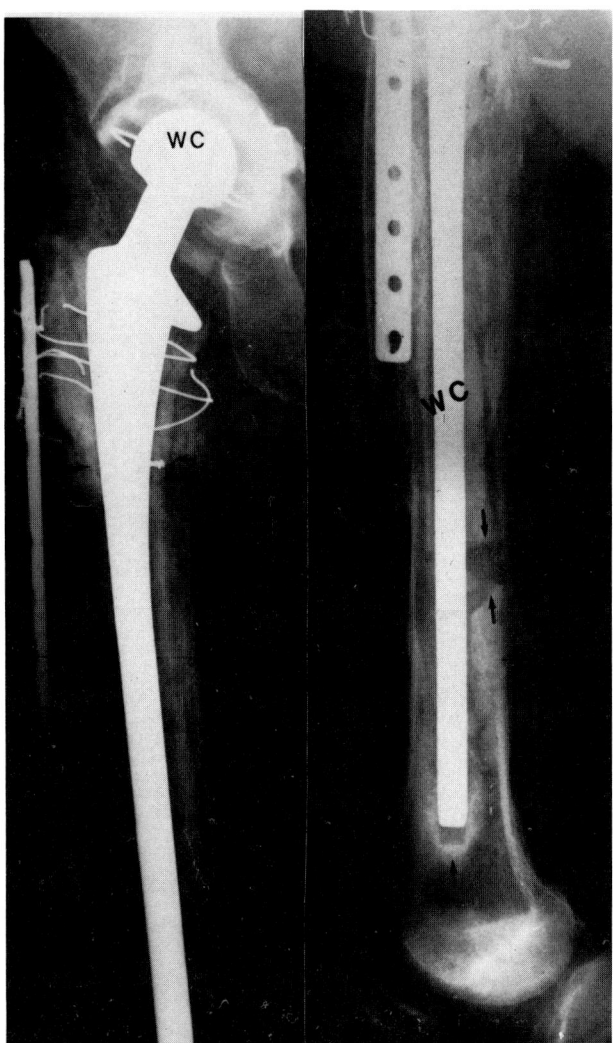

Figure 6-24A. This 57-year-old man had a loose acetabular component with a combined medial and superior intra-acetabular defect, as well as a loose femoral component. Because of a malunited fracture and cemented long stem disease, the proximal femur was absent and the remaining medullary canal was over 26mm. in diameter. Note the fracture of the cement mantle on the lateral view with evidence of pistoning of the femoral stem.

should be routinely used. It is not necessary to remove a well fixed component and even with a loose component, the surgeon's decision as to the length of the stem used for revision should not be affected by the fracture. Long stem components are not necessary in treatment of the fracture.

A fracture or loss of position at the junction of a proximal allograft replacement and the recipient femur, should also be treated with a massive medial allograft cortical strut that encompasses at least one half of the diameter of the femur. If the canal of the distal fragment is too large to provide distal fixation of a larger stem, a supracondylar DCP plate (Synthes, Ltd., Wayne, PA) should be added to act as a tension band. If proximal screw holes over lie the prosthesis and/or cement, cerclage wires can be used in these areas rather than screws. Supplemental autologous strips from the iliac crest are routinely added.

Circumferential Deficiencies of the Metaphysis and Proximal Diaphysis

If a thin shell of the diaphysis remains, a proximal ipsilateral femur can be used. This allograft femur should be large enough so that the recipient femur can fit within it, and still provide enough bone for a long distal fixation strut as well.

If there is complete loss of the proximal femur, an ipsilateral femur that is large enough to provide a butt joint and a distal fixation strut should be used. The stem of the uncemented component should extend at least 6cm. within the recipient femur for fixation. In most situations, this can be accomplished by means of a standard length component; but if the proximal allograft segment should extend below a conventional stem, this is the one instance where we might consider a longer uncemented stem. A tension band DCP plate (Synthes, Ltd, Wayne, PA) is an alternative to a longer stem.

Cement used within the proximal and distal fragment is undesirable and can cause distraction and nonunion. Autogenous strips should be routinely used.

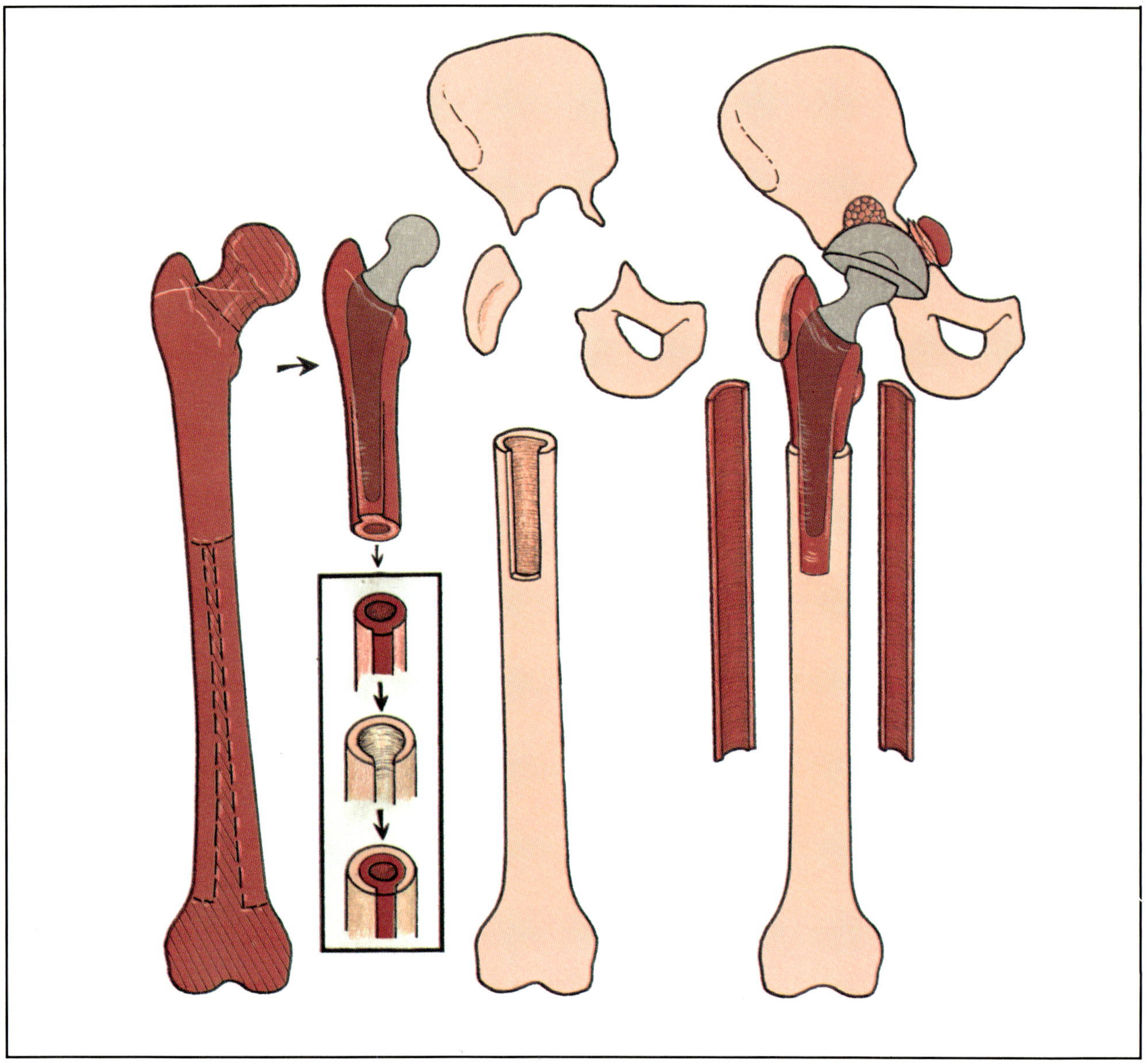

Figure 6-24B. The proximal 12cm. of the femur was absent and there was a large anterior defect on the remaining femur. An uncemented femoral component was used with a smaller allograft proximal femur which in turn was placed within the very large medullary canal of the patient's femur. A ridge of bone was left anteriorly in the allograft proximal femur. This filled the anterior defect and provided rotational stability. Two additional allograft cortical struts reinforced the junction of the allograft and the patient's femur. The medial acetabular defect was reconstructed by means of an allograft disc and autogenous strips from the iliac crest. The superior intra-acetabular defect was grafted with a mixture of morsellized autologous and allograft bone. An uncemented acetabular component was used.

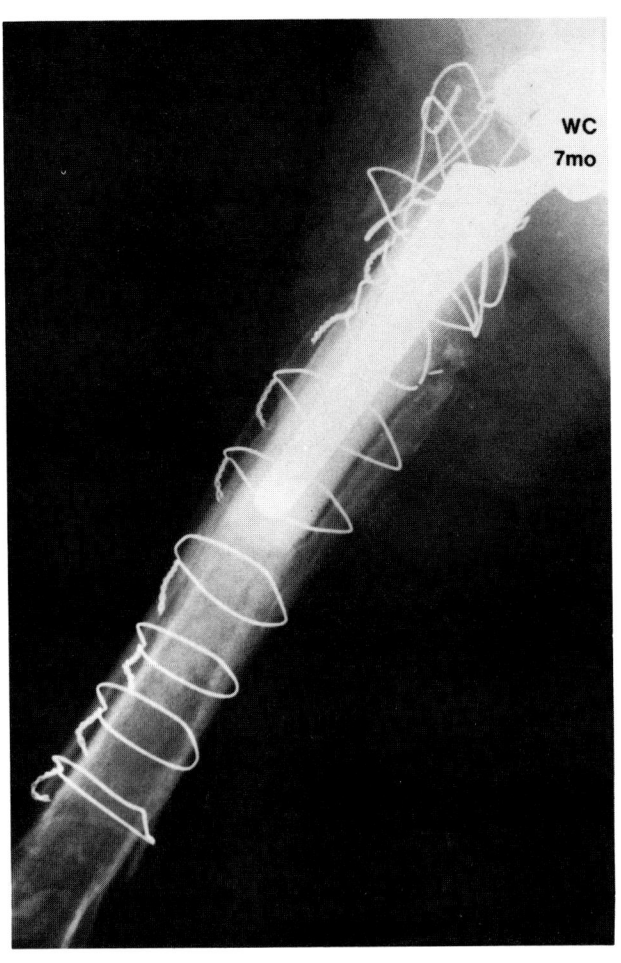

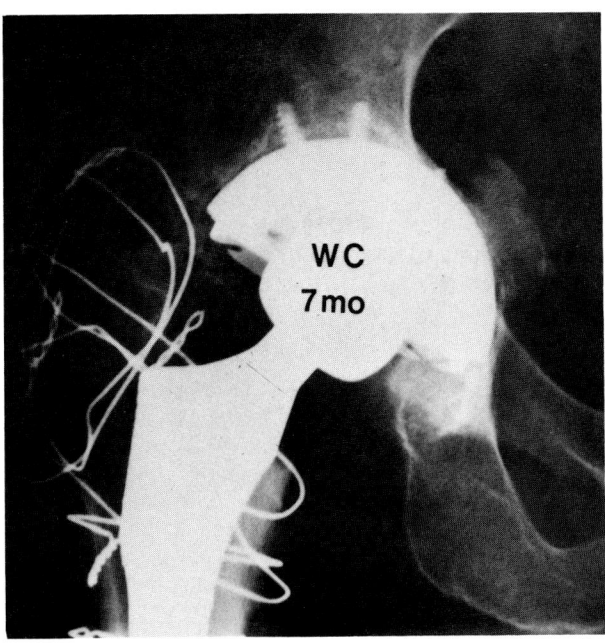

Figure 6-24C. The reconstruction appears to be doing well at seven months. The patient uses a cane only for long walks outside, has minimal discomfort and rates 87.

References

1. Turner, R.H., Emerson, R.H.: Femoral revision total hip arthroplasty, p. 97, in Turner, R.H., Scheller, A.O. (eds.): Revision total hip arthroplasty, Grune and Stratton, NY, 1982.
2. Johnson, R.C., Crowninshield, R.D.: Roentgenologic results of total hip arthroplasty. A ten year follow-up study. Clin Orthop 181:92-98, Dec. 1983.
3. Harris, W.H., Allen, J.R.: The calcar replacement femoral component for total hip arthroplasty. Clin Orthop 157:215-224, June 1981.
4. Calandruccio, R.A.: Arthroplasty, in Edmonson, A.S., Crenshaw, A.H. (eds.): Campbell's Operative Orthopaedics, 6th edition, The C.V. Mosley Co., p. 2274, 1980.
5. Bargar, W.L., Paul, H.A., Merritt, K., et al.: The calcar bone graft. Clin Orthop 202:269-277, 1986.
6. Chandler, H.P., Penenberg, B.L.: Autografts and allografts in total hip replacement. Sci. exhibit, AAOS, 1984.
7. Pauwels, F.: Funktionelle anpassung des knochens durch Langenwachstum. Verh Dtsch Orthop Ges 45:400-427, 1965.
8. Calandruccio, R.A., McConnell, J.C.: The use of a circumferential femoral head graft to compensate for deficiency of the proximal femur in patients requiring total hip arthroplasty. AAOS exhibit, 1982.
9. Krengel, W.G., Turner, R.H.: Trochanteric revision, in Turner, R.H., Scheller, A.O. (eds.): Revision Total Hip Arthroplasty, Grune and Stratton, NY. p.269, 1982.
10. Scott, R.D., Turner, R.H.: Avoiding complications with long stem total hip replacement arthroplasty. J Bone Joint Surg 57A:722, 1975.
11. Turner, R.H.: Revision arthroplasty in the U.S.A., in Caldwell, A.O., Elson, R.A. (ed.): Proceedings of the international Revision Arthroplasty Symposium. Oxford Eng. Med. Educ. Services, p. 85-88, Mar. 1979.
12. Bartel, D.: Theoretical Modeling: Stress analysis effect of geometry proceedings of the workshop mechanical failure of total joint replacement. AAOS, document 916-78, p. 141, June 1978.
13. Haiskes, R.: Some fundamental aspects of human joint replacement: Analysis of stresses and heat conduction in bone prosthesis structures. Acta Orthop Scand Suppl 185, 1980.
14. Scott, R.D., Turner, R.H., Leitzes, S.N., et al.: Femoral fractures in conjunction with total hip replace-

ment. J Bone Joint Surg 57A:494-501, 1975.

15. Taleb, Y.A., States, J.D., Evarts, C.N.: Femoral shaft perforations. Clin Orthop 141:158-165, 1979.

16. Scott, R.D., Turner, R.H., Leitzes, S.N., et al.: Femoral fractures in conjunction with a total hip replacement, J Bone Joint Surg 57A:494-501, 1975.

17. McElfresh, E.C., Coventry, M.B.: Femoral and pelvic fractures after a total hip arthroplasty. J Bone Joint Surg 56A:483-492, 1974.

18. Johansson, J.E., McBroom, R., Barrington, T.W., et al.: Fracture of the ipsilateral femur in patients with total hip replacement. J Bone Joint Surg 63A:1435-1442, 1981.

19. Scott, R.D., Schilz, J.P.: Femoral Fracture and Revision Arthroplasty. in Turner, R.H., Scheller, A.D. (ed.): Revision total hip arthrccl.asty, Grune and Stratton, NY, 1982, p. 141.

20. Sim, F.H. Chao, E.Y.S.: Hip salvage by proximal femoral replacement. J Bone Joint surg 63A:1228-1239, Oct. 1981.

21. Scheller, A.D., D'Erreico, J.: Hip biomechanics and prosthetic design and selection. p. 67 in Turner, R.H.,

Scheller, A.D. (eds.): Revision Total Hip Arthroplasty, Grune and Stratton, NY, 1982.

22. Mankin, H.J., Gebhardt, M.C., Tomford, W.W.: The use of frozen cadaveric allografts in the management of patients with bone tumors of the extremities. Ortho Clin No Am 18:275-289, 1987.

23. McGann, W. Mankin, H.J., Harris, W.H.: Massive allografting for severe failed total hip replacement. J Bone Srug 68A: 1-12, Jan. 1986.

24. Makley, J.T.: The use of allografts to reconstruct intercalary defects of long bones. Clin Orthop 197:58-75, 1985.

25. Mnaymneh, W. Malinin, T. Head, W.C. et al.: Massive osteo-articular allografts in non-tumorous conditions. Sci. exhibit, AAOS, 1986.

26. Gross, A.E., Lavoie, M.V., McDermott, P. et al.: The use of allograft bone in revision of total hip arthroplasty. 197:115-122, 1985.

27. Head, W.C., Malinin, T.I., Berlacich, F.: Freeze-dried proximal femur allografts in revision total hip arthroplasty. Clin Orthop 215:109-120, 1987.

SEVEN

Hugh P. Chandler, M.D.
Brad L. Penenberg, M.D.

Postoperative Management

When making the decision as to how vigorously to institute an exercise program and especially how rapidly to progress to weightbearing after major reconstructions involving bone grafting procedures, the surgeon must consider two factors. The first concerns the biomechanical aspects of bone autografts and allografts. The second involves the strength of the fixation methods used to secure the grafts to the recipient bone.

Biomechanical Aspects

Dead bone initially is as strong as living bone but preservation methods can affect its biomechanical properties. Freezing to $-80°C$ does not significantly affect the mechanical properties of bone as far as compression, torsion or bending is concerned. Freeze drying does not affect compression strength but torsional strength is decreased by 39% and bending strength is diminished by 55% to 90%.[1] In our series, all allografts have been frozen to $-80°C$.

"Creeping substitution" also changes the mechanical properties of bone. Cancellous and cortical bone differ in their strengths as they are replaced by creeping substitution. With autogenous cancellous bone, apposition of new bone occurs before old trabeculae are resorbed so that the graft may actually become stronger as substitution occurs.[2] Since bone is two times as stronger in compression than it is in tension, cancellous grafts that are subjected to compression forces (as with acetabular reconstruction) are capable of accepting early weightbearing.[3,4] Autogenous cortical bone is initially very strong but as it becomes revascularized, resorption of necrotic trabeculae take place before apposition and the graft becomes weaker.[5,6] It has been estimated that autogenous cortical grafts are weakest at 12 to 24 weeks and do not reach their original strength for at least two years.[2] Since cortical grafts are commonly used on the lateral femur, and in this application are subjected to tension forces, they should be protected longer by external support or ideally by other load bearing structures— the recipient femur, the stem of a femoral prosthesis, or metal plates used to provide tension reinforcement. Allograft cancellous and cortical grafts respond in a similar fashion but the process is slower and complete substitution with living bone may never occur.[7]

Methods of Fixation of Bone Grafts

Acetabular grafts subjected to weight-bearing forces must be buttressed against areas of recipient bone strong enough to support these forces. Fixation devices are used to hold the graft against the buttress and in themselves should not be subjected to weight-bearing forces. Cancellous bone screws must be oriented in the weight-bearing axis, should be roughly parallel, and should have lag screw fixation only in the recipient bone so the graft is not prevented from maximal impaction against the buttress. Transverse screws or bolts can hold the graft distracted and prevent the graft from incorporating to the host bone or can break if impaction occurs. Such transverse devices can also prevent the graft from remodeling, even if union occurs.

Femoral grafts subjected to compression forces (total calcar replacement, intramedullary calcar replacements, and medial cortical struts) must also be allowed to impact to a position of stability. Transverse screws are not necessary and are undesirable. Number 16 cerclage wires are more than adequate to hold cortical allograft struts in place, even on the tension (lateral) side of the femur. Cerclage wires used for this purpose are subjected only to hoop stresses and do not have the flexion and extension stresses present with trochanteric reattachment.[8] Despite the frequency of wire breakage with trochanteric reattachment, we have never seen breakage of a cerclage wire used to hold cortical grafts to the femur.

Cement also can prevent optimal impaction of the graft to the host bone. We now feel that cement is almost never necessary in conjunction with acetabular prostheses. Although we prefer to use uncemented femoral components, there may be a place for cement fixation of a femoral stem within an allograft that replaces the proximal femur. However, if the stem extends into the medullary canal of the recipient femur, cement should not be used in the distal fragment as well because it can prevent impaction of the graft to the host and can cause nonunion (Figures 7-1A and 7-1B).

Early weightbearing has been shown to be beneficial in fracture healing, in part because of impaction forces and perhaps because of the effect of electrical potentials.[9] As with fractures, we feel that weightbearing is beneficial in the union of a bone graft to the host and to later remodeling of the graft. Some years ago we placed a femoral head allograft within the acetabulum at the time of resection arthroplasty in the hope that it would incorporate and could

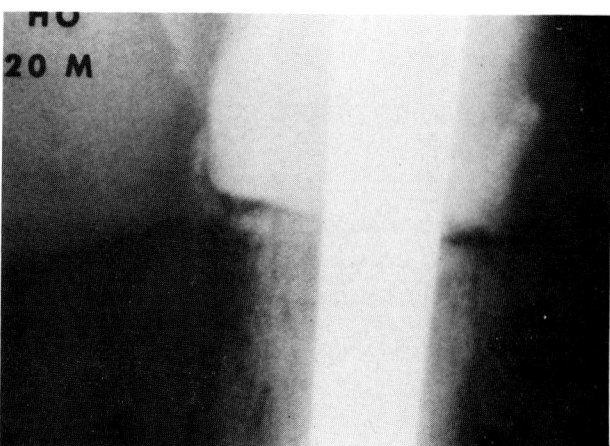

Figure 7-1B. At one and a half years there is a nonunion, presumably because the allograft and the recipient femur are kept distracted by the prosthesis and cement.

be used at a later date for acetabular reconstruction (Figure 7-2A). The graft almost completely resorbed and the screws migrated (Figures 7-2B and 7-2C). We have seen this occur in several other patients who have been referred to us. We are convinced that grafts must be subjected to at least some weightbearing forces if they are to incorporate.

Review of Literature

There is great variation in the postoperative programs advocated by different authors. Turner recommended three weeks of bed rest in balanced suspension for all patients who have had revision surgeries.[10] Harris and Crothers reported that the average time in bed for their patients after autograft reconstruction of acetabular defects was four weeks.[11] Engh recommended a fiberglass spica for four weeks.[12]

The recommended time on crutches has also varied. Heywood protected his patients for eight weeks.[13] Engh, Gordon and McCollum advocated 12 weeks, Mendes recommended 12 to 16 weeks, Coventry six months and Harris one year.[11,12,14-17] Harris has recommended the permanent use of a cane in all patients with autograft or allograft reconstructions.[18]

Authors' Preferred Treatment

Because we make every effort to assure that every graft subjected to compression forces is mechanically stable and is buttressed against solid bone and that every graft subjected to bending stresses is protected by either a femoral stem, the patient's femur or a tension band plate, we are guided only by the soft tissues and by the prosthetic bone interface in making decisions concerning exercise or ambulation. Since these operations are lengthy with extensive soft tissue dissections, patients are kept in balanced suspension for a few days longer than with primary hips. The average time in suspension in our series was five days

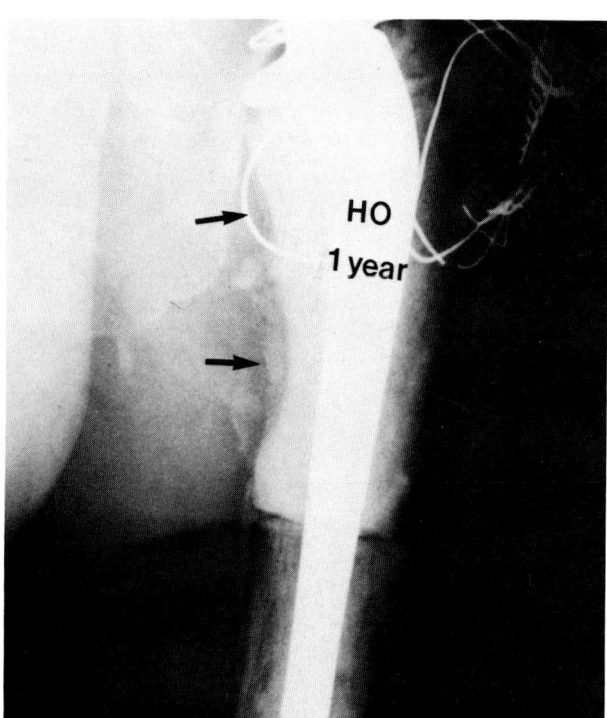

Figure 7-1A. A long stem femoral prosthesis cemented at both sides of the junction between an allograft and the recipient femur can prevent the graft from impacting. The etiology of the proximal medial scalloping is not clear.

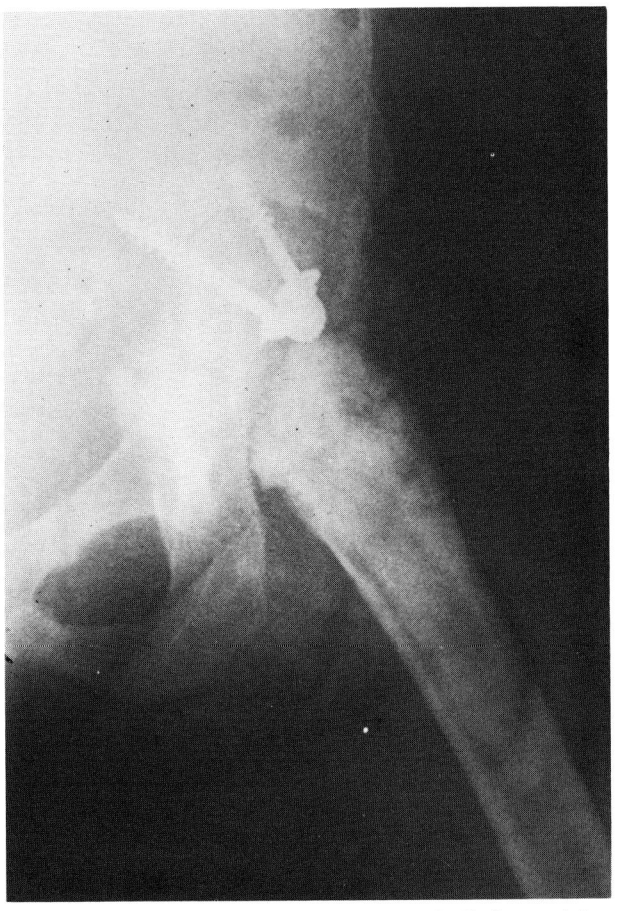

Figure 7-2A. A femoral head allograft was inserted in the acetabulum at the time of resection arthroplasty because of aseptic loosening in a 250 lb. female.

muscle strength and prosthesis fixation and is not affected by the fact that the patient has a graft.

Patients who have lateral femoral grafts loaded in tension theoretically should be protected longer; however, this type of graft may not be at maximum strength for two to five years. It seems unreasonable to protect these hips for this length of time. We therefore have tried to supplement the graft with either an intramedullary prosthesis, a metal tension band plate or by the patient's femur, if it is strong enough, and have allowed full weightbearing at six to eight weeks as with grafts that bear compression loads.

Therefore, at eight weeks all patients are encouraged to

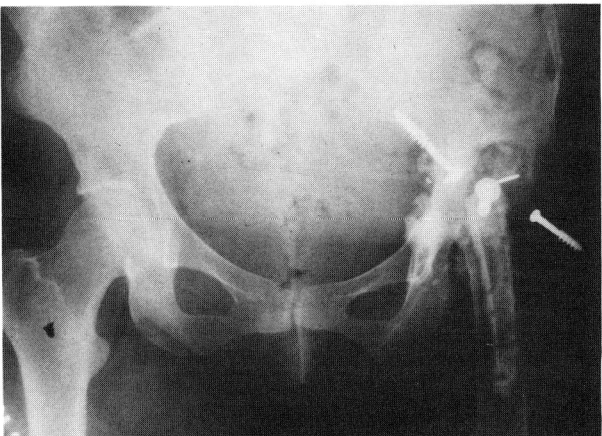

Figure 7-2B. Four years later, the graft has resorbed and the screws have migrated.

(range two to eight days). In past years we were more cautious and kept patients in bed longer, but now most patients are walking at two days. An ace bandage spica is applied in the operating room and is left in place for two to four days. Hemovac drains are used deep and superficial to the fascia lata for 24 hours and then are removed without disturbing the ace bandage spica. Partial weightbearing using a walker is begun on the first day the suspension is removed and the majority of our patients progress to two axillary crutches within a few days. They are encouraged to put 50 to 60 pounds of weight on the involved extremity and to walk with a normal heel-toe gait. Most patients are taught a fairly extensive exercise program including the use of a stationary bicycle. The average hospital stay in our series was 14 days (range four to 27 days). Patients are encouraged to use crutches for six to eight weeks and then are evaluated clinically and by radiographs.

At six to eight weeks, if the patient has a graft that is loaded in compression (all acetabular grafts and femoral grafts involving total calcar, calcar intramedullary grafts or medial femoral cortical struts) or a graft that is not subject to weight-bearing stresses (small intra-acetabular, all central acetabular defects and femoral trochanteric augmentation) full weightbearing is encouraged and is limited only by

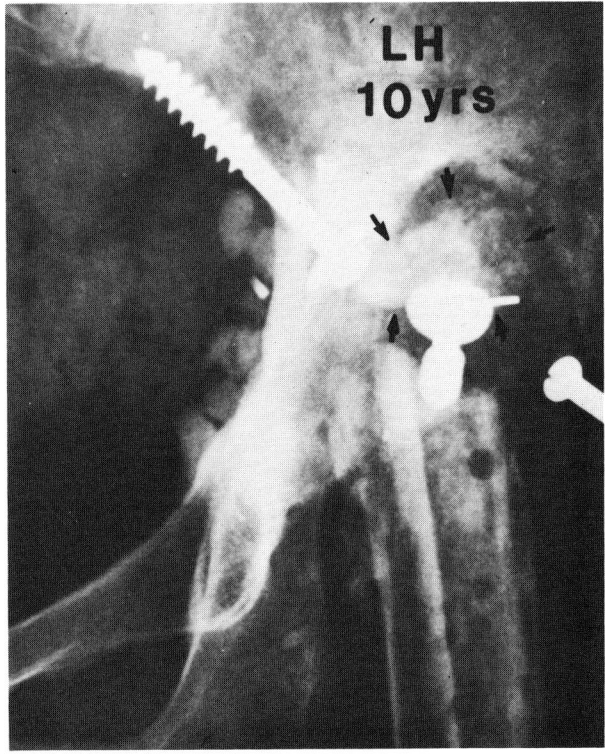

Figure 7-2C. At ten years, the graft has not united and has been almost completely resorbed.

use whatever support is necessary to avoid pain or limp. In our series, for the patients that were able to give up support completely, the average time to discard the cane was slightly over four months from the time of surgery (range six weeks to 48 months).

References

1. Pelker, R.R., Friedlander, G.E.: Biomechanical aspects of bone autografts and allografts. Orth Clin No Am 18(4):235-239, 1987.
2. Springfield, D.S.: Massive autogenous bone grafts. Orth Clin No Am 18(4):249-256, 1987.
3. Evans, F.G.: Mechanical Properties of Bone. Springfield, IL, Charles C. Thomas, 1973.
4. Bright, R., Burstein, A.: Material properties of preserved cortical bone. Trans Orthop Res Soc 3:210, 1968.
5. Burchardt, H.: The biology of bone graft repair. Clin Orthop 174:28-42, 1983.
6. Burchardt, H., Busbee, G.A. III, Enneking, W.F.: Repair of experimental autologous grafts of cortical bone. J Bone Joint Surg 57A:814-819, 1975.
7. Burchardt, H.: Biology of bone transplantation. Orth Clin No Am 18(4):187-196, 1987.
8. Turner, R.H., Scheller, A.D.: Revision Total Hip Arthroplasty, Grune and Stratton, Inc., NY, 1982.
9. Basset, C.A.L., Becker, R.O.: Generation of electrical potentials by bone in response to mechanical stress, Science, 137:1063, 1962.
10. Turner, R.H., Scheller, A.D.: Revision Total Hip Arthroplasty, Grune and Stratton, Inc., NY, 1982.
11. Harris, W.H., Crothers, O., Oh, I.: Total hip replacement and femoral head bone grafting in severe acetabular deficiency in adults. J Bone Joint Surg 59A:752, 1977.
12. Engh, C., Bobyn, J.: Biological Fixation in Total Hip Arthroplasty. Slack, Thorofare, NJ, 1985.
13. Heywood, A.W.B.: Arthroplasty with a solid bone graft for protrusio acetabuli. J Bone Joint Surg 62B:332-339, 1980.
14. Gordon, S.G., et al.: Assessment of bone grafts used for acetabular augmentation in total hip arthroplasty; A study using roentgenograms and bone scintigraphy. Clin Orthop 201(12):18-25, 1985.
15. McCollum, D.E., Nunley, J.A., Harrelson, J.M.: Bone grafting in total hip replacement for acetabular protrusio. J Bone Joint Surg 62A(10):1065-1073, 1980.
16. Mendes, D.G., Roffman, M., Silbermann, M.: Reconstruction of the acetabular wall with bone graft in arthroplasty of the hip. Clin Orthop 186:29, 1984.
17. Coventry, M.B.: Hip arthroplasty in older patients with hip dysplasia. In Evarts, C.M. (ed.): Surgery of the Musculoskeletal System, vol. 3, Churchill Livingstone, NY, 1983.
18. Jasty, M., Harris, W.H.: Total hip reconstruction using frozen femoral head allografts in patients with acetabular bone loss. Orth Clin No Am 18(4):291, 1987.

Charles P. Capito, M.D.
Hillel D. Skoff, M.D.
Steven A. Bohmer, M.D.

Hugh P. Chandler, M.D.
Brad L. Penenberg, M.D.

Results and Complications

Our series now consists of 119 grafts in 92 hips (83 patients) that were followed for an average of 42 months (range six months to 15 years). There were 19 primary and 73 revision total hip replacements. Forty-nine had only acetabular grafting, 16 had isolated femoral grafts and 27 required both femoral and acetabular grafts.

This unique group of patients presented with formidable problems that were considerably more complex than those seen with most primary or revision total hip replacement arthroplasty. Only 17 patients had no previous hip surgery and of the remaining patients, there had been an average of two prior ipsilateral hip procedures, including total hip arthroplasty (range one to 16 prior procedures). These operations were major and lengthy, averaging 7.2 hours. Blood loss was also greater than that seen with routine total hip replacement and averaged 6.75 units.

After discharge, all patients were seen in follow up by the senior author and were assessed according to the Harris hip scale. Postoperative visits were scheduled at six to eight weeks, at six months and then at yearly intervals.

The radiographs of cemented components were analyzed according to the criteria of Stauffer with special attention to component migration and to progressive lucency of greater than 2mm.[1] The radiographs of non-cemented components were examined using the methods described by Tullos et al., but with special emphasis on evidence of component migration.[2] The bone grafts themselves were evaluated for evidence of union, remodeling, resorption, migration, or fracture.

Results

Using the Harris hip rating system, we considered ratings of 90-100 as excellent, 80-89 good, 70-79 fair and below 70 as failures.[3] We compared our results with and without the use of cement and found no statistical difference (Tables 8-1 and 8-2). The average Harris rating for the series was improved from a mean of 44 preoperatively to 88 postoperatively. At follow up, there were 46 hips (50%) that rated excellent, 23 good (25%), 13 fair (14%) and there were ten failures (11%).

Primary Hips

There were 19 primary hip replacements. The average preoperative rating was 44 and the postoperative rating was 91 with a mean follow-up time of six years (range three to 12 years). There were 80% good or excellent results and there were no failures or impending failures. These results compare favorably with published reports of 66% to 88% good or excellent results in primary total hip replacement without grafts.[4-7] They are better than the 24% failure and depending failure reported by Christie et al. in primary dysplastic

Table 8-1
Hips With Cemented Components

	# Hips	Average Harris Rating		Follow-Up (mos.)	
		Pre-op	Post-op	Average	Range
ACETABULUM					
Autografts	23*	44	91	73	36-184
Allografts	23*	48	87	54	15-106
FEMUR					
Autografts	2*	44	91	39	37-41
Allografts	12*	43	80	54	27-77
*Includes hips with both acetabular and femoral grafts.					

Table 8-2
Hips With Uncemented Components

	# Hips	Average Harris Rating		Follow-Up (mos.)	
		Pre-op	Post-op	Average	Range
ACETABULUM					
Autografts	3	46	94	27	18-34
Allografts	26*	40	86	12	6-34
FEMUR					
Autografts	none	—	—	—	—
Allografts	29*	44	85	12	6-34
*Includes hips with both acetabular and femoral grafts.					

hips treated with femoral head grafts.[8] They are also better than the average postoperative rating of 74 that was reported by Harris et al. in primary dysplastic hips treated with autografts in which the rate of failure was 20% with minimum five years follow-up.[9]

Revision Hips

The other 73 hips in the series were revisions. The average preoperative rating was 44 and the postoperative rating was 87. There were 34 hips that rated excellent, 18 good, 11 fair and there were ten failures. Of the eleven patients in the fair category, four had unrelated factors that adversely affected their ratings. One of these patients had severe Parkinson's disease, another had extrapyramidal athetoid movements, a third used a walker because of poor balance and a fear of falling, and the last used two crutches because of weakness secondary to polio. Of the ten patients with failed hips, four had resection arthroplasties for sepsis and six had aseptic loosening. Nine have been revised or are scheduled for revision and one patient refuses further surgery.

These revision results (72% good or excellent and 14% failures) compare favorably with other published series

concerning revision total hip surgery without the use of grafts that report less than 65% good or excellent results and failure rates of nine to 29%.[10-12] They are also comparable to other series of revision hip replacements using autografting and allografting techniques which have reported mean Harris scores of 89 to 91 and failure rates of 0 to 25%.[13-21]

Complications

These operations were major procedures and the incidence of complications was significant. These included intra-operative complications, postoperative complications, complications related to the graft and complications relating to loosening or migration of the component. It should be noted that any individual patient could appear as a statistic in several different categories.

Intra-operative Complications

Fractures.. There were six fractures of the femoral shaft (6.6%) that occurred during cement removal or during reconstruction of the femur. This figure is slightly greater than the 3% to 4% reported in the literature.[22,23] In the

early part of our series, five of these fractures were treated with long stem cemented prostheses. The last (Figure 6-19) was stabilized by means of onlay cortical grafts and a short stem uncemented prosthesis. One patient had a probable stress fracture of his femur distal to allograft struts (Figure 6-23I). The patient used crutches for six weeks and subsequently was pain free without support.

Perforation of the Femoral Shaft. There were four known perforations of the femur (4.4%), which inadvertently occurred while removing cement. This incidence is comparable to reports in the literature of 0.4 to 4.4%.[24,25] Because of our confidence with femoral onlay grafts to reinforce cortical defects, we now have a low threshold for windowing the femur anteriorly to remove distal cement and have abandoned the technique of using high-speed burrs under image intensifier control. The window is replaced, grafted with autogenous bone and then reinforced by a cortical onlay graft and no attempt is made to bypass the window with a longer stem.

Neurological Problems. There were three nerve injuries (3.3%). All were in revision cases. One patient had a laceration of the femoral nerve at the time of acetabular exposure. It was not possible to repair this and the patient has a permanent quadriceps paralysis. Two other patients were noted to have complete peroneal palsies the morning after surgery. These probably occurred because of local pressure on the peroneal nerve at the neck of the fibula. One patient recovered completely and the other had a partial recovery.

Neurologic injuries, particularly to the peroneal division of the sciatic nerve have been reported by other authors to occur at a frequency of up to 7% during revision surgery.[26-30]

Vascular Problems. One patient (the same who had the femoral nerve laceration) had a laceration of the femoral artery and vein (1.1%) during exposure for an acetabular defect. The acetabular reconstruction was terminated, the vein was tied off and the artery was repaired. The patient had no residual vascular sequellae and has subsequently had a successful graft to the acetabulum (Figure 5-37). This patient had undergone four previous procedures through an anterior (Smith-Petersen) approach and the iliopsoas had been destroyed. The artery was encountered over the anterolateral aspect of the acetabulum. Since then we have had one other patient with a laterally positioned neurovascular bundle after multiple previous anterior approaches and are now particularly cautious with patients who have had previous anterior approaches. Vascular injuries during revision surgery are rare but have been reported.[31-33]

Excessive Blood Loss. Two patients (2.2%) had excessive blood loss that eventually required greater than 20 units of blood replacement. One of these was secondary to injury to the branches of the obturator artery from intrapelvic dissection. The other was most likely related to a coagulopathy. Both responded to compression dressings,

platelet transfusions and fresh frozen plasma. The use of arteriograms and arterial embolus to control excessive bleeding after total hip replacement has been described, but we have no experience with this technique.[34,35]

Postoperative Complications

Dislocations. A total of ten patients had component dislocations (10.8%). Two were anterior and the rest were posterior. All were in revision cases. One required open reduction and the rest were reduced by closed means. Two dislocations resulted from malposition of the acetabular component, two from weak musculature (one trochanteric avulsion and another with paralysis of the hip muscles), one because of impingement of heterotopic bone, one patient because of severe Parkinson's disease, and one patient because of major trauma. The other patients with well positioned components, dislocated in their early postoperative period because of inadvertent positioning of their extremities in adduction, flexion and internal rotation. Three patients were temporarily treated by abduction braces, one patient had excision of impinging heterotopic bone and the patient with Parkinson's disease has been stable after anterior obturator neurectomy and adductor tenotomy. No hips have required revision of the components because of recurrent dislocation.

Although dislocation was the most frequent postoperative complication in this series, the incidence was not excessive when compared to reports in the literature of dislocation rates ranging from 1.8% in primary hips to 27.3% with revision surgery.[36-39]

Infections. There were no superficial infections. There were two acute deep infections (2.2%). One patient with *Staphylococcus aureus* infection had five previous operations following traumatic dislocation. These included an open reduction, an attempt at surgical arthrodesis, a total hip replacement, and two revisions. However, he had no previous infection prior to the insertion of an allograft femoral head to reconstruct the lateral acetabular rim. This patient responded to resection arthroplasty, removal of the graft, extensive debridement, and six weeks of intravenous antibiotics. He has subsequently undergone a second allograft reconstruction of his acetabulum and femur without difficulty and remains infection free at two years, nine months (Figures 5-49 and 6-18). *Pseudomonas* was the infecting organism in the second patient with an acute deep infection. He had undergone ten previous hip operations. The initial procedure was an open reduction of a fracture dislocation which was complicated by a *Pseudomonas* infection. He then underwent seven debridements and finally a successful hip fusion before his first total hip replacement. He presented to us with a loose acetabular component, four years after his arthroplasty. He was dry at the time of reconstruction of his acetabular rim using an allograft femoral head and intra-operative cultures were negative. However, aspiration three weeks after his surgery proved that he had a *Pseudomonas* infection, the same organism that had been present after his original open reduction many years previously. This patient has refused further surgery and continues to drain copiously. His graft has migrated proximally and shows significant resorption (Figure 8-1). At followup of 11 years, he has minimal pain but requires two crutches for all steps and rates 65.

There were two other late hematogenous infections. One *Escherichia coli* infection occurred two years, four months after a successful revision of a total hip replacement that required an acetabular allograft. This patient rated 90 prior to the acute onset of hip pain associated with fever. Four days prior to presentation with hip pain he had symptoms of a urinary tract infection and subsequent hip aspiration and urine cultures grew the same organism. The second patient had a *Staphylococcus aureus* hematogenous infection four years after successful allograft reconstruction of his femur (Figure 6-6D). Prior to the onset of this infection he rated 96. The source of this infection was never determined. Both patients required resection arthroplasty, extensive debridement and treatment with intravenous antibiotics. At present both are dry and are awaiting revision.

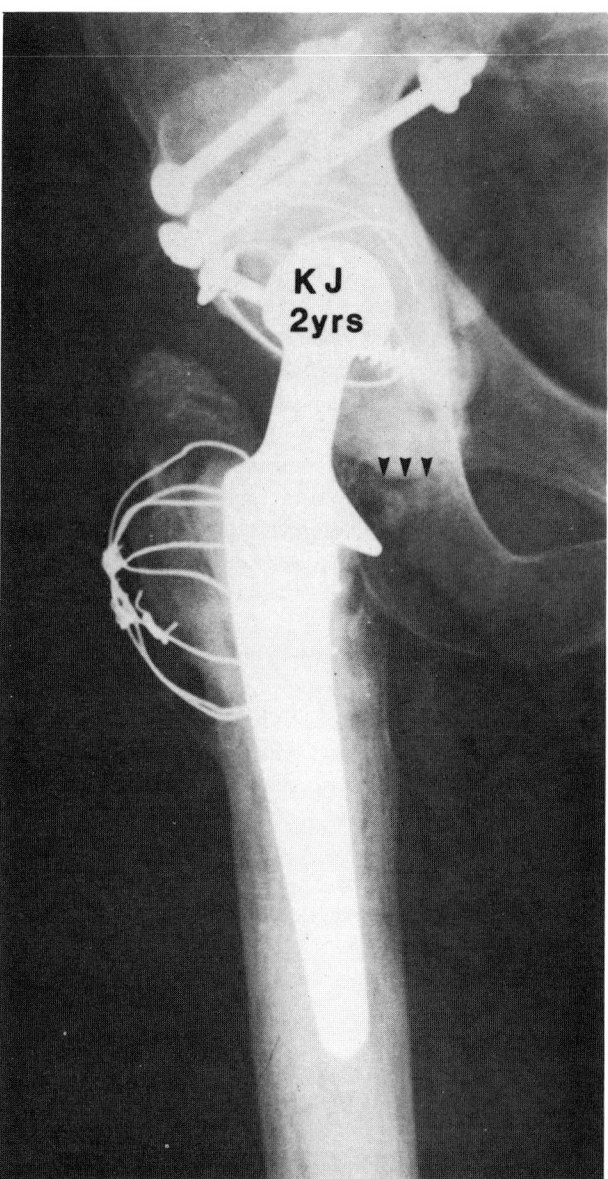

Figure 8-1B. Two years later, the graft has migrated proximally. The patient has copious drainage with persistent growth of *Pseudomonas*.

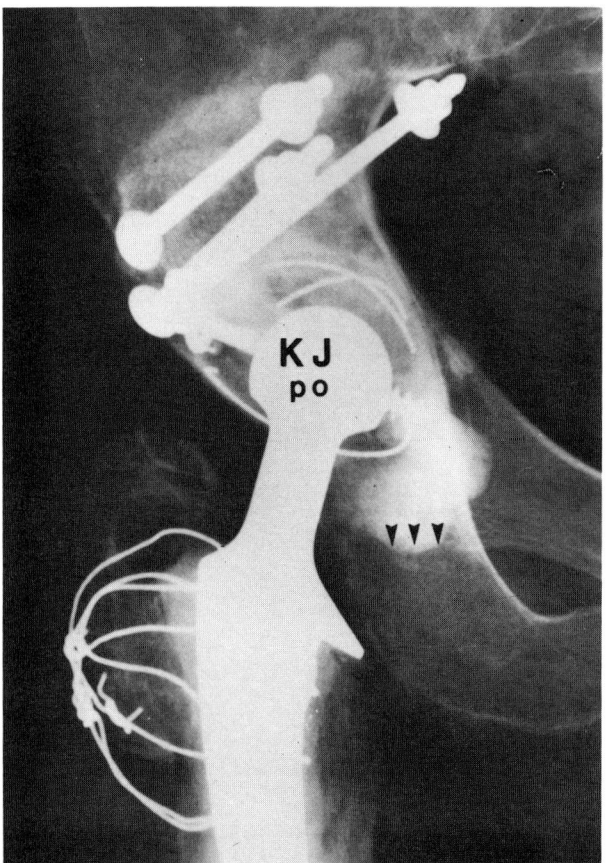

Figure 8-1A. This 55-year-old man had a *Pseudomonas* infection 11 years previously. He had ten subsequent operations but was dry at the time this femoral head allograft was used to reconstruct a superior rim defect. Aspiration three weeks later grew *Pseudomonas* but the patient refused resection arthroplasty.

In our series, there were nine patients (9.9%) who had a previous history of major infection of their hip that had required surgical and antibiotic intervention prior to their bone grafting procedure. All had negative preoperative aspirations and negative intra-operative cultures. Only one of these patients had recurrence of his infection (the patient with *Pseudomonas*, Figure 8-1).

If both acute and late hematogenous infections are combined, the incidence of deep infection in the entire series was 5.5%. There were no infections in the 19 primary hips. This infection rate is not excessively high if compared with that reported for primary hips with grafting (2.1% to 5%), with revision series without grafting (2% to 32%), or with the high rate reported in immunocompromised tumor patients with allograft reconstruction (13.2%).[13,17,40-44] It

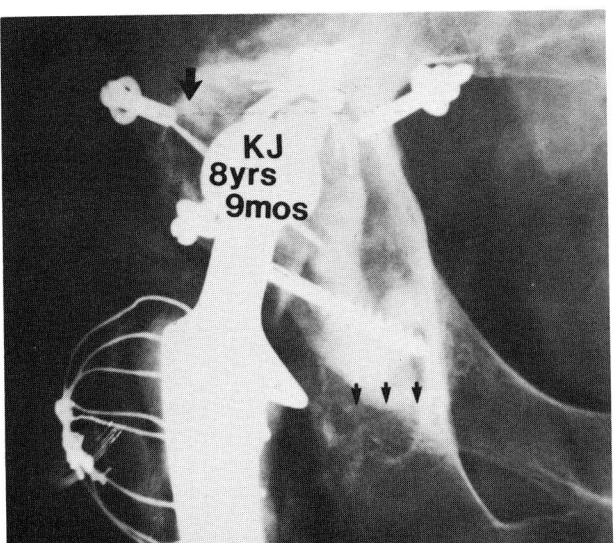

Figure 8-1C. At eight years, nine months, further proximal migration and resorption have occurred and the bolts have fractured.

is of interest that all four infections in our series (two primary and two hematogenous) occurred in patients where cement was used. There were no infections in patients with uncemented allografts or autografts but followup of these is shorter than that of the grafts used with cement.

Heterotopic Ossification. Heterotopic bone that significantly affected motion occurred in four patients (4.4%). One patient had excision of the bone and the others elected to accept somewhat limited motion. This incidence of heterotopic bone compares favorably with that reported in both primary and revision total hip replacement (2% to 53%).[45-47]

We have treated high-risk patients (mesomorphic men, hypertrophic arthritis, ankylosing spondylitis) with indomethacin (75mg per day) if they have not had a previous history of heterotopic ossification.[48] If a patient has previously demonstrated heterotopic bone formation we have used radiation (1000 rads).[49] In recent years, the radiation therapy department at the Massachusetts General Hospital routinely has shielded the acetabular and femoral components with a lead template so that only the area between the femur and the pelvis receives radiation. To our knowledge this has caused no adverse effects on bone ingrowth in the patients with uncemented sintered prostheses.

Trochanteric Avulsion. Trochanteric avulsion that required reattachment occurred in three patients (3.3%). One other patient with trochanteric avulsion did not have further surgery (Figure 5-36E). These figures compare favorably with the 5% to 17.5% reported in the literature for both primary and revision surgery.[50,51]

Thromboembolic Disease. Unless there was a clinical suspicion of phlebitis, venograms were not obtained routinely and therefore it is possible that there were instances of phlebitis that were missed. There were, however, four cases of deep vein thrombosis proven by venogram (4.4%). There were no known pulmonary

emboli. Both male and female patients were treated prophylactically with aspirin (600mg. po twice per day) unless they were considered high risk (a previous history of phlebitis or pulmonary embolus, stasis dermatitis or prominant peripheral veins). Such high-risk patients were treated with low dose Coumadin for prophylaxis. Patients who had postoperative phlebitis proximal to the popliteal vein, proven by venogram, were discharged on Coumadin for six months. Patients without phlebitis, even those with high risk, were sent home on aspirin, which they were encouraged to continue for six weeks.

In the literature, it has been reported that up to 70% of patients without prophylaxis develop deep venous thrombosis.[52-54] With various methods of prophylaxis (aspirin, coumadin, heparin, dextran, pneumatic boots), the incidence of deep vein thrombosis has been reduced to 13% to 30%.[55-57]

Medical Complications

Seven patients had urinary tract infections that responded to appropriate antibiotics. Five patients had transient electrocardiogram changes that returned to their baseline status. There were no known myocardial infarctions. One patient had erosive gastritis with bleeding that required two units of blood replacement and responded to conservative therapy. One patient had acute renal failure. Although she had also had an episode of hypotension during the operation, the etiology was possibly hydronephrosis because she was not catherized and her surgery took longer than anticipated. She recovered normal renal function without dialysis. We now routinely insert a Foley catheter prior to grafting procedures and remove this on the morning after surgery.

Complications Related to the Graft

Nonunion. In our series there was only one patient (1.1%) with a definite nonunion of the graft-host interface. This patient had a recurrent *Pseudomonas* infection (previously described) and the femoral head allograft used for reconstruction of the superior rim migrated proximally (Figure 8-1). Although 100% union rate has been reported by others to occur between three months and one year, we have found it very difficult to tell if or when a graft has united.[9,13,16,17,19,21] Recovery room x-rays frequently show no interface between the graft and the host bone if the fit is accurate (Figures 5-24B, 5-33B, and 8-1A). If there was an obvious space by x-ray, this frequently had disappeared at the time of the six month x-rays (Figures 5-19D, 5-19F, 5-22C and 5-22D). We have not routinely obtained bone scans and agree with Berggren et al. that bone scanning is not reliable in determining union of a graft or in determining its viability.[58]

Migration of the Graft. There were four hips (4.4%) with migration of a graft. All were femoral heads used to reconstruct the rim and/or the superior intra-acetabular area. One was an autograft and three were allografts. One patient has a septic nonunion (Figure 8-1) and the other three grafts have probably united in their final position (Figures 8-2C, 5-34D, and 5-41E). Fixation devices were oriented in a transverse position and fractured in two of these patients when the grafts migrated. We have not found reports in the literature describing migration of a graft.

Resorption of the Graft. Minor resorption occurred at the periphery of acetabular grafts in 14 patients (15.2%). This resorption was associated with medial migration of the washers and did not appear to be ominous or progressive (Figures 5-10C, 5-11B, and 5-45E). It occurred with equal frequency in autografts and allografts. We have interpreted such peripheral resorption as representing remodeling of revascularized bone in areas that were not stressed.

Major resorption of a graft occurred in five of 119 grafts (3.3%). Four of these were acetabular grafts and one was a femoral graft. Of the acetabular grafts, three were allografts (Figures 5-38D, 8-1C, and 8-3C) and one was an autograft (Figure 8-4B). In all four cases, the screws were placed too transversely and may have prevented the grafts from impacting or remodeling. Major resorption occurred in one femoral graft. One patient had complete resorption of an allograft femoral head used to reconstruct the calcar and greater trochanter (Figure 6-7E). This may have occurred because the graft was not stressed. In the literature, an incidence of up to 55% of some degree of graft resorption has been reported with major resorption occurring in 4.3% to 5.9% of cases.[8,15,18,20]

Graft Fracture. Three hips had fractures of the graft (2.5%). All were allografts. One patient had a fracture at the periphery of an acetabular graft because of impaction and proximal migration of the graft. Fixation of the acetabular component did not appear to be compromised (Figure 5-34D). Two patients had fractures of an allograft cortical strut used on the lateral side of the femur. One patient is doing well following the application of a lateral plate and further grafting (Figure 6-17D). The other patient is currently in a cast brace and has minimal pain but will probably

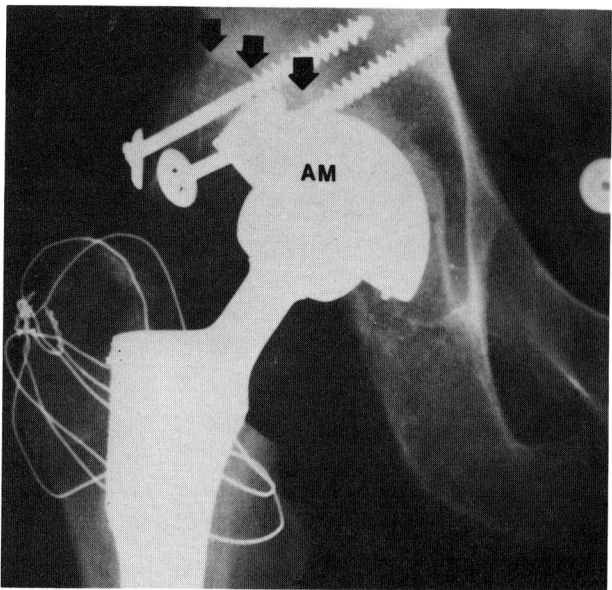

Figure 8-2B. In retrospect it is debatable whether he needed a graft but his femoral head was used to augment the lateral rim. The screws are oriented transversely and are not in the line of weight-bearing.

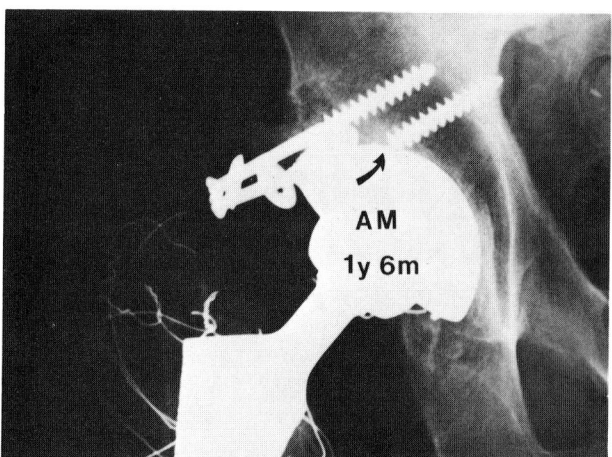

Figure 8-2C. At one year, six months, the graft has migrated proximally and has probably united. One of the screws has fractured.

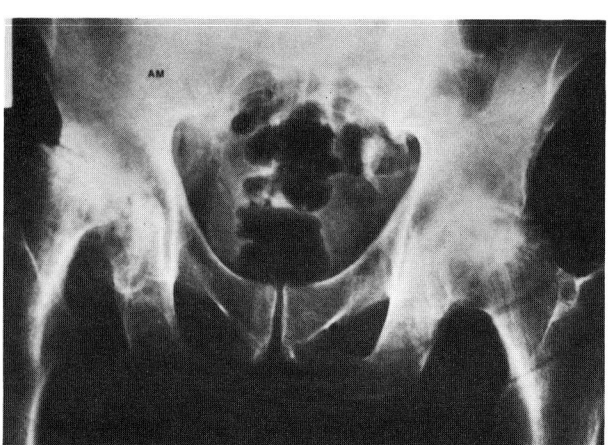

Figure 8-2A. This 67-year-old man has palindromic arthritis.

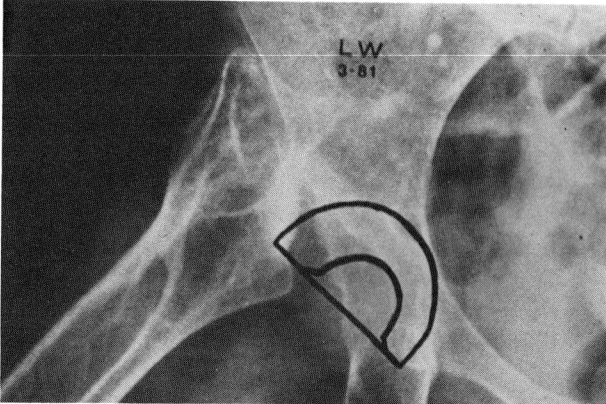

Figure 8-3A. This 62-year-old woman had a resection arthroplasty performed four years previously because of a septic hip. She had a major femoral perforation which was previously discussed (Figure 6-11).

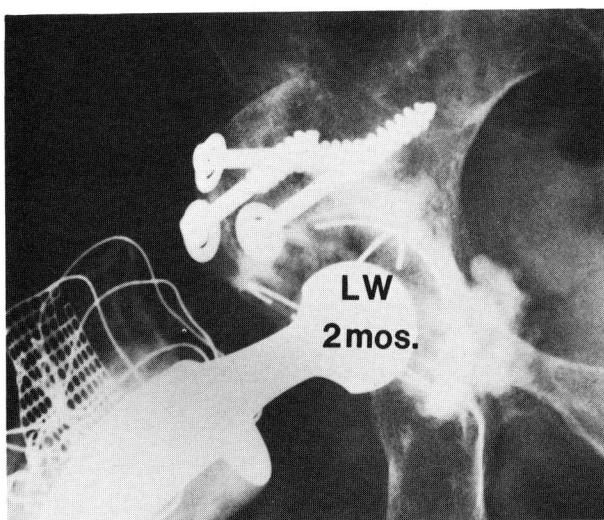

Figure 8-3B. A femoral head allograft was used to reconstruct the superior rim and superior intra-acetabular defect. Intra-operative cultures were negative. At least one of the screws is oriented transversely and could prevent the graft from impacting and/or remodeling.

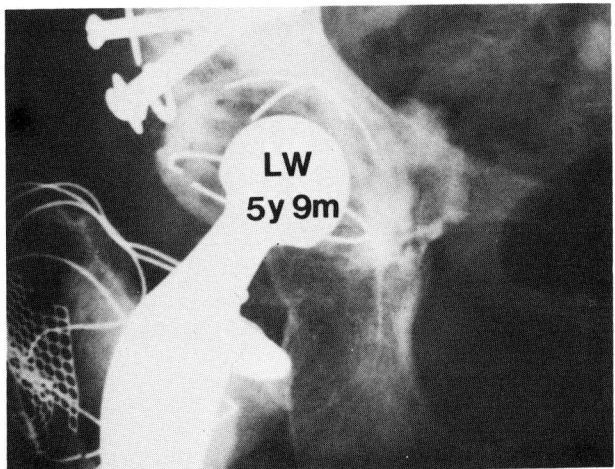

Figure 8-3C. X-rays at five years and nine months show worrisome resorption of the graft. However, at followup of six years, four months, the patient still rates 100.

need further surgery. We have not found reference to graft fracture in the literature.

Complications Related to the Components

Radiolucent Lines. Of the 57 cemented components, radiolucent lines between the cement mantle and the graft occurred in ten (17.5%). All were associated with acetabular grafts. In seven patients, these radiolucent lines were less than 2mm. in width, not continuous and not associated with loosening. In two, the radiolucent line did progress entirely about the component but despite these worrisome x-rays, both patients are asymptomatic (Figures 5-23C, 8-5A, and 8-5B). Radiolucent lines about cemented

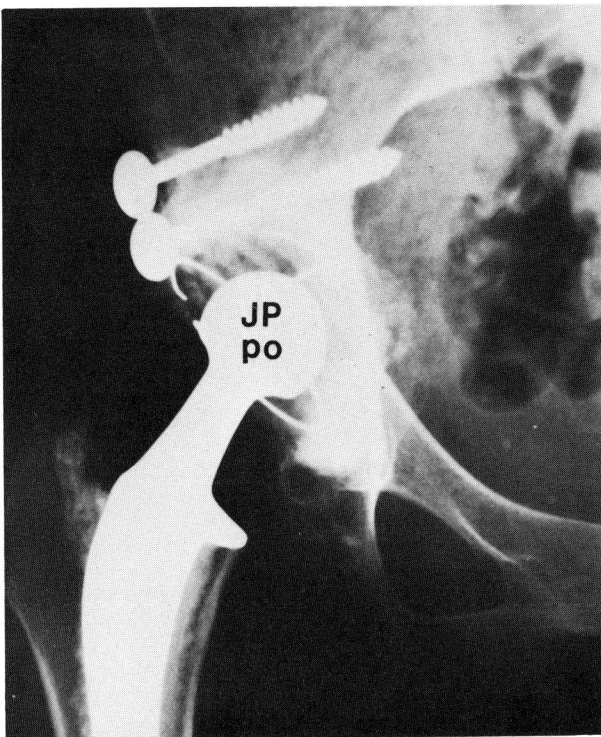

Figure 8-4A. This 31-year-old woman had an autograft femoral head used to reconstruct a deficient superior rim after a failed surface replacement arthroplasty. The head may have had avascular necrosis. The screws are poorly oriented in a transverse portion.

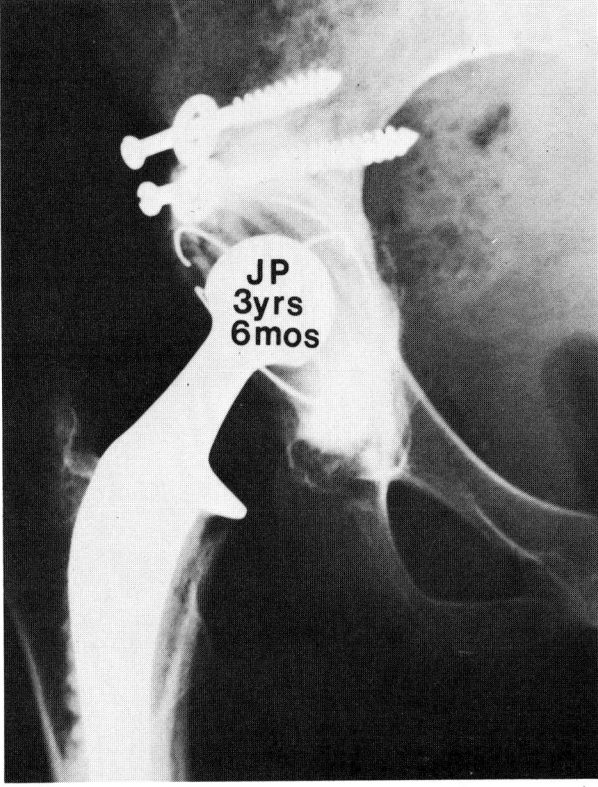

Figure 8-4B. After only three and one half years, there was major resorption of the graft and a radiolucent line has formed entirely about the cement-bone interface.

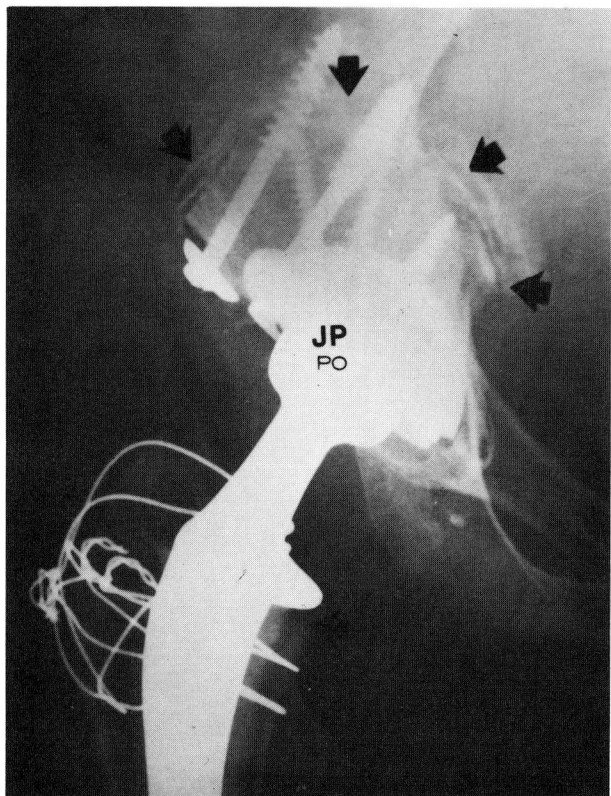

Figure 8-4C. At revision very little of the autograft remained and there was now a significant combined superior rim and superior intra-acetabular defect as well as a central perforation. An allograft femoral head was used to reconstruct the superior rim and superior intra-acetabular defects and the central defect was grafted with autogenous iliac crest strips. The screws are now correctly oriented. Note the resorption of the calcar.

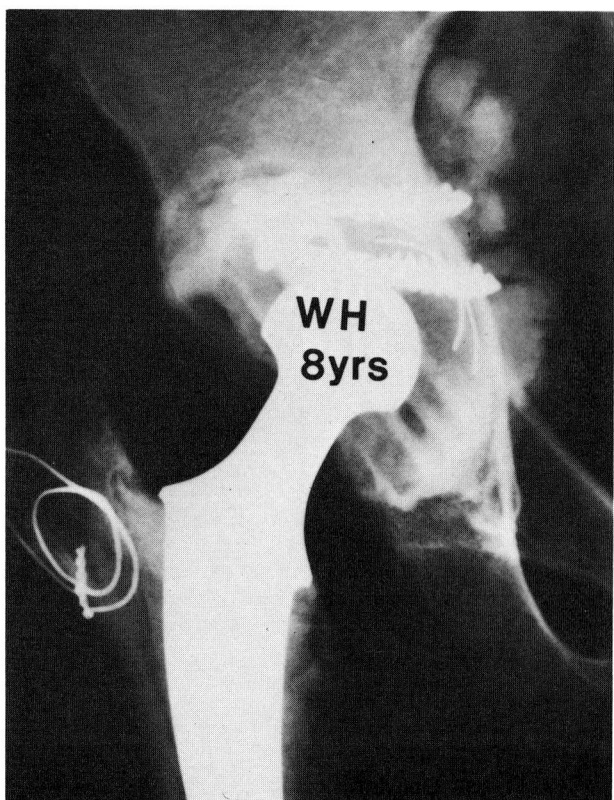

Figure 8-5A. This 39-year-old man presented with a painful mold arthroplasty. A superior rim defect was reconstructed with the femoral head that was within the cup. There may have been avascular necrosis. The screws are poorly oriented in a transverse position. At eight years, there is a worrisome radiolucent line about the acetabular component.

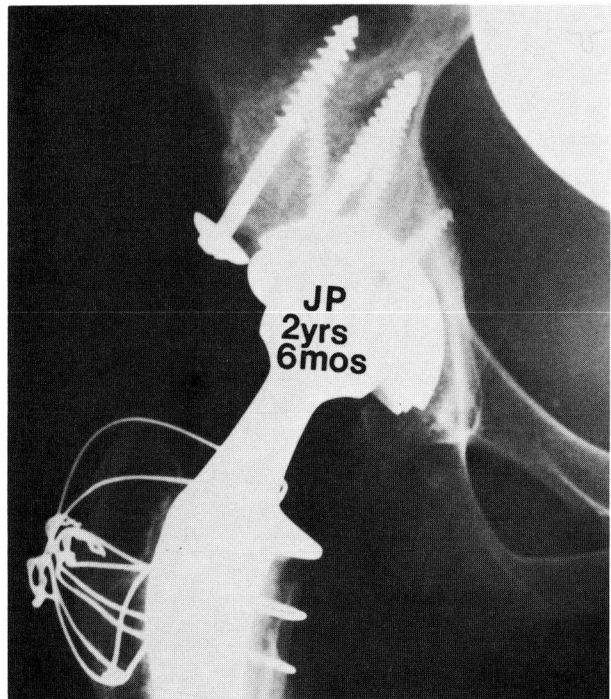

Figure 8-4D. At two and one half years, the allografts appear to have incorporated. The patient rates 90.

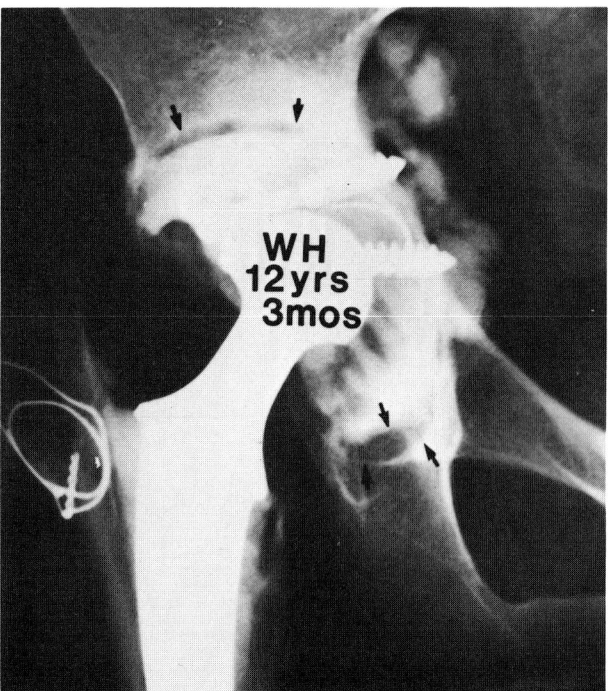

Figure 8-5B. At twelve years, three months, this line has progressed and is now circumferential and more than 2mm. in some areas. Despite this worrisome x-ray, the patient rates 100.

components, not associated with grafts, are common and have been reported as being present in up to 100%.[1,5,59] The relatively low incidence in our series is probably because the membrane formation at the cement-bone interface requires a blood supply from the bone and until the graft is revascularized, this membrane does not occur.

Loosening of a Component. Definite loosening of eight components occurred in seven hips (7.7%), at an average postoperative time of 31 months (range nine to 62 months). Four had migrated by x-ray and four were proven to be loose at revision but had not migrated. There were five loose acetabular components (6.8%) and three loose femoral components (7.2%).

Acetabular loosening occurred in two uncemented and in three cemented components. Four were allografts and one was an autograft. Three of the loose cemented components have been revised to uncemented components (Figures 8-4A, 8-4B, 8-4C, 5-38D, 5-38E, 6-7E, and 6-7F), one is scheduled for revision (Figures 5-49C and 5-49D), and one is asymptomatic after probable proximal migration of an uncemented acetabular component which now appears stable (Figure 5-41E).

Femoral loosening occurred in two cemented and one uncemented components. All were allografts. One patient with definite subsidence of a femoral component (Figures 6-16C, 6-16D, and 6-16E) functions at a high level and does not require revision. Another patient was explored to revise an acetabular component (not grafted) and was foundd to have a loose femoral component in a femur that had been grafted. The final patient with a loose acetabular component (proved by arthrogram), was also found to have a loose femoral component at revision (Figure 6-7E).

This loosening rate compares favorably with other published series of total hip replacements used without bone grafts where loosening of 6% to 30% for primary hip replacement and 9% to 29% for revision surgery have been reported.[4-7,10] They are also comparable with other series of total hip replacements used with bone grafts where loosening of 0% to 25% has been reported.[8,13-21]

Conclusion

Although these procedures are complex and require a longer operative time, our results and complications are comparable with reports in the literature of total hip replacement when primary hips that have required bone grafting are compared with primary hips both with and without bone grafting. They are also comparable when revision hips that required bone grafting are compared with other series of revision hips that have and have not required grafting procedures.

We have not seen a statistical difference between the results of cemented and uncemented components except with regard to the complication of infection where uncemented components have fared better. For this reason we now tend to use uncemented components in most situations.

It is obvious that followup is short in many of the cases in this series. However, we still feel that the bone grafting techniques that have been described offer the best solution to these very difficult examples of major bone stock deficiency in total hip replacement.

References

1. Stauffer, R.N.: Ten-year follow-up study of total hip replacement. J Bone Joint Surg 64A:983, 1982.
2. Tullos, H.S., et al.: Total hip arthroplasty with a low modulus porous coated femoral component: A progress report. J Bone Joint Surg 66A:888, 1984.
3. Harris, W.H.: Traumatic Arthritis of the hip after dislocation and acetabular fracture: Treatment by mold arthroplasty. An end-result study using a new method of result evaluation. J Bone Joint Surg 51A(6):737-755, 1969.
4. Salvati, E., et al.: A ten-year follow-up study of our first 100 consecutive Charnley total hip replacement. J Bone Joint Surg 63A:753, 1981.
5. Sutherland, C., et al.: A ten-year follow-up of 100 consecutive Muller curved stem total hip replacement arthroplasties. J Bone Joint Surg 64A:970, 1982.
6. Thomas, B.J., Salvati, E., Small, R.: The CAD hip arthroplasty: Five to ten year follow-up. J Bone Joint Surg 68A:640, 1986.
7. Gunmunur, G., Hedeboe, J., Kjaer, J.: Mechanical loosening after hip replacement. Acta Orthop Scand 56:314, 1985.
8. Christie, M., et al.: Total hip arthroplasty in congenital dislocation of the hip. Orthop Trans 9:449, 1985.
9. Gerber, S., Harris, W.: Femoral head autografting to augment acetabular deficiency in patients requiring total hip replacement. J Bone Joint Surg 68A:1241, 1986.
10. Pellicci, P., et al.: Long term results of revision total hip replacement. J Bone Joint Surg 67A:513, 1985.
11. Kavanagh, B., Ilstrup, D., Fitzgerald, R.: Revision total hip arthroplasty. J Bone Joint Surg 67A:517, 1985.
12. Murray, M., et al.: Function after revision of failed total hip arthroplasty. Acta Orthop Scand 55:59, 1984.
13. Ritter, M., Trancik, T.: Lateral acetabular bone graft in total hip arthroplasty. Clin Orthop 193:156, 1985.
14. Autografting and allografting in aseptic failure of total hip replacement. In The Hip: Welsh, R.B., (ed): St. Louis, C.B. Mosby Co., p. 286, 1984.
15. Trancik, T., et al.: Allograft reconstruction of the acetabulum during revision total hip arthroplasty. J Bone Joint Surg 68A:527, 1986.
16. Sloof, T., et al.: Bone grafting in total hip replacement for acetabular protrusion. Acta Orthop Scand 55:593, 1984.
17. Gross, A., et al.: The use of allograft bone in revision of total hip arthroplasty. Clin Orthop 197:115, 1985.
18. Borja, F., Mnaymneh, W.: Bone allografts in salvage

of difficult hip arthroplasties. Clin Orthop 197:123, 1985.

19. Mendes, D., Roffman, M., Silbermann, M.: Reconstruction of the acetabular wall with bone graft in arthroplasty of the hip. Clin Orthop 186:29, 1984.

20. Mankin, H., Doppelt, S., Tomford, W.: Clinical experience with allograft implantations. Clin Orthop 174:69, 1983.

21. Eaton, R., Capello, W.: Reconstruction of acetabular deficiency utilizing iliac bone graft. Orthopedics, 6:973, 1983.

22. Taylor, M., Meyers, M., Harvey, J.: Intra-operative femur fractures during total hip replacement. Clin Orthop 137:96, 1978.

23. Scott, R., et al.: Femoral fractures in conjunction with total hip replacement. J Bone Joint Surg 57A:494, 1975.

24. Pellicci, P., Inglis, A., Salvati, E.: Perforation of the femoral shaft during total hip replacement. J Bone Joint Surg 62A:234, 1980.

25. Talab, Y., States, J., Evarts, L.M.: Femoral shaft perforation. Clin Orthop 141:158, 1979.

26. Amstutz, H., et al.: Revision of aseptic loose total hip arthroplasties. Clin Orthop 170:21, 1982.

27. Johanson, N., et al.: Nerve injury in total hip arthroplasty. Clin Orthop 179:214, 1983.

28. Stone, R., et al.: Evaluation of sciatic nerve compromise during total hip arthroplasty. Clin Orthop 201:26, 1985.

29. Eftekhar, N., Stinchfield, F.: Experience with low friction arthroplasty. Clin Orthop 95:60, 1973.

30. Stillwell, W.T.: Sciatic Neurolysis: An adjunct to complex total hip arthroplasty, In The Art of Total Hip Arthroplasty, Stillwell, W.F., (ed): Grune and Stratton, Orlando, Florida, pp. 437-444, 1987.

31. Reiley, M., et al.: Vascular complications following total hip arthroplasty. Clin Orthop 186:23, 1984.

32. Aust, J., Bredenberg, L., Murry, P.: Mechanisms of arterial injuries associated with total hip replacement. Arch Surg 116:345, 1981.

33. Salama, R., Stavorsky, M., Itellin, A.: Femoral artery injury complicating total hip replacement. Clin Orthop 85:143, 1972.

34. Athansoulis, C.A., et al.: Arterial embolism to control pelvic hemorrhage. In The Hip: Sledge, L., (ed): C.V. Mosby Co., St. Louis, MO, p. 247, 1979.

35. Stock, J., et al.: Transcatheter embolization for the control of wound hemorrhage following hip surgery. J Bone Joint Surg 62A:1000, 1980.

36. Fackler, C., Poss, R.: Dislocation in total hip arthroplasties. Clin Orthop 151:169, 1980.

37. Lewinnek, G., et al.: Dislocations after total hip replacement arthroplasties. J Bone Joint Surg 60A:217, 1978.

38. Roberts, J., et al.: A comparison of the posterolateral and anterolateral approaches to total hip arthroplasty. Clin Orthop 187:205, 1984.

39. Woo, R., Morrey, B.: Dislocations after total hip arthroplasty. J Bone Joint Surg 64A:1295, 1982.

40. Bucholz, H., et al.: Management of deep infection of total hip replacement. J Bone Joint Surg 63B:342, 1981.

41. Wilson, P.: Joint replacement. Southern Med J 70:55, 1977.

42. Surin, V., Sundholm, K., Backman, L.: Infection after total hip replacement. J Bone Joint Surg 65B:412, 1983.

43. Tomford, W., Starkweather, R., Goldman, M.: A study of the clinical incidence of infection in the use of banked allograft bone. J Bone Joint Surg 63A:244, 1981.

44. Speller, D.C.E.: Microbiology of infected joint prostheses. Semin Orthop 1:1, 1986.

45. Reigler, H., Harris, C.: Heterotopic bone formation after total hip arthroplasty. Clin Orthop 117:209, 1976.

46. Nollen, A., Sloff, T.: Para-articular ossification after total hip replacement. Acta Orthop Scand 44:230, 1973.

47. Parkinson, J., Evarts, C.M.: Heterotopic bone formation after total hip arthroplasty. Adv Orthop Surg 8:18, 1984.

48. Ritter, M., Gioe, T.: The effect of Indomethacin on para-articular ectopic ossification following total hip arthroplasty. Clin Orthop 167:113, 1982.

49. Coventry, M., Scanlon, P.: The use of radiation to discourage ectopic bone. J Bone Joint Surg 63A:201, 1981.

50. Boardman, K., Bocco, F., Charnley, J.: An evaluation of a method of trochanteric fixation using 3 wires in the Charnley low friction arthroplasty. Clin Orthop 132:31, 1978.

51. Thompson, R., Culver, J.: Role of trochanteric osteotomy in total hip replacement. Clin Orthop 106:102, 1975.

52. Hull, R.D., Raskob, G.E.: Prophylaxis of venous thromboembolic disease following hip and knee surgery: Current concepts review. J Bone Joint Surg 68A:146, 1986.

53. Harris, W.H., et al.: Detection of pulmonary emboli after total hip replacements using serial C15 (SP) 02 (SB) pulmonary scans. J Bone Joint Surg 66A:1388, 1984.

54. Sikorski, J., Hampson, W., Staddon, S.: The natural history and aetology of deep vein thrombosis after total hip replacement. J Bone Joint Surg 63B:171, 1981.

55. Gallus, A., Raman, K., Darby, T.: Venous thrombosis after elective hip replacerent. The influence of preventative intermittent calf compression and of surgical technique. Br J Surg 70:17, 1983.

56. Harris, W., et al.: High and low dose aspirin pro-

phylaxis against venous thromboembolic disease in total hip replacement. J Bone Joint Surg 64A:63, 1982.

57. Leyvraz, P., et al.: Adjusted versus fixed dose subcutaneous Heparin in the prevention of deep vein thrombosis after total hip replacement. N Engl J Med 309:954, 1983.

58. Berggren, A., Weiland, A., Ostrup, L.: Bone scintigraphy in evaluating the viability of composite bone grafts revascularized by microvascular anastamosis, conventional autogenous bone grafts, and free non-revascularized periosteol grafts. J Bone Joint Surg 64A:799, 1982.

59. Ranawat, C.S., Dorr, L.D., Inglis, A.E.: Total hip arthroplasty in protrusio acetabuli of rehematoid arthritis. J Bone Joint Surg 62A:1059, 1980.

AATB (American Association of Tissue Banks), 13-14
Acetabular component, 31-32
  loosening, 177
  sintered, 55
Acetabular defects
  autogenous bone grafts, 33-34
  classification, 48-49
  column defects
    clinical examples, 98-101
    treatment, preferred, 96
  combined protrusio and perforation of medial wall, 73-75
  global deficiency
    clinical examples, 91-96, 97
    treatment, preferred, 89-91
  intra-acetabular, 62-67
  perforation of acetabular medial wall
    clinical examples, 72
    literature review, 70-71
    treatment, preferred, 71-72
  protrusio acetabulum, 67-70
  superior and posterior rim, 57-58
    clinical examples, 59-62
    literature review, 58
    treatment, preferred, 58-59
  superior rim
    clinical examples, 56-57
    graft decision, 49-50, 51
    grafting technique, 51, 53-56
    literature review, 49
    no grafting, preferred technique for, 50-51, 52
  superior rim defects with superior intra-acetabular defects
    clinical examples, 76-79
    treatment, preferred, 75-76
Acetabular grafts, fixation methods, 165
Acetabular reconstruction
  materials, 47
  methods, 47
  postoperative management, 47-48
Acetabulum. See also Acetabular entries
  computer assisted modeling, 29, 30
Acquired immunodeficiency syndrome (AIDS), 7
Allografts. See also specific allograft sites
  biology of, 4-5
  bone, 34-39
    experimental studies results, 6
    immune response to, 5-6
  bone banking, 6-7

cartilage
  experimental studies results, 6
  immune response to, 5-6
cortical onlay, 38
future of implants, 8-9
history of, 2-3
procurement, 6-7
surgery, special problems with, 7-8
American Association of Tissue Banks (AATB), 13-14
Arthrogram, preoperative hip, 27, 28
Autografts
  biology of, 3-4
  bone, 33-34

Billing, in bone bank, 16
Blood cultures, 15
Blood-donor program, autologous, 20
Blood loss, excessive intra-operative, 171
Bolts, vs. screws, 30-31, 55
Bone bank, organization, 13-14
Bone banking
  allograft procurement, 6-7
  billing, 16
  freeze drying, 13
  networking of bones, 16-17
  record keeping, 16
  use of banked bones, 17
Bone culture, 15
Bone grafts, autogenous, 33-34
Bone procurement, techniques and storage, 14-16
Bone tumors, malignant, survival, 1

Calcar deficiency
  clinical examples, 105-106
  literature review, 104-105
  total, clinical examples, 106-110
  treatment, 106, 160
Calcar intramedullary deficiency, 105
  allograft femoral heads for augmentation, 36
  clinical examples, 105-106
Cavitary defects, 49
Cell surface antigens, 5
Cement, 55-56, 166
Central segmental defects, 49
Chondrocytes, 5, 6
Chondrosarcoma, 1
Collagen, 5
Commercial bone banks, organization, 13-14

Complications, 170
  component related, 175-177
  graft related, 173-175
  intra-operative, 170-171
  medical, 173
  postoperative, 171-173
  of primary hip replacement, 170
  of revision hip surgery, 170
Components
  complications from, 175-177
  loosening, 177
Computer assisted modeling of acetabulum and pelvis, 29, 30
Computer assisted tomography, preoperative, 28-29
Cortical onlay grafts, 38
Cortical perforation
  clinical examples, 121-123
  literature review, 120
  treatment, 120-121
Cortical thinning, 116
  clinical examples, 117-120
  literature review, 117
  treatment, 117
Coumadin prophylaxis, 173
Creeping substitution, 3
  allograft, 4
  mechanical properties of bone, 165
Cryopreservatives, 6
Culture methods, 15
Cutting cones, 3, 4

Dimethylsulfoxide (DMSO), 5
Direct lateral surgical approach, 42, 43
Dislocations, postoperative, 171
Dissolution of donor site, in allograft, 4
DMSO (dimethylsulfoxide), 5
Donors, allograft, criteria, 7
Escherichia coli infection, 172
Ewing's tumor, 1

Femoral component loosening, 177
Femoral defects
  calcar deficiency
    clinical examples, 105-106
    literature review, 104-105
    total, clinical examples, 106-110
    treatment, 105, 160
  calcar intramedullary deficiency, 105
    allograft femoral heads for augmentation, 36
    clinical examples, 105-106

circumferential deficiencies of meta-
    physis and diaphysis
        clinical examples, 134-158
        literature review, 133-134
        treatment, 134, 161
    cortical perforation
        clinical examples, 121-123
        literature review, 120
        treatment, 120-121
    cortical thinning, 116
        clinical examples, 117-120
        literature review, 117
        perforation, 160
        treatment, 117, 160
    deficiency of metaphysis and trochanter
        clinical examples, 134-137
        treatment, 134
    fatigue fracture of allograft, 129-130
        clinical examples, 130-133
    fractures above or below stem of compo-
        nent, 123-124
        clinical examples, 127-129
        literature review, 124
        treatment, 125-127, 160-161
    total deficiency of proximal femur
        clinical examples, 138-158
        treatment, 137-138
        treatment summary, 158-161
    trochanteric deficiencies
        clinical examples, 111-116
        literature review, 110
        treatment, preferred, 110-111, 160
Femoral grafts, fixation methods, 165-166
Femoral head
    allografts, 34-36
        indications, 35-38
    autogenous grafts, indications, 34, 35
    procurement and storage, 16
Femoral reconstruction
    material, 103
    methods, 103-104
Femur. *See also* Femoral entries
AP and rotational views, 23, 26, 27
fractures, intra-operative, 170-171
proximal, massive bone loss, 38
Fixation methods for bone grafts, 165-166
Fracture(s)
    fixation, cortical onlay allografts for, 38
    graft, 174-175
    intra-operative, 170-171
    postallograft, 8
Freeze drying
    mechanical properties of bone, 165
    method, 15

Gastrointestinal system, preoperative
    assessment, 20
Genitourinary system, preoperative assess-
    ment, 20
Glycoproteins, surface membrane, 5
Graft. *See also* Allograft; Autograft
    migration, 173-174
    nonunion, 173
    resorption, 174
Graft fracture, 174-175
Graft incorporation, biology of, 3-5

Graft related complications, 173-175

Harris hip rating system, 19
Healing, allograft, 4
Hepatitis, 7
Heterotopic ossification, postoperative, 173
Hip, true lateral film of, 22-26
Hip aspiration, 26-27
Hip replacement
    preoperative period
        medical assessment, 20
        radiographic assessment, 20-29
    primary
        complications, 170
        treatment results, 169-170
Hip revision surgery
    complications, 170
    treatment results, 170

Iliac crest grafts, full thickness, 33-34
Immune response, to bone and cartilage
    allografts, 5-6
Incisions, old, 41
Infections, postoperative, 7-8, 171-173
Intra-acetabular defects, 62
    clinical examples, 62-67
    femoral head allografts, 35, 36
    femoral head autogenous graft, 35, 36
    literature review, 62
    superior, with perforation of medial
        wall, 85-89
    superior, with superior rim defects
        clinical examples, 76-79
        treatment, preferred, 75-76
    superior, with superior rim defects and
        perforation of medial wall
        clinical examples, 80-84
        treatment, preferred, 79-80
    treatment, preferred, 62-63
Intra-operative complications
    fractures, 170-171
    perforation of femoral shaft, 171

Kirschner wires, 29, 31

Leg length discrepancy, assessment, 21
Long bones
    packaging, 14-15
    procurement, 14

Mandibular mesh, 35
Medical complications, 173
Midas Rex, 29, 31
Migration of graft, 173-174
Modeling, computer assisted of acetabulum
    and pelvis, 29, 30

Neurological problems, intra-operative, 171
Nonunion, 173

Organ procurement agencies, 14
Ossification, heterotopic postoperative, 173
Osteoclastic resorption, 6
Osteoconduction, 3
Osteoconductive system, 4
Osteoinduction, 3, 4

Osteosarcoma, 1

Patient evaluation, preoperative
    medical assessment, 20
    orthopedic assessment, 19-20
    radiographic assessment, 20-29
Pelvis
    computer assisted modeling, 29, 30
    oblique view, 22, 23, 24
Peripheral segmental defects, 49
Posterior surgical approach, 41-42
Postoperative period
    acetabular reconstruction management,
        47-48
    biomechanical management aspects,
        165
    complications, 171-173
    fixation methods for bone grafts,
        165-166
    literature review, 166
    treatment, preferred, 166-168
Preoperative period
    medical assessment, 20
    orthopedic assessment, 19-20
    radiographic assessment, 20-29
        computer assisted modeling of ace-
            tabulum and pelvis, 29, 30
        computer assisted tomography,
            28-29
        scanograms, 27
        tomograms, 27-28
Protrusio acetabulum
    clinical examples, 68-70
    combined with perforation of medial
        wall
        clinical example, 74-75
        treatment, preferred, 73-74
    literature review, 67-68
    treatment, preferred, 68
Proximal femoral bone, massive loss, 38
Proximal tibial allograft, 37
Pseudomonas infection, 171-172

Radiography
    patient positioning, 21
    preoperative
        AP and rotational views of femur,
            23, 26, 27
        AP of pelvis and hips in neutral rota-
            tion and neutral abduction, 20-22
        arthrogram, 27, 28
        hip aspiration, 26-27
        obliques of pelvis, 22, 23, 24
        true lateral of involved hip, 22-26
    x-ray procedure for bone allografts,
        15-16
Radiolucent lines, from graft components,
    175-177
Record keeping, in bone banks, 16
Resistantiae minoris, 8
Resorption of graft, 174

Scanograms, 27
Sciatic nerve complications, 171
Screws
    chrome cobalt, 29-30

vs. bolts, 30-31, 55
Smith-Petersen approach, 42
Staphylococcus aureus infection, 171, 172
Staphylococcus epidermidis, 15
Sterilization of bone, 15
Storage of bone, temperatures, 15
Surgical approaches
    anterior, 42
    dealing with old incisions, 41
    direct lateral, 42, 43
    posterior, 41-42
    transtrochanteric, 44-46
    trochanteric slide, 46
    vastus slide, 42, 44
Surgical reconstruction

acetabular component, 31-32
femoral component, 32, 33
special equipment, 29-30

Table vise, 29, 30
Thromboembolic disease, postoperative, 173
Tibial allograft, proximal, 37
Tomograms, 27-28
Total calcar deficiency, 106-108
    clinical examples, 108-110
Transtrochanteric surgical approach, 44-46
Treatment results. *See also* under specific condition
    for primary hip replacements, 169-170

for revision hip surgery, 170
Trochanteric augmentation, femoral head allograft, 36
Trochanteric avulsion, postoperative, 173
Trochanteric deficiencies
    clinical examples, 111-116
    literature review, 110
Trochanteric slide, 46

Vascular problems, intra-operative, 171
Vastus slide, 42, 44

Watson-Jones approach
WeiWatson-Jones approach
Weightbearing, early, 166